T0265274

Hospital Acquired Infections: Causes, Diagnosis and Treatment

Hospital Acquired Infections: Causes, Diagnosis and Treatment

Editor: Ezra Axon

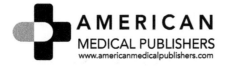

AMERICAN
MEDICAL PUBLISHERS
www.americanmedicalpublishers.com

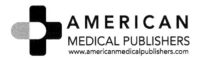

Cataloging-in-Publication Data

Hospital acquired infections : causes, diagnosis and treatment / edited by Ezra Axon.
    p. cm.
Includes bibliographical references and index.
ISBN 978-1-63927-692-9
1. Nosocomial infections. 2. Infection. 3. Nosocomial infections--Diagnosis.
4. Nosocomial infections--Treatment. 5. Nosocomial infections--Etiology.
6. Hospital buildings--Sanitation. I. Axon, Ezra.
RA969 .H67 2023
614.44--dc23

American Medical Publishers,
41 Flatbush Avenue,
1st Floor, New York,
NY 11217, USA

ISBN 978-1-63927-692-9 (Hardback)

Contents

Preface

Over the recent decade, advancements and applications have progressed exponentially. This has led to the increased interest in this field and projects are being conducted to enhance knowledge. The main objective of this book is to present some of the critical challenges and provide insights into possible solutions. This book will answer the varied questions that arise in the field and also provide an increased scope for furthering studies.

Hospital acquired infection (HAI) is a type of infection acquired while receiving healthcare services in a hospital. The common forms of hospital acquired infections are bacterial infections, fungal infections and viral infections. Fever, cough, burning sensation while urinating, extreme weakness or tiredness are a few of the most common symptoms associated with these infections. Hospital acquired infections can be prevented by disinfecting equipment and skin, wearing protective equipment, like gloves and face masks, and washing hands regularly. Treatment for these infections includes antibiotics, rest and consuming sufficient water. Diagnostic tests like taking blood sample, taking sample from lungs or undertaking other specific tests is helpful in determining the specific infection. The topics included in this book on hospital acquired infections are of utmost significance and bound to provide incredible insights to readers. It picks up individual infections and explains their significance in the context of the modern healthcare system. The book will serve as a valuable source of reference for graduate and post graduate students.

I hope that this book, with its visionary approach, will be a valuable addition and will promote interest among readers. Each of the authors has provided their extraordinary competence in their specific fields by providing different perspectives as they come from diverse nations and regions. I thank them for their contributions.

Editor

Biofilm Formation and Antimicrobial Susceptibility of *Staphylococcus epidermidis* Strains from a Hospital Environment

Robert D. Wojtyczka [1], Kamila Orlewska [1], Małgorzata Kępa [1], Danuta Idzik [1], Arkadiusz Dziedzic [2], Tomasz Mularz [1], Michał Krawczyk [1], Maria Miklasińska [1] and Tomasz J. Wąsik [1,*]

[1] Department and Institute of Microbiology and Virology, School of Pharmacy with the Division of Laboratory Medicine, Medical University of Silesia, ul. Jagiellońska 4, 41-200 Sosnowiec, Poland; E-Mails: rwojtyczka@sum.edu.pl (R.D.W.); kamila_orlewska@o2.pl (K.O.); mkepa@sum.edu.pl (M.K.); didzik@sum.edu.pl (D.I.), tomekmularz@aol.com (T.M.), michalk1988@interia.pl (M.K.), mariii89@o2.pl (M.M.)

[2] Department of Conservative Dentistry with Endodontics, School of Medicine with the Division of Dentistry, Medical University of Silesia, Pl. Akademicki 17, 41-902 Bytom, Poland; E-Mail: adziedzic@sum.edu.pl

* Author to whom correspondence should be addressed; E-Mail: twasik@sum.edu.pl

---

Abstract: The hospital environment microflora comprise a wide variety of microorganisms which are more or less pathogenic and where staphylococci are one of the most common types. The aim of the presented study was to evaluate the prevalence of the biofilm forming coagulase-negative staphylococci (CoNS) in a hospital environment as a risk factor for nosocomial infections. Among 122 isolated and tested strains of CoNS the most frequent were: *S. epidermidis*—32 strains, *S. haemolyticus*—31 strains, *S. capitis* subsp. *capitis*— 21 strains, *S. hominis*—11 strains, *S. cohnii* subsp. *cohnii*—nine strains. In case of CoNS, the main molecule responsible for intercellular adhesion is a polysaccharide intercellular adhesin (PIA), encoded on the *ica* gene operon. The analysis revealed the presence of the *icaADBC* operon genes in 46.88% of *S. epidermidis* isolates. *IcaA* and *icaD* were present in 34.38% and 28.13% of strains respectively while *IcaC* gene was present in 37.50% of strains. *IcaB* gene was found in 21.88% of *S. epidermidis* strains. In 15 (63%) strains all *icaADBC* operon genes were observed. The assessment of antibacterial drugs susceptibility demonstrated that analyzed CoNS strains were highly resistant to macrolides and lincosamides and more sensitive to rifampicin and linezolid. Our data indicates that the hospital environment can be colonized by biofilm forming coagulase-negative staphylococci and transmission of these strains can cause an increased risk of serious nosocomial infections.

Keywords: biofilm; nosocomial infections; *icaADBC* operon; *Staphylococcus epidermidis*

1. Introduction

According to The European Centre for Disease Prevention nosocomial infection are identified in approximately three million people in the European Union each year and about 50,000 of them are fatal [1]. These infections can also affect medical personnel, patient's visitors and hospital support staff [2]. Approximately 60%–70% of nosocomial infections are associated with the use various types of medical-devices with surfaces contaminated with pathogenic bacteria [3] and what is more, the contaminated hands of medical personnel are also considered as one of the pathways of nosocomial infection spread. It has been shown that proper use of disinfectants can significantly reduce microorganism content and thus reduce the risk of hospital associated nosocomial infections by more than 40% [4]. Due to the reduced susceptibility of biofilm forming microorganisms to antibiotics [5,6] and some disinfectants [7] commonly used skin disinfection techniques seems to be inefficient. Therefore to reduce the risk of infection associated with these microorganisms it is important to introduce more rigorous disinfection procedures to remove biofilm strains from the general hospital environment.

Many microorganisms in the natural environment are organized in biofilm structures [8]. Biofilms can be defined as multicellular communities of bacteria, immobilized by an extracellular polymeric matrix produced by the bacteria, which can be attached to various biotic and abiotic surfaces [9,10]. This three-dimensional biofilm structure is made up in 85% by the extracellular matrix which comprises polysaccharides, proteins, enzymes, DNA, bacterial glycolipids, water, and in 15% by aggregates of microorganism cells [8]. Biofilm development depends on many physical, chemical and biological factors [3]. In staphylococci, the main molecule responsible for intercellular adhesion is a polysaccharide intercellular adhesin (PIA), also known as a poly-N-acetylglucosamine (PNAG) [11]. It is a partially deacylated polymer of β-1,6-N-acetylglucosamine, which with the other polymers such as teichoic acids and proteins can form a major part of the extracellular matrix. Recently, PIA homologs were identified in many pathogens with biofilm formation ability, what points out that the three-dimensional matrix formation plays a crucial role in bacterial virulence in biofilm-associated infections [12–14].

PIA biosynthesis is carried out by the proteins encoded by the *ica* gene operon: N-acetylglucosamine transferase (*icaA* and *icaD*), PIA deacylase (*icaB*), PIA exporter (*icaC*) and the regulatory gene (*icaR*) [15,16]. *Ica* locus expression is regulated by a variety of environmental factors and internal regulatory proteins. Biosynthesis and deacetylation of PIA are recognized as crucial virulence factors in *Staphylococcus epidermidis*- associated infections [15,17,18].

Biofilms protects microorganisms, such as coagulase-negative staphylococci (CoNS), against both antibiotics used to treat infections and host immune system responses. Medical implants contaminated by biofilm-forming bacteria may lead to the development of inflammatory foci where implant removal is frequently the only effective treatment of such infections [19–21]. Since *Staphylococci* are part of the resident microbiological flora of the skin the presence of the biofilm-forming strains among them may be associated with an increased risk of transmission of virulent biofilm-forming strains in the hospital environment.

CoNS colonization in humans occurs as early as at birth and many strains inhabit the skin and mucous membranes till death [9]. Among many coagulase-negative staphylococci *Staphylococcus epidermidis* is the most frequently isolated species and accounts for more than 90% of the aerobic flora [22]. Although, this very common species of the cutaneous microflora is believed to be generally innocuous in nature, the last 20 years have pointed at *S. epidermidis* as a very frequent cause of hospital-acquired infections [23]. Therefore, we made an effort to evaluate the prevalence of biofilm-forming *S. epidermidis* and other CoNS strains present in the hospital environment by both phenotypic and molecular methods. Acquired data, together with the antimicrobial susceptibility profile of the isolated strains, may provide important epidemiological information which can be implemented in hospital infection prevention and control plans.

2. Experimental Section

A total of 122 coagulase-negative staphylococci strains isolated from a hospital environment were included to the presented study. The samples were collected from air and surfaces in the hospital. The sedimentation method was used for the air sample collection, where Petri dishes containing nutrient growth medium were exposed to the environment for one hour [24].

Standard Replicate Organism Detection and Counting (RODAC) contact plates (BTL, Łódź, Poland) contained neutralizing agents which inactivated any residual disinfectants were used for collection of bacteria from surfaces. The convex agar meniscus allowed direct application to the tested surfaces e.g. walls, floors, medical equipment, equipment for hygiene control [25].

Routine microbiological methods with a semi-automatic MICRONAUT identification system (Merlin-Virotech, Bornheim-Hersel, Germany) were used for bacterial species identification. Samples were stored for future analysis in TBE medium with 20% glycerol, at −86 °C.

2.1. Analysis of Biofilm Production by the Congo Red Agar (CRA).

Phenotypic characterization of biofilm production was performed by culture of the CoNS isolates on CRA plates as previously described by Freeman *et al.* [26]. A specific brain-heart infusion broth (BHI) medium supplemented with 5% sucrose and Congo Red was prepared. The medium was comprised BHI (37 g/L), sucrose (50 g/L), No. 1 agar (10 g/L) and Congo Red stain (0.8 g/L). Plates were inoculated and incubated in aerobic environment for 24 h at 37 °C. Under such condition, biofilm producers form black crusty colonies on CRA, whereas non-producers form red colonies. A darkening of the colonies with the absence of a dry crystalline colonial morphology indicated an intermediate result [27].

2.2. Microtiter Plate Assay (TCP)

To evaluate the biofilm formation we performed the modified microtiter plate assay described by Christensen et al. [27]. Bacteria were suspended in Muller-Hinton Broth (MHB-BTL, Łodź, Poland) in density equivalent to 0.5 McFarland standard and 100 μL from each bacterial suspension was inoculated onto 96-well tissue microculture plates. The plates were incubated at 37 °C for 24 h in a normal atmosphere. To remove the free floating planktonic bacteria the medium was removed and the wells were washed 3 times with phosphate saline buffer (PBS, pH = 7.2). Then 150 μL of 1% crystal violet (Sigma) was added to each well and incubated for 30 min at room temperature. The dye was removed, by 4× wash with sterile deionized water. The samples were incubated with 200 μL of 95% isopropanol in 1 M HCl for 5 min. Finally, 100 μL of colored isopropanol from each well was transferred to a fresh microtiter plate. The optical density (OD) of suspension was measured at wave length of 490 nm with a Multitec SX microplate reader.

The negative control comprised all reagents but without bacterial inoculums. According to Christensen et al. [27], the samples with the OD > 0.11 should be considered as positive. The assay was performed in triplicates. Mean $A_{490} \pm$ SD values were calculated.

In the present study, bacterial strains were considered non-adherent when the OD was equal or lower than 0.11; weakly adherent when the OD was higher than 0.11 or equal or lower than 0.17 and strongly adherent when the OD was higher than 0.17.

2.3. Detection of icaADBC Genes S. epidermidis Strains

Bacterial DNA was isolated using Genomic DNA Mini Kit (BLIRT SA, Gdańsk, Poland). Briefly, all isolates stored at −86 °C were thawed and expanded in vitro on blood agar plates and checked for strain purity prior to the DNA isolation. In the next step 3–4 bacterial colonies were suspended in 100 μL TRIS buffer with 10 μL of lysostaphine (1 mg/mL; BLIRT SA, Gdańsk, Poland) and incubated at 37 °C for 30 min. The mix was treated with proteinase K and LT Buffer at 37 °C for overnight than incubated at 75 °C for 5 min. The DNA samples were purified according to the protocol with the use of ethanol and wash buffer supplied in the kit, and finally diluted to 200 μL with TRIS buffer. Purified DNA samples were stored at −20 °C for future analysis.

A standard PCR technique was used for icaA, icaD, icaB and icaC genes detection in the S. epidermidis strains as earlier described by Ziebuhr et al. [28] and de Silva et al. [29]. The primer sequences for icaA (f) were 5'-GAC CTC GAA GTC AAT AGA GGT-3' and icaA (r) 5'-CCC AGT ATA ACG TTG GAT ACC-3'; icaD (f) were 5'-AGG CAA TAT CCA ACG GTA A-3' and icaD (r) 5'-GTC ACG ACC TTT CTT ATA TT-3' (reverse); icaB (f) 5'-ATA AAC TTG AAT TAG TGT ATT-3' and icaB (r) 5'-ATA TAT AAA ACT CTC TTA ACA-3' icaC (f) 5'-AGG CAA TAT CCA ACG GTA A-3' and icaC (r) 5'-GTC ACG ACC TTT CTT ATA TT-3'.

The PCR reactions were performed using 10× PCR RED master mix kit (BLIRT SA). The PCR mix contained 2 μL of PCR red mix, 0.2 μL of each primer, 16.6 μL of PCR water and an average of 75 ng of DNA per 20 μL of reaction mix. The PCR reaction was performed in 30 cycles with 30 s of denaturation at 95 °C and 3 min of elongation at 72 °C for all reactions, and with annealing for 1 min at 60 °C (icaA), 59 °C (icaD, icaB), 45 °C (icaC). The PCR was performed using a MJ Mini Personal thermal cycler (Bio-Rad, Hercules, CA, USA). PCR products were electrophoresed in 1.5% agarose gel containing 0.5 µg/mL ethidium bromide. The bands were visualized by ultraviolet illumination by an UVP Bioimaging System (UVP Inc., Upland, CA, USA) and checked for size against molecular weight markers using 1 Kb HyperLadder IV (BLIRT SA)

2.4. Antimicrobial Susceptibility Testing

The antimicrobial susceptibility to cefoxitin (FOX), erythromycin (E), clindamycin (DA), tetracycline (T), chloramphenicol (C), ciprofloxacin (CIP), gentamicin (CN), rifampicin (RIF), linezolid (LIN) and trimethoprim/sulphamethoxazole (SXT) was tested by disk-diffusion method and interpreted according EUCAST guidelines [30]. Commercial antibiotic discs (EMAPOL, Gdańsk, Poland) and Mueller-Hinton agar medium (BTL, Łódź, Poland) were used in this tests.

2.5. Statistical Analysis

The two-sided Fisher's exact tests was use to assess the relationship between the capacity of the biofilm formation and drug resistance. The Pearson chi-square was used to measure the concordance between *ica* genes, CRA positivity and TCP positivity. *P*-value was two-tailed and was considered significant at a level of ≤ 0.05. The descriptive statistic was used to calculate mean values and standard deviation. Data were analyzed by use of STATISTICA v 9.0 (StatSoft Inc., Tulsa, OK, USA) on the Windows platform.

3. Results and Discussion

Microbiological samples from hospital environments were collected between November 2011 and May 2012. Samples were collected from air and flat surfaces of the both surgical operating theater (50 samples) and general surgery hospital ward (20 samples), as described in Experimental section. In the operating surgery theater samples were collected from: floor, sterile lock, corridor, cleaning room, preparation room, sterile materials room, post-surgery care room. In the general surgery ward samples were collected from: patients' facilities, day-operating surgery, baths, nursery office. From each of the aforementioned areas samples were collected twice a day, in the morning and in the afternoon. In the surgical operating theater 83 (35.8%) out of total 236 isolated strains were CoNS while in the general surgery ward that percentage was lower—39 (22.5%) CoNS strains out of a total of 173 strains isolated. The species distribution of the 122 analyzed CoNS strains isolated from hospital environment was as follows: *S. epidermidis*—32 strains, *S. haemolyticus*—31 strains, *S. capitis subsp. capitis*—21 strains, *S. hominis*—11 strains, *S. cohnii subsp. cohnii*—9 strains, *S. saprophyticus*—5 strains, *S. warneri* and *S. kloosii*—4 strains, *S. cohnii subsp. urealyticum*—2 strains and *S. lugdunensis*, *S. hyicus*, and *S. chromogenes*—1 strain each. Isolated CoNS strains demonstrated various susceptibility to tested chemotherapeutics (Table 1).

Table 1. The number/percentage of CoNS strains susceptible to selected chemotherapeutics.

Strain (No. of Strains)	[a] FOX	[a] E	[a] DA	[a] T	[a] C	[a] CIP	[a] CN	[a] RIF	[a] LNZ	[a] SXT
S. epidermidis (32)	25/78.1	18/56.3	26/81.3	25/78.1	32/100	32/100	31/96.9	32/100	31/96.9	23/71.9
S. haemolyticus (31)	26/83.9	14/45.2	19/61.3	26/83.9	25/80.6	27/87.1	28/90.3	31/100	31/100	18/58.1
S. capitis subsp. capitis (21)	17/81	9/42.9	15/71.4	19/90.5	21/100	10/47.6	10/41.6	19/90.5	21/100	17/81
S. hominis (11)	10/90.9	4/36.4	9/81.8	6/54.5	9/81.8	11/100	11/100	11/100	11/100	8/72.7
S. cohnii subsp. cohnii (9)	7/77.8	5/55.6	5/55.6	5/55.6	9/100	9/100	9/100	9/100	9/100	5/55.6
S. saprophyticus (5)	5/100	1/20	4/80	5/100	5/100	5/100	5/100	5/100	5/100	3/60
S. kloosii (4)	4/100	2/50	3/75	1/25	3/75	4/100	4/100	4/100	4/100	4/100
S. warneri (4)	3/75	1/25	1/25	3/75	3/75	4/100	4/100	4/100	4/100	3/75
S. cohnii subsp. urealyticum (2)	2/100	0/0	1/50	1/50	2/100	2/100	2/100	2/100	2/100	1/50
S. lugdunensis (1)	1/100	1/100	1/100	1/100	1/100	1/100	1/100	1/100	1/100	1/100
S. hyicus (1)	1/100	1/100	1/100	1/100	1/100	1/100	1/100	1/100	1/100	0/0
S. chromogenes (1)	1/100	0/0	1/100	0/0	1/100	1/100	1/100	1/100	1/100	1/100
Total (122)/%	10/83.6	56/45.9	86/70.5	93/76.2	112/91.8	107/87.7	107/87.7	120/98.4	121/99.2	84/68.9

[a] FOX—cefoxitin, E—erythromycin, DA—clindamycin, T—tetracycline, C—chloramphenicol, CIP—ciprofloxacin, CN—gentamicin, RIF—rifampicin, LIN—linezolid and SXT trimethoprim/ sulphamethoxazole.

CoNS strains isolated from hospital environment were highly susceptible to linezolid (99.2% sensitive strains) rifampicin and chloramphenicol (98.4% and 91.85% sensitive strains respectively) while erythromycin (45.9% sensitive strains), clindamycin (70.5% sensitive strains) and trimethoprim in combination with sulphamethoxazole (68.9%) showed low antistaphylococcal activity (Figure 1).

Figure 1. The proportion of susceptible and resistant CoNS strains to the tested chemotherapeutics.

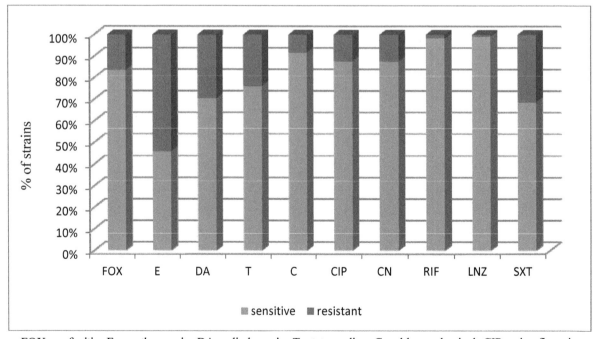

FOX—cefoxitin, E—erythromycin, DA—clindamycin, T—tetracycline, C—chloramphenicol, CIP—ciprofloxacin, CN—gentamicin, RIF—rifampicin, LIN—linezolid and SXT trimethoprim/ sulphamethoxazole.

What is more, the susceptibility profile for all CoNS strains was very similar for *S. epidermidis* strains alone (Figure 2). *S. epidermidis* strains were highly susceptible to chloramphenicol, rifampicine and ciprofloxacine (100% strains), with lesser susceptibility to erythromycin (56.3% stains) and trimetoprime in combination sulphamethoxazole—71.9% isolated and tested strains.

Figure 2. The proportion of susceptible and resistant *S. epidermidis* strains to the tested chemotherapeutics.

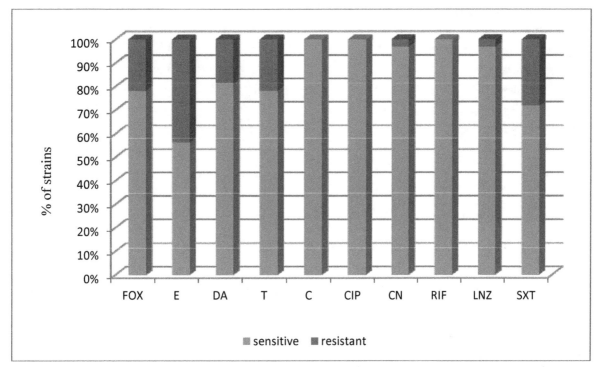

FOX—cefoxitin, E—erythromycin, DA—clindamycin, T—tetracycline, C—chloramphenicol, CIP—ciprofloxacin, CN—gentamicin, RIF—rifampicin, LIN—linezolid and SXT trimethoprim/ sulphamethoxazole.

Only nine (7.4%) out of 122 tested strains were considered as biofilm-formers by CRA method and what is more, not a single *S. epidermidis* strain was among them.

The biofilm production analysis by TCP method showed 12 (9.8%) biofilm-forming strains ($A_{490} > 0.17$), and 13 (10.7 %) strains with intermediate biofilm forming ability with A_{490} ranging from 0.11 to 0.16 (Table 2). Among 32 analyzed *S. epidermidis* strains, 12 (37.5%) were assessed as a biofilm formers by this method.

Genetic analysis of 32 *S. epidermidis* strains showed the presence of *icaADBC* operon genes in 15 (46.9%) isolates (Figure 3A–C). *IcaA* and *icaD* were present in 34.4% and 28.1% of strains respectively and *icaC* gene in 37.5% of strains (Figure 3A,3C). The lowest frequency (21.9%) showed *icaB* gene (Figure 3B). The presence of all *icaADBC* operon genes was found in five (15.6%) *S. epidermidis* strains, while in four (12.5%) isolates we found coexistence of *icaA/icaC*. The frequencies of *icaB/icaD*, *icaA/icaD/icaB*, and *icaA/icaB/icaC* genotypes were on the same level (3.1%)

Table 2. Assessment of biofilm formation ability of CoNS strains determined by CRA and TCP methods.

Strain (No. of strains)	No (%) of Positive Strains, CRA Method	No (%) of Positive Strains, TCP Method OD > 0.17,—Strong Biofilm Production	No (%) of Positive Strains, TCP Method 0.11 > OD >0.16—Weak Biofilm Production
S. epidermidis (32)	0	9 (28.1)	3 (9.4)
S. haemolyticus (31)	1 (3.2)	1 (3.2)	3 (3.2)
S. capitis subsp. capitis (21)	3 (14.3)	0	1 (4.8)
S. hominis (11)	1 (9.1)	0	2 (18.2)
S. cohnii subsp. cohnii (9)	2 (22.2)	0	0
S. saprophyticus (5)	0	0	0
S. kloosii (4)	1 (25)	1 (25)	1 (25)
S. warneri (4)	0	0	1 (25)
S. cohnii subsp. urealyticum (2)	0	1 (50)	1 (50)
S. lugdunensis (1)	0	0	0
S. hyicus (1)	1 (100)	0	0
S. chromogenes (1)	0	0	1 (100)
Total: (122)	9 (7.4)	12 (9.8)	13 (10.7)

Figure 3. Detection of operon *icaADBC* genes in *Staphylococcus epidermidis* strains. (**A**) PCR results with primer for *icaA*, positive probe—the presence of the 814-bp product; (**B**) PCR results with primer for *icaB* and *icaD*, positive probe—the presence of the 526-bp product to *icaB* and 371-bp product to *icaD*; and (**C**) PCR results with primer for *icaC* genes, positive probe—the presence of the 989-bp product. Line 1—molecular size maker 100-1000-bp, line 2-9 different *S. epidermidis* strains.

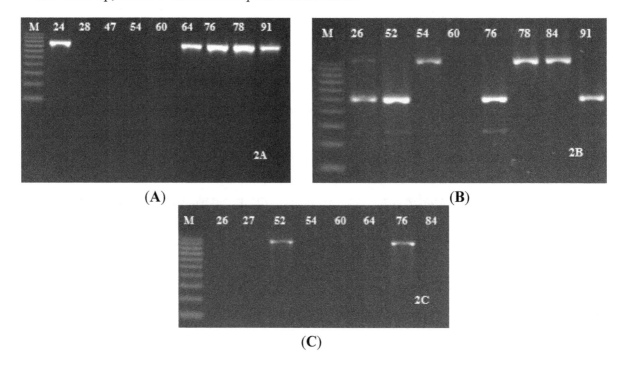

(A)

(B)

(C)

Among the 5 *S. epidermidis* strains with all *icaADBC* operon genes, only three isolates showed biofilm formation ability (A_{490} = 0.66 ± 0.25). Among four *icaC/icaA* positive *S. epidermidis* strains, three showed phenotypic ability to biofilm formation (A_{490} = 0.54 ± 0.2). All *S. epidermidis* strains with *ica* genes yielded negative results for biofilm production assessed by the CRA method while 12 strains were considered as biofilm positive in by the TCP method.

There were no significant differences in antimicrobial susceptibility between biofilm forming and non-biofilm strains, neither in the magnitude nor in the resistance pattern (Table 3). This observation suggest that diminished susceptibility to antibiotics of biofilm-forming strains, described previously by some authors [5,6,22] may be due to impaired penetration of the drug across the biofilm rather than to any other biochemical or genetic mechanisms.

Table 3. *S. epidermidis* strains susceptibility to chemotherapeutics with correlation to phenotypic biofilm production ability.

	[a]FOX	[a]E	[a]DA	[a]T	[a]C	[a]CIP	[a]CN	[a]RIF	[a]LNZ	[a]SXT
S. epidermidis (32)										
No. of susceptible strains	25	18	26	25	32	32	31	32	31	23
% of susceptible strains	78.1%	56.3%	81.3%	78.1%	100%	100%	96.9%	100%	96.9%	71.9%
biofilm strains (12)										
No. of susceptible strains	9	6	9	9	12	12	11	12	11	10
% of susceptible strains	75%	50%	75%	75%	100%	100%	91.7%	100%	91.7%	83.3%
non biofilm strains (20)										
No. of susceptible strains	16	12	17	16	20	20	20	20	20	13
% of susceptible strains	80%	60%	85%	80%	100%	100%	100%	100%	100%	65%
[b]*P*	1.000	0.718	0.647	0.535	[c]NA	NA	0.375	NA	0.375	0.205

[a] FOX—cefoxitin, E—erythromycin, DA—clindamycin, T—tetracycline, C—chloramphenicol, CIP—ciprofloxacin, CN—gentamicin, RIF—rifampicin, LIN—linezolid and SXT trimethoprim/ sulphamethoxazole [b] *p*: the two-sided Fisher's exact test for biofilm forming strains *vs.* non biofilm forming strains; all presented *P* values are two-sided, $p \leq 0.05$ was considered as statistically significant. [c] NA—not applicable.

Biofilm formation is a relatively common phenomenon among many microorganisms. The balance between biofilm-type and planktonic-type growth is influenced by a vast variety of regulatory mechanisms. To date many factors which exert significant influence on biofilm formation have been identified. Environmental factors such as oxygen and iron ions availability and high osmotic pressure can influence extracellular matrix biosynthesis, thus the biofilm formation as a whole [31].

In our study we have analyzed the prevalence of coagulase-negative staphylococci with biofilm formation ability isolated from hospital environment. We applied three widely used methods, such as: the growth rate on the CRA, evaluation of the biofilm formation ability by TCP method and PCR-based detection of *icaADBC* operon genes associated with biofilm formation.

We showed that only 7.4% of all analyzed CoNS strains yielded positive reactions in the CRA method. Among *S. epidermidis* none of strains showed the ability to form biofilms when assessed by this method, while the presence of *icaABCD* operon genes associated with the biofilm formation was found in 15 (46.9%) *S. epidermidis* isolates. The biofilm production by hospital environment CoNS strains estimated by TCP method showed that 20.5% of isolates were able to produce biofilm. Our data strongly suggest that the use of TCP method together with the PCR-based techniques should be used as a gold standard for the evaluation of biofilm formation ability by CoNS strains isolated from hospital environments. This methodological problem was also addressed by Mathur *et al.* [32] who compared three phenotypic methods used for determination of biofilm formation. The authors evaluated 152 clinical isolates of *Staphylococcus* spp. by CRA, TCP and tube (TM) methods. Their results showed that 97.1% of strains were assessed as biofilm producers with the use of TCP method, 73.6% by TM, and only 6.8% in the case of CRA method, thus the authors concluded that the most sensitive method for biofilm formation analysis was the TCP method. The low effectiveness of the CRA method in evaluation of biofilm production, was also shown by de Silva *et al.* [29]. In these studies they analyzed strains of coagulase-negative staphylococci isolated from blood and skin of neonatal patients and healthy newborns. Among the 180 strains, 122 (68%) was *S. epidermidis, S. capitis* (29), *S. haemolyticus* (11), *S. hominis* (9), *S. warneri* (8), and *S. auricularis* (1). The majority of analyzed strains have not demonstrated the phenotypic ability of biofilm formation in TCP and CRA methods, with the exception of *S. hominis* isolates, where four out of nine strains were positive in the CRA method. The authors concluded that the quantification of biofilm formation by absorbance measurement on titrate plates is significantly higher than using the CRA method.

Oliveira and Cucha confirmed the relatively high efficiency of the microplate method [21]. Analysis of 100 CoNS strains isolated from clinical specimens obtained from newborns and tested with the method described by Christensen *et al.*, showed that 46% of isolated were characterized by strong phenotypic capacity for biofilm production, while 35% of them were weak biofilm producers. The most frequently isolated strain from clinical specimens identified in this study was *S. epidermidis* (81%) with *S. cohnii, S. saprophyticus, S. warneri, S. haemolyticus, S. xylosus, S. capitis,* and *S. lugdunensis* composing the remaining 19%.

Our data have shown that among coagulase-negative staphylococci from hospital environments, the most frequent were *S. epidermidis* (26.2%), *S. haemolyticus* (25.4%), *S. capitis* (17.2%), which indicates that these strains may be transferred from the hospital environment to the patient and may be responsible for hospital-acquired infections. A study carried out in the hospital environment by Wojtyczka *et al.* [33] showed that among 85 isolated strains of *Staphylococcus* spp. most common species of CoNS were *S. epidermidis* (17.7%), *S. hominis* (15.3%), *S. cohnii* (14.1%) and *S. haemolyticus* (12.9).

It is worth mentioning that the results presented here indicate a strong predominance of *S. epidermidis* isolates over other CoNS strains isolated from the clinical samples wereas such a phenomenon is less notable among CoNS strains isolated from the general hospital environment. This observation reinforces the notion that biofilm-forming *S. epidermidis* strains colonizing the hospital environment are responsible for an increased risk of nosocomial infections.

It is believed that the presence of *icaABCD* operon genes in the staphylococcal genome s associated with biofilm formation ability. Fredheim *et al.* [34], suggested a strong similarity between *ica* operons in different species of staphylococci. Phylogenetic analysis showed a substantial likeness of *ica* operon primary structure in such species as *S. haemolyticus* and *S. epidermidis*. Oliveira and Cucha's study [21] on the prevalence of *icaA, icaC* and *icaD* genes in CoNS strains showed that the *icaA* and *icaD* genes were present in 40% of isolates, and *icaA, icaC* and *icaD* in 42% of strains. In our study only 18% of analyzed strains lacked all *icaABCD* genes. In studies carried out by Arciola *et al.* [35] 101 *S. aureus* and *S. epidermidis* clinical isolates were checked for the presence of *icaA* and *icaD* genes. Sixty strains of *S. epidermidis* and 23 strains of *S. aureus* were isolated from infections associated with the implementation of vascular catheter and 10 strains of *S. epidermidis* were isolated from the skin and mucous membranes of healthy subjects. The presence of both genes (*icaA* and *icaD*) were confirmed in 48.5% (33) of *S. epidermidis* clinical strains. The remaining 35 strains of *S. epidermidis* and 10 strains isolated from the skin and mucous membranes, lacked *ica* operon genes. The results coincided with the phenotypic assessment of biofilm formation by CRA method. On the other hand, many experiments have shown the low usefulness of the CRA method for biofilm production analysis and this was also confirmed in the presented work where such a coincidence was not observed. Phenotypic methods for biofilm formation detection are among the easy and cheap techniques available for routine laboratory use, but may cause some difficulties in result interpretation since they can be influenced by variations in medium composition and cultivation conditions and are prone to subjective errors [36].

Our analysis of CoNS strains isolated from hospital environment showed the coexistence of all *icaADBC* operon genes in eight (6.6%) of all isolates and among them in five (15.63) *S. epidermidis* strains.

Only two strains *S. epidermidis* and *S. cohnii subsp. urealyticum* had the ability to produce biofilm when assessed by the TPC method but lacked *icaADBC* operon genes, which is in accordance with an observation presented by Qin *et al.* [37]. The authors showed that the *aap* and *bhp* genes may be involved in an alternative PIA-independent mechanism of biofilm formation, thus indicating that the absence of *icaABCD* operon genes does not exclude biofilm formation. Assessing the ability of biofilm production by two groups of *S. epidermidis* strains isolated from nosocomial infections and skin of healthy subjects, Eftekhar and Mirmohamadi [38] showed that the prevalence of biofilm-forming strains in the TPC method was at the 52% and 56% level for the analyzed groups, respectively. The application of molecular techniques with single pair of primers for the *icaA*, *icaB* and *icaD* yielded positive results in 30% *S. epidermidis* isolates from nosocomial infections and in 8% of the isolates from the skin of healthy volunteers.

The increased frequency of strains resistant to many antibiotics and chemotherapeutics is responsible for a substantial number of infections in hospital environments. The resident hospital microflora is relatively dynamic and susceptibility and resistance patterns of microorganisms isolated from clinical environmental samples can vary significantly [39].

Our study demonstrated that CoNS strains isolated from hospital environment showed high susceptibility towards the majority of tested chemotherapeutics, and susceptibility to resistance patterns only slightly varied among investigated CoNS species.

Many studies showed that resistance of CoNS to selected antibiotics can vary among strains within a broad range [39–46]. It has been shown that proportion of susceptible to resistant strains to erythromycin varied from 29.5% to 73.4%, to clindamycin from 34% to 70.3% strains, to ciprofloxacin from 6.4% to 59.4%, and to gentamicin from 15% to 42.3% strains. The proportion of resistant Staphylococci strains to trimethoprim/sulphamethoxazole varied from 24% to 40.7%, to chloramphenicol from 0% to 60.9%, to tetracycline from 13.1% to 51.9%, and to rifampicin from 7% to 39.1% [39–42]. Our study confirmed high resistance of CoNS to lincosamides and macrolides. On the contrary to data presented by others [43,44], ciprofloxacin was substantially more effective towards CoNS and, what is worth mentioning, all analyzed *S. epidermidis* strains were susceptible to that drug. What is more, analyzed *S. epidermidis* strains were highly susceptible to rifampicin. This observation is in accordance with previous findings describing rifampicin as a potent agent against biofilm forming CoNS strains [45,46] thus it may be used in therapies against infections associated with biofilm forming *S. epidermidis* strains.

4. Conclusions

Our results have confirmed previous data presented by other authors that the molecular presence of *icaADBC* operon genes in the bacterial genome is associated with the ability to form biofilms, but the absence of these genes does not preclude this phenomenon phenotypically. Therefore, it seems appropriate to use both genotypic and phenotypic methods to improve the identification of the ability to produce biofilms by CoNS strains isolated from the hospital environment. Despite the fact that the analyzed CoNS strains were in the majority susceptible to the tested chemotherapeutics, a substantial contribution of biofilm-forming strains among them may cause problems in chemotherapy of hospital infections, particularly in the dose assessment. In this light, it is obvious that the information about bacterial species prevailing in hospital environment, their susceptibility and resistance patterns and on their biofilm formation ability is vital for both health care providers for the implementation of hospital infection prevention and control plans and for physicians in building up adequate antibacterial therapies.

Acknowledgments

This study was supported by the research grant from Medical University of Silesia No. KNW 1-003/N/3/0.

Author Contributions

Robert D. Wojtyczka and Kamila Orlewska conceived the study idea, designed the experiments, analyzed the data, and wrote the manuscript. Małgorzata Kępa, Danuta Idzik,Tomasz Mularz and Michał Krawczyk conceived the study idea, designed the experiments, and critically revised the manuscript. Arkadiusz Dziedzic, Maria Miklasińska and Tomasz J. Wąsik organized the data and revised the manuscript. All authors read and approved the final manuscript.

References

1. European Centre for Disease Prevention and Control (ECDC). *Annual Epidemiological Report on Communicable Diseases in Europe*; ECDC: Stockholm, Sweden, 2007.
2. Lis, D.O.; Pacha, J.Z.; Idzik, D. Methicillin resistance of airbiorne coagulase-negative staphylococci in homes of persons having contact with a hospital environment. *Am. J. Infect. Control* **2009**, *37*, 177–182.
3. Bryers, J.D. Medical biofilms. *Biotechnol. Bioeng.* **2008**, *100*, 1–18.
4. Kampf, G.; Löffler, H.; Gastmeier, P. Hand hygiene for the prevention of nosocomial infections. *Dtsch. Ärztebl. Int.* **2009**, *106*, 649–655.

5. Høiby, N.; Bjarnsholta, T.; Givskovb, M.; Molinc, S.; Ciofub, O. Antibiotic resistance of bacterial biofilms. *Int. J. Antimicrob. Agents* **2010**, *35*, 322–332.

6. Nieshimura, S.; Tsurumoto, T.; Yonekura, A.; Adachi, K.; Shindo, H. Antimicrobial susceptibility of *Staphylococcus aureus* and *Staphylococcus epidermidis* biofilms isolated from infected total hip arthroplasty case. *J. Orthoped. Sci.* **2006**, *11*, 46–50.

7. Presterl, E.; Suchomel, M.; Eder, M.; Reichmann, S.; Lassnigg, A.; Graninger, W.; Rotter, M. Effects of alcohols, povidone-iodine and hydrogen peroxide on biofilms of *Staphylococcus epidermidis*. *J. Antimicrob. Chemother.* **2007**, *60*, 417–420.

8. Costerton, J.W.; Stewart P.S.; Greenberg, E.P. Bacterial biofilms: A common cause of persistent infections. *Science* **1999**, *284*, 1318–1322.

9. Izano, E.; Amarante, M.; Kher, W.; Kaplan, J. Differential roles of poly-*N*-acetylglucosamine surface polysaccharide and extracellular DNA in *Staphylococcus aureus* and *Staphylococcus epidermidis* biofilms. *Appl. Environ. Microbiol.* **2008**, *74*, 470–476.

10. Otto, M. *Staphylococcus epidermidis*—the "accidental" pathogen. *Nat. Rev. Microbiol.* **2009**, *7*, 555–567.

11. Mack, D.; Fischer, W.; Krokotsch, A.; Leopold, K.; Hartmann, R.; Egge, H.; Laufs, R. The intercellular adhesin involved in biofilm accumulation *Staphylococcus epidermidis* linear beta-1,6-linked glucosaminoglycan: purification and structural analysis. *J. Bacteriol.* **1996**, *178*, 175–183.

12. Darby, C.; Hsu, J.W.; Ghori, N.; Falkow, S. *Caenorhabditis. elegans*: Plague bacteria biofilm blocks food intake. *Nature* **2002**, *16*, 243–244.

13. Kaplan, J.B.; Velliyagounder, K.; Ragunath, Ch.; Rode, H.; Mack, D.; Knobloch, J.K.; Ramasbbu, N. Genes involved in the synthesis and degradation of matrix polysaccharide in *Actinobacillus. actinomycetemcomitans* and *Actinobacillus. pleuropneumoniae* biofilms. *J. Bacteriol.* **2004**, *186*, 8213–8220.

14. Wang, X.; Preston, J.F.I.; Romeo, T. The *pgaABCD* locus of *Escherichia coli* promotes the synthesis of a polysaccharide adhesin required for biofilm formation. *J. Bacteriol.* **2004**, *186*, 2724–2734.

15. Vuong, C.; Kocianova, S.; Voyich, J.M.; Yao, Y.; Fishcer, E.R.; DeLeo, F.R.; Otto, M. A crucial role for exopolysaccharide modification in bacterial biofilm formation, immune evasion, and virulence. *J. Biol. Chem.* **2004**, *279*, 54881–54886.

16. Gerke, C.; Kraft, A.; Sussmuth, R.; Schweitzer, O.; Götz, F. Characterization of the N-acetylglucosaminyltransferase activity involved in the biosynthesis of the *Staphylococcus epidermidis* polysaccharide intercellular adhesion. *J. Biol. Chem.* **1998**, *273*, 18586–18593.

17. Rupp, M.E.; Fey, P.D.; Heilmann, C.; Götz, F. Characterization of the importance of *Staphylococcus epidermidis* autolysin and polysaccharide intercellular adhesin in the pathogenesis of intravascular catheter-associated infection in a rat model. *J. Infect. Dis.* **2001**, *183*, 1038–1042.

18. Fluckiger, U.; Ulrich, M.; Steiuhuber, A.; Döring, G.; Mack, D.; Landmann, R.; Goerke, Ch.; Wolz, Ch. Biofilm formation, *icaADBC* transcription, and polysaccharide intercellular adhesin synthesis by staphylococci in a device-related infection model. *Infect. Immun.* **2005**, *73*, 1811–1819.

19. Costa, F.S.; Miceli, M.H.; Anaissie, E.J. Mucosa or skin as source of coagulase-negative staphylococcal bacteraemia. *Lancet Infect. Dis.* **2004**, *4*, 278–286.

20. Klingenberg, C.; Aarag, E.; Ronnestad, A.; Sollid, J.E.; Abrahamsen, M.D.; Kjeldsen, G.; Flaegstad, T. Coagulase-negative staphylococcal sepsis in neonates—Association between antibiotic resistance, biofilm formation and the host inflammatory response. *Pediatr. Infect. Dis. J.* **2005**, *24*, 817–822.

21. Oliveira, A.; Cunha, M.L.R.S. Comparison of methods for the detection of biofilm production in coagulase-negative staphylococci. *BMC Res. Notes* **2010**, *3*, doi:10.1186/1756-0500-3-260.

22. O'Gara, J.; Humphreys, H. *Staphylococcus epidermidis* biofilms: Importance and implications. *J. Med. Microbiol.* **2001**, *50*, 582–587.

23. Cogen, A.L.; Nizet, V.; Gallo, R.L. Skin microbiota: A source of disease or defence? *Brit. J. Dermatol.* **2008**, *158*, 442–455.

24. Hart, J.B.; French, M.L.V.; Eitzen, H.E.; Ritter, M.A. Rodac plate-holding device for sampling surfaces during surgery. *Appl. Microbiol.* **1973**, *26*, 417–418.

25. Lemmen, S.W.; Häfner, H.; Zolldann, D.; Amedick G.; Lutticken, R. Comparison of two sampling methods for the detection of Gram-positive and Gram-negative bacteria in the environment: Moistened swabs *versus* Rodac plates. *Int. J. Hyg. Environ. Health* **2001**, *203*, 245–248.

26. Freeman, D.J.; Falkiner, F.R.; Keane, C.T. New method for detecting slime production by coagulase negative staphylococci. *J. Clin. Pathol.* **1989**, *42*, 872–874.

27. Christensen, G.D.; Simpson, W.A.; Younger, J.J.; Baddour, L.M.; Barrett, F.F.; Melton, D.M.; Beachey, E.H. Adherence of coagulase-negative staphylococci to plastic tissue culture plates: A quantitative model for the adherence of staphylococci to medical devices. *J. Clin. Microb.* **1985**, *22*, 996–1006.

28. Ziebuhr, W.; Krimmer, V.; Rachid, S.; Lößner, I.; Götz, F.; Hacker, J. A novel mechanism of phase variation of virulence in *Staphylococcus epidermidis*: Evidence for control of the polysaccharide intercellular adhesin synthesis by alternating insertion and excision of the insertion sequence element IS256. *Mol. Microbiol.* **1999**, *32*, 345–356.

29. De Silva, G.D.I.; Kantzanou, M.; Justice, A.; Massey, R.C.; Wilkinson, A.R.; Day, N.P.J.; Peacock, S.J. The *ica* operon and biofilm production in coagulase-negative staphylococci associated with carriage and disease in a neonatal intensive care unit. *J. Clin. Microbiol.* **2002**, *40*, 382–388.

30. European Committee for Antimicrobial Susceptibility Testing (EUCAST) of the European Society of Clinical Microbiology and Infectious Diseases (ESCMID). Terminology relating to methods for the determination of susceptibility of bacteria to antimicrobial agents. EUCAST definitive document E. Def 1.2. *Clin. Microbiol. Infect.* **2000**, *6*, 503–508.

31. Otto, M. Staphylococcal biofilms. *Curr. Top. Microbiol. Immunol.* **2008**, *322*, 207–228.

32. Mathur, T.; Singhal, S.; Khan, S.; Upadhyay, D.J.; Fatma, T.; Rattan, A. Detection of biofilm formation among the clinical isolates of staphylococci: An evaluation of three different screening methods. *Ind. J. Med. Microbiol.* **2006**, *24*, 25–29.

33. Wojtyczka, R.D.; Krakowian, D.; Marek, Ł.; Skiba, D.; Kudelski, A.; Jasik K.; Pacha, J. Analysis of the polymorphism of *Staphylococcus* strains isolated from a hospital environment. *Afr. J. Microbiol. Res.* **2011**, *5*, 4997–5003.

34. Fredheim, E.G.A.; Klingenberg, C.; Rohde, H.; Frankenberger, S.; Gaustad, P.; Flægstad T.; Solid, J.E. Biofilm Formation by *Staphylococcus haemolyticus*. *J. Clin. Microbiol.* **2009**, *47*, 1172–1180.

35. Arciola, C.R.; Baldassarri, L.; Montanaro, L. Presence of *icaA* and *icaD* genes and slime production in a collection of staphylococcal strains from catheter-associated infections. *J. Clin. Microbiol.* **2001**, *39*, 2151–2156.

36. Růžička, F.; Holá, V.; Vota, M.; Tejkalová, R.; Horvát, R.; Heroldová M.; Woznicową, V. Biofilm detection and the clinical significance of *Staphylococcus epidermidis* isolates. *Folia Microbiol.* **2004**, *49*, 596–600.

37. Qin, Z.; Yang, X.; Yang, L.; Jiang, J.; Ou, Y.; Molin S.; Qu, D. Formation and properties of *in vitro* biofilms of ica-negative *Staphylococcus epidermidis* clinical isolates. *J. Med. Microbiol.* **2007**, *1*, 83–93.

38. Eftekhar, F.; Mirmohamadi, Z. Evaluation of biofilm production by *Staphylococcus epidermidis* isolates from nosocomial infections and skin of healthy volunteers. *Int. J. Med. Med. Sci.* **2009**, *1*, 438–441.

39. Kochman M. Susceptibility of the bacteria isolated from samples of clinical material in Poland in 1998 to selected chemotherapeutics and antibiotics. The analysis of the questionnaire findings. I. Susceptibility of staphylococci. *Przegl. Epidemiol.* **2005**, *59*, 679–694.

40. Michnowska-Swincow, E.; Szychlińska, I. Drug resistance of methicillin resistant coagulase-negative staphylococci (MRCNS) isolated from hospital environment. *Diag. Labor.* **2001**, *37*, 437–444.

41. Piette, A.; Verschraegen, G. Role of coagulase-negative staphylococci in human disease. *Vet. Microbiol.* **2009**, *134*, 45–54.

42. Tunger, O.; Ozbakkaloglu, B.; Aksoy, H. Trends in antimicrobial resistant staphylococci in an university hospital over a 6-year period. *Int. J. Antimicrob. Agents* **2001**, *18*, 93–96.

43. Olivares, M.J.; Orozco, R.H.; Garrido, S.R.; Rodríguez-Vidigal, F.F.; Tomé, A.V.; Marcos, M.R. Activity of vancomycin, ciprofloxacin, daptomycin and linezolid against coagulasenegative staphylococci bacteremia. *Rev. Esp. Quimioter.* **2011**, *24*, 74–78.

44. Sarathbabu, R., Rajkumari, N., Ramani, V. Characterization of Coagulase negative Staphylococci isolated from urine, pus, sputum and blood samples. *Int. J. Pharma. Sci. Inv.* **2013**, *2*, 37–46.

45. Zheng, Z., Stewart PS. Penetration of Rifampin through *Staphylococcus epidermidis* Biofilms *Antimicrob. Agents Chemother.* **2002**, *46*, 900–903.

46. Leite, B.; Gomes, F.; Teixeira, P.; Souza, C.; Pizzolitto, E.; Oliveira, R. *In vitro* activity of daptomycin, linezolid and rifampicin on *Staphylococcus epidermidis* biofilms. *Curr. Microbiol.* **2011**, *63*, 313–317.

2

Pseudomonas aeruginosa Genome Evolution in Patients and under the Hospital Environment

Céline Lucchetti-Miganeh [1], **David Redelberger** [2], **Gaël Chambonnier** [2], **François Rechenmann** [1], **Sylvie Elsen** [3], **Christophe Bordi** [2], **Katy Jeannot** [4], **Ina Attrée** [3], **Patrick Plésiat** [4] **and Sophie de Bentzmann** [2,*]

[1] Genostar, 60 rue Lavoisier, Montbonnot 38330, France;
E-Mails: miganeh@genostar.com (C.L.-M.); rechenmann@genostar.com (F.R.)

[2] UMR7255-Laboratoire d'Ingénierie des Systèmes Macromoléculaires,
CNRS—Aix Marseille University, Marseille 13402, France; E-Mails: redel@imm.cnrs.fr (D.R.);
gchambonnier@imm.cnrs.fr (G.C.); bordi@imm.cnrs.fr (C.B.)

[3] INSERM, UMR-S 1036, Biology of Cancer and Infection, Grenoble 38054, France;
E-Mails: sylvie.elsen@cea.fr (S.E.); ina.attree-delic@cea.fr (I.A.)

[4] Laboratoire de Bactériologie, Faculté de Médecine-Pharmacie, Université de Franche-Comté,
Besançon 25030, France; E-Mails: katy.jeannot@univ-fcomte.fr (K.J.);
patrick.plesiat@univ-fcomte.fr (P.P.)

* Author to whom correspondence should be addressed; E-Mail: bentzman@imm.cnrs.fr;

Abstract: *Pseudomonas aeruginosa* is a Gram-negative environmental species and an opportunistic microorganism, establishing itself in vulnerable patients, such as those with cystic fibrosis (CF) or those hospitalized in intensive care units (ICU). It has become a major cause of nosocomial infections worldwide and a serious threat to Public Health because of overuse and misuse of antibiotics that have selected highly resistant strains against which very few therapeutic options exist. Herein is illustrated the intraclonal evolution of the genome of sequential isolates collected in a single CF patient from the early phase of pulmonary colonization to the fatal outcome. We also examined at the whole genome scale a pair of genotypically-related strains made of a drug susceptible, environmental isolate recovered from an ICU sink and of its multidrug resistant counterpart found to infect an ICU patient. Multiple genetic changes accumulated in the CF isolates over the disease time course including SNPs, deletion events and reduction of whole genome size. The strain isolated from the ICU patient displayed an increase in the genome size of 4.8% with major genetic rearrangements as compared to the initial environmental strain. The annotated genomes are given in free access in an interactive web application WallGene designed to facilitate large-scale comparative analysis and thus allowing investigators to explore homologies and syntenies between *P. aeruginosa* strains, here PAO1 and the five clinical strains described.

Keywords: *Pseudomonas aeruginosa*; microevolution; genome; virulence; resistance; cystic fibrosis; ventilator-associated pneumonia; ICU

---

1. Introduction

Genome sequencing capabilities have expanded exponentially in the last 10 years and the number of finished or draft genomes has considerably enriched databases [1]. This growing bulk of data has already proven to be useful for strain-to-strain comparisons, to obtain novel information on pathogen diversity, as well as to rapidly identify bacterial genes that play a role in infection and SNPs or other mutational events that shape the virulence in clonal expansion of strains. Several sequencing techniques are now available at low cost that can address all these issues. However, access to bioinformatic tools that rapidly provide a user-friendly way to compare neo-sequenced genomes with references available in databases is required for microbiologists.

Pseudomonas aeruginosa, a Gram-negative environmental species and an opportunistic pathogen, is a major cause of infections in vulnerable patients with cystic fibrosis (CF) or admitted to intensive care units (ICUs). With ca. 10% nosocomial infections incurred, this pathogen is now considered as serious problem to Public Health worldwide. In September 2013, the US Centers for Disease Control and Prevention (CDC) announced that the threat level associated with *P. aeruginosa* was "serious" because of high number of untreatable infections. Thus, an expanding number of genome sequencing projects have been launched to unravel the complex genetic changes occurring in *P. aeruginosa* during long-term chronic infections such as those encountered in CF [2-9] or to investigate the multiple resistance determinants of ICU strains [10]. In the present work, we sequenced and annotated genomes of *P. aeruginosa* isolates sequentially collected from a single CF patient as well as of two clonally-related isolates recovered in a same ICU (sink and patient) but having several different phenotypic traits. Draft genome versions were obtained by using Illumina Hiseq 2000 system, Genostar suite software and WallGene facilities allowing to track possible genetic events that could sustain their phenotypes. The clinical strains were compared to reference strain PAO1. Applied to CF (chronic evolution) and ICU (fast evolution) *P. aeruginosa* strains, our data provide new insights into the genomic diversification of clones, the potential role of prophages in shaping bacterial genomes in specific environments and key interesting genetic or genomic events that point out mechanisms that need further investigation.

2. Results and Discussion

2.1. Strains

2.1.1. Description of KK Related-Strains

Three related isolates, named KK, belonging to a same lineage A were sequentially collected from the sputum samples of a CF patient followed at the CF clinic of Hannover (Germany) who exhibited a *cftr* ΔF508/ΔF508 genotype associated with an exocrine pancreatic insufficiency.

The KK1 strain corresponds to the primo-colonization strain isolated when the patient was 16.2 year-old, the second KK14 strain was isolated 18 months later, and the third strain KK72 was recovered 156 months after the KK1 strain. The patient died shortly after this latest sampling.

2.1.1.1. Growth Characteristics

Under laboratory conditions, strains KK1 and PAO1 grew better than KK14 and KK72 (Figure 1B). Only KK14 produced mucoid colonies, a phenotype associated with alginate production (Figure 1A).

2.1.1.2. Motility and Biofilm Capacities

In addition to being mucoid, KK14 is non-flagellated and known to promote a higher IL6 and TNFα release from monocytes as compared to PAO1 reference strain [11]. None of the KK strains displayed a swarming phenotype, and the twitching motility of KK1 strain was identical to that of PAO1, whereas KK14 and KK72 did not twitch at all (Figure 1C). Under static growth conditions *in vitro*, KK1 and KK14 formed biofilm while KK72 did not (Figure 1D).

2.1.1.3. Proteolytic Activity, T3SS and T6SS

We previously showed that KK1 strain produced a phosphate limitation-like secretome [12] very different from the PAO1 one, including production of the Type 6 secretion system (T6SS HSI-I) marker protein Hcp1, that is part of the cell-puncturing device allowing the translocation of effectors into other bacterial species [13], but lacking T2SS-dependent substrates such as elastase. Proteolysis halo observed on TSA milk plates mainly indicating recovery of LasB in the extracellular medium, was strongly and statistically attenuated in KK strains as compared to PAO1, although KK14 displayed the highest activity among the KK strains (Figure 1E). Proteolytic halos were significantly different in size between KK strains.

Figure 1. Phenotypic characterization of KK cystic fibrosis (CF) strains. From the top left to the bottom right panels: (**A**) Aspect of KK strains plated on PIA agar plates (M for mucoid aspect and NM for non mucoid aspect); (**B**) Growth curves of KK strains in LB medium at 37 °C (n = 3); (**C**) Swarming and twitching behaviors of KK strains; (**D**) Biofilm biomass formed by KK strains evaluated by $OD_{570\,nm}$ measurement normalized by the $OD_{600\,nm}$ (growth) after crystal violet staining; (**E**) Proteolytic activity (highly dependent on T2SS) of extracellular products produced by KK strains. The mean and standard deviation of proteolytic halo measurements were presented (n = 9); T3SS production of KK strains evaluated in non induced or induced conditions (Ca^{2+} chelation) by the synthesis and secretion of the translocon proteins PopB and PcrV of the needle apparatus and the exotoxin ExoS, the cytosolic (Cytos) production of the positive regulator protein ExsA of the *P. aeruginosa* T3SS regulon [14] and of the anti-ExsA protein ExsD [15]; T6SS (HSI-1) production of KK strains evaluated by the synthesis (WC) and secretion (SN) of the Hcp1 protein; (**F**) Activity of *rsmY* and *rsmZ* promoters in KK strains.

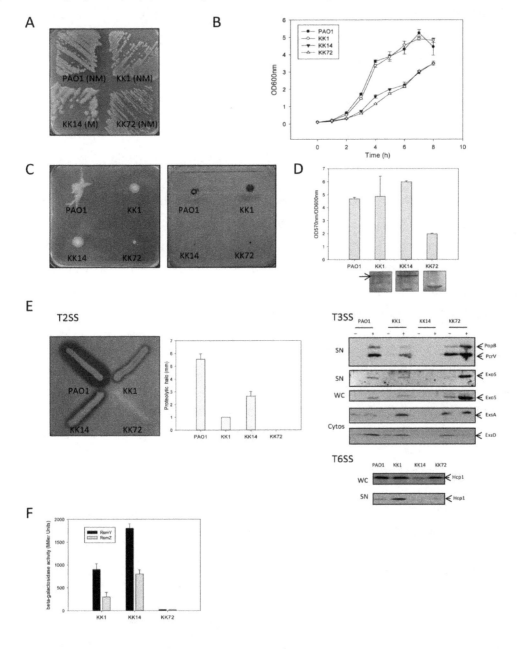

Type 3 secretion system (T3SS) is a secretion machinery looking like a molecular needle able to deliver cytotoxic effectors into host cells and thus which initiates and maintains infection by manipulating host cell biology such as cell signaling, secretory trafficking, cytoskeletal dynamics, and the inflammatory response (for review, see [16–18]). Clearly the KK strains were not equivalent T3SS producers. While KK1 produced and secreted T3SS proteins (here, the translocator proteins PopB and PcrV, and the effector protein ExoS) under calcium-depleted conditions similarly to PAO1, KK14 did not produce any of the T3SS proteins under both T3SS-induced and non-induced conditions. The transcriptional activator ExsA and its anti-activator, the ExsD protein were not detected in the KK14 strain, reflecting a strong defect or lack of T3SS gene expression. On the contrary, increased synthesis of ExoS and PopB/PcrV was observed in KK72 whatever the growth conditions used compared to KK1, in accordance with upregulated synthesis of ExsA even under high calcium concentrations. High amounts of ExoS were present in the supernatant of calcium-depleted cells, while PopB and PcrV appeared to be secreted under both conditions, in agreement with the absence of calcium control on translocator secretion [19] (Figure 1E). Transcription of genes (data obtained from transcriptomes of KK strains) encoding T3SS machinery and regulators as well as T3SS effectors was in complete agreement with our translation data (not shown).

T6SS production was effective in KK1 [12], strongly reduced in KK14, and similar to KK1 and PAO1 in KK72. Recovery of Hcp1 in supernatants was maximal in KK1, attenuated in KK72 and PAO1, and undetectable in KK14 (Figure 1E).

2.1.1.4. sRNA Rsm

The mutually exclusive biofilm-T3SS phenotypes, hallmarks of small non-coding RNA (sRNA) RsmY and RsmZ-dependent regulation [20,21] were investigated by monitoring the levels of *rsmY* and *rsmZ* transcriptional fusions. The *rsmY* and *rsmZ* promoter activities were found to be the highest in KK14, at intermediate level in KK1, and under the detection limit in KK72 (Figure 1E). Unexpectedly, T6SS production in KK strains (and transcript levels as well, data not shown) were not correlated with Rsm sRNA levels as already reported in other studies, suggesting that in KK strains, another level of T6SS regulation is operating that should be examined in the future.

2.1.2. Description of ST395 Related-Strains

Two genotypically identical isolates belonging to an epidemic clone, ST395, previously implicated in hospital outbreaks [22] were isolated from a sink (ST395E) and from a mechanically ventilated patient (ST395P) in a same intensive care unit (ICU) at the teaching Hospital of Besançon (France).

2.1.2.1. Growth Characteristics

The environmental isolate ST395E grew slightly faster than the clinical one, ST395P, (Figure 2A) though the difference was minimal after 8 h incubation.

Figure 2. Phenotypic characterization of ST395 ICU-related strains. (**A**) Growth curves of the ST395 strains in LB medium at 37 °C (n = 3); (**B**) Antibiograms of ST395 strains (FEP: cefepim, PIP: piperacillin, TZP: piperacillin+tazobactam, CTX: cefotaxime, TIC: ticarcillin, TCC: ticarcillin+clavulanic acid, CAZ: ceftazidime, MEM :meropenem, IPM: imipenem, GM: gentamicin, TM: tobramycin, ATM: aztreonam, K: kanamycin, CS: colistin, CIP: ciprofloxacin, AN: amikacin); (**C**) Swarming behaviour of ST395 strains grown on M8 medium supplemented with 0.5% agar for 48 h at 37 °C; Twitching behavior of ST395 strains grown on LB medium supplemented with 1.5% agar for 48 h at 37 °C.

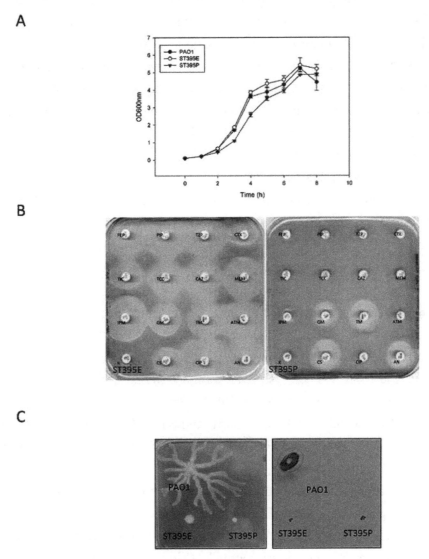

2.1.2.2. Antibiotic Resistance

While ST395E was susceptible to antipseudomonal antibiotics, ST395P exhibited panresistance to ß-lactams (including carbapenems imipenem and meropenem, penicillins ticarcillin ± clavulanic acid and piperacillin ± tazobactam, cephalosporins ceftazidime, cefepime, and cefotaxime, monobactam aztreonam) and fluoroquinolones (ciprofloxacin) (Figure 2B). A low level of resistance to aminoglycosides (amikacin, tobramycin and gentamicin) was also noted while ST395P remains susceptible to colistin thus fitting the definition of extremely drug resistance (XDR) [23]. Both ST395 strains turned out to be defective in swarming and twitching motility (Figure 2C).

2.2. Genome Examination

We obtained the assembled draft genomes of these five strains and compared them with reference strain PAO1, a primary analysis that will be completed by using other published annotated genomes as comparators [24].

We investigated the overall genomic differences between PAO1 and KK strains by aligning the genomes using MAUVE 2.3.1 software (Figure 3A). Alignment of the assembled contig sequences of draft genomes of KK strains with PAO1 suggests a high level of conservation along the chromosome. The KK strains have their chromosomes organized in a very similar way than in PAO1 except one inversion of two physically close syntenic blocks colored in green and yellow in Figure 3A (highlighted by arrows). Based on the total length of KK assembled contig sequences, as well as on the size of the PAO1 genome (6,264,404 bp), we could estimate the percentages of genome covered to be 97% for KK1 and KK14, and 96.6% for KK72. KK1 has an estimated genome size of 6,759,575 bp (6219 ORF with a GC% of 63.7), KK14 of 6,690,898 bp (6,157 ORF with a GC% of 64.1) and KK72 of 6,657,327 bp (6132 ORF with a GC% of 63.9) (Table 1), suggesting a slight reduction in the genome size during the pulmonary colonization timescale.

The draft genomes of the three KK strains were compared with that of PAO1 using the WallGene software. KK1, KK14 and KK72 were thus found to share 5308 genes with PAO1 and to contain 911,849,824 specific genes in their accessory genome, respectively. The KK strains shared a core of 6019 genes and had 84, 22 and 57 genes of difference between them, respectively (Figure 3C), while 222, 225 and 251 genes of PAO1 were absent in KK1, KK14 and KK72, respectively.

We investigated the overall genomic differences between PAO1 and ST395 strains by aligning the three genomes using the MAUVE 2.3.1 software (Figure 3B). Based on the total length of ST395 assembled contigs, as well as on the size of the PAO1 genome, we could estimate the percentages of genome covered to be 97.5% and 97.7% for ST395E and ST395P genomes, respectively. ST395E has a genome size of 6,993,173 bp (6,507 ORF with a GC% of 65.9) while ST395P has a genome of 7,133,660 bp (6,604 ORF with a GC% of 63.1) (Table 2).

The draft genomes of these two ICU strains were compared with that of PAO1 using WallGene. From these results, it appeared that ST395E and ST395P shared 5322 genes with PAO1 but contained 1185 and 1282 additional accessory genes, respectively. ST395 strains had 6135 genes in common but differed by 192 and 289 specific genes, respectively (Figure 3C). On the other hand, 189 and 181 genes present in PAO1 were lacking in ST395E and ST395P genomes, respectively. We next focused our analysis on regions of genome plasticity (RGP) in KK and ST395 strains.

2.2.1. KK Strain Microevolution and Phenotypic Consequences

The regions differing in KK strains as compared to PAO1 strain but also, changes that have occurred in the different KK genomes (summarized in Table 3 and Figure S1) were further examined.

Figure 3. Alignment of genomes using MAUVE. Pairwise alignment between the three KK strains (**A**) and the ST395 strains (**B**) and the complete genome of *P. aeruginosa* PAO1 using the MAUVE software. Colored blocks outline genome sequences that align to part of another genome, and is presumably homologous and internally free of genomic rearrangement (Locally Colinear Blocks or LCBs). White regions correspond to sequences that are not aligned and probably contain sequence elements specific to a particular genome. Blocks below the center line indicate regions that aligned in the reverse complement (inverse) orientation. The height of the profile within each LCB demonstrates the average degree of sequence conservation within an aligned region; (**C**) Venn diagrams of KK and ST395 strains.

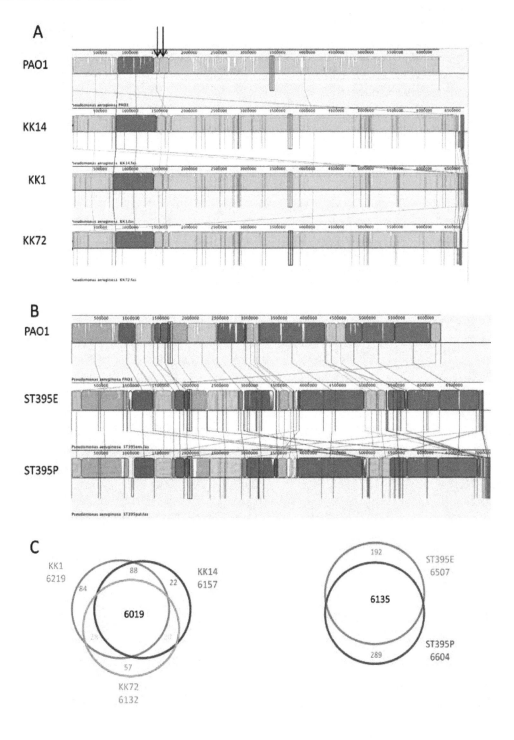

Table 1. Statistics and features of the sequenced *P. aeruginosa* KK strains.

Strains	PAO1	KK1	KK14	KK72
Numbers of reads	NA	10,357,778	10,357,778	10,357,778
Average read length (bp)	NA	90	90	90
Sequence coverage	NA	138	140	140
DNA scaffolds	NA	95	78	125
DNA total number bases	6,264,404	6,759,575	6,690,898	6,657,327
ORF	5571	6219	6157	6132
Genes with EC number (enzymes)	NA	978	978	974

NA: Non available.

Table 2. Statistics and features of the sequenced *P. aeruginosa* ST395 strains.

Strains	PAO1	ST395E	ST395P
Numbers of reads	NA	9,422,224	9,880,000
Average read length	NA	90	90
Sequence coverage	NA	121	125
DNA scaffolds	NA	55	86
DNA total number bases	6,264,404	6,993,173	7,133,660
ORF	5571	6507	6604
Genes with EC number (enzymes)	NA	982	982

NA: Non available.

Table 3. Regions of genome plasticity of the sequenced *P. aeruginosa* KK strains.

	Location in PAO1 genome	Phagic origin	KK1	KK14	KK72
Region KK_1	PA3357-PA3391 (24 kb)	no	+ (33.119 kb)	+ (33.119 kb)	-
Region KK_2	PA0632-PA0649	yes	-	-	-
Region KK_3 Prophage KK_1	PA0729.1	yes ΦCTX	+ (38.859 kb)	+ (38.859 kb)	-
Region KK_4 Prophage KK_2	PA0820-PA0826.1	yes F10	+ (>54.093 kb)	+ (>54.074 kb)	+ (>54.093 kb)
Region KK_5	PA1087-PA1094	no	+ (12.703 kb) Novel locus	+ (12.703 kb) Novel locus	+ (12.703 kb) Novel locus
Region KK_6 Prophage KK_3	PA1796.1-PA1796.4	yes Φ297	+ (51.617 kb)	-	+ (51.625 kb)
Region KK_7 Prophage-like_KK_4	PA4673.1	??	+ (>24.424 kb)	+ (22.616 kb)	+ (24.664 kb)
Region KK_8	PA2593-PA2594	no	+ (31.824 kb)	+ (34.971 kb)	+ (31.814 kb)
Region KK_9	PA2819.1-PA2819.3	no	+ (123.358 kb)	+ (122.554 kb)	+ (122.566 kb)
Region KK_10	PA2583.1	no	+ (102.482 kb)	+ (>83.975 kb)	+ (102.482 kb)
Region KK_11	PA3768-3769	no	+ (6.955 kb)	+ (6.955 kb)	+ (6.955 kb)
Region KK_12	Upstream PA2077	no	+ (57.2 kb)	+ (57.2 kb)	+ (57.2 kb)

2.2.1.1. Major Genomic Changes between KK Strains

A region consisting of 33 genes, named KK_1, was present in the KK1, KK14 and PAO1 genomes but absent in KK72. In KK1 and KK14, this locus contains additional ORF genes covering approximately 8 kb, compared with PAO1.

The region named KK_2 of PAO1 genome which overlaps the RGP4 previously identified (PA0641-PA0648) [25] was absent in all KK strains, at least at that location and in the covered sequences.

The region KK_3 of 38,859 kb (prophage KK_1 corresponding to 50 ORF with a GC% of 61.4, Figure 4) was identified in KK1 and KK14 strains but not in KK72 strain. This region displays high homology with bacteriophage ΦCTX.

The region KK_4 of 56.3 kb (prophage KK_2 corresponding to 81 ORF with a GC% of 60.6, Figure 4) replaced the locus PA0820-PA0826.1 of PAO1 in all the KK strains. This region displays a high homology with bacteriophage F10 although the full region was unavailable in all the KK strains due to overlapping of this region with ends of contigs.

The 12.3 kb-long region KK_5 located between PA1087 (*flgL*) and PA1094 (*fliD*), that in the PAO1 genome contains the *fgtA* and the *fliC* genes encoding the flagellar glycosyltransferase FgtA and the type B flagellin, respectively, was found to be replaced in all the KK strains by a locus of 9 genes identical to RGP9 of strain PAC2, encoding among others, a type A flagellin [25].

The region KK_6 (prophage KK_3 corresponding to 38 ORF with a GC% of 61.1, Figure 4) was identified in KK1 and KK72. This region displays high homology with bacteriophage Φ297. In KK14, the prophage sequence was missing except 2 genes indicating a partial excision.

The region KK_7 (prophage-like KK_4 corresponding to 38 ORF with a GC% of 61.1) occurring in all the KK strains appeared to be incomplete since present at the ends of contigs in all these bacteria. PHAST software was unable to ascertain the phage origin of this region, probably because of incomplete sequences of the draft genomes.

Region KK_8 (31.5 kb, 20 ORF) was present in all the KK strains while absent from PAO1. This region carries the *pltLABCDEFGMR* locus involved in biosynthesis of antifungal product pyoluteorin, a hybrid polyketide-nonribosomal peptide molecule of *Pseudomonas fluorescens* Pf-5 [26] also produced by LESB58 and M18 strains of *P. aeruginosa*. Whether it contributes to antifungal defence in the CF lungs has to be elucidated.

Region KK_9 (125 kb) was found to be inserted in all the KK strains between gene PA2818 encoding the aminoglycoside response regulator Arr [27] and the PA2820 gene in place of the tRNA-Gly, Gly and Glu PA2819.1 to PA2819.3 of the PAO1 strain. KK_9 is part of the RGP29 identified in PA2192 strain [25] (from PA2G_02184 to PA2G_02073) with particularities of this region in KK strains since it possesses a gene encoding a supplementary heavy metal RND efflux pump of the CzcABC type, several genes encoding putative copper resistance proteins and putative regulatory proteins.

The region KK_10 of 106 kb in length detected in all the KK strains between PA2583 and PA2584 in place of the tRNA-Gly PA2583.1 of PAO1 genome exhibited high homologies with the PA_01003088 to PA_01003140 genes of RGP27 of from *P. aeruginosa* strain PAC2 strain [25]. This region was incomplete in KK14 since ending a contig (Figure S1).

Figure 4. Prophages identified in KK strains. The identification has been performed using PHAST software; each arrow represents a gene predicted by PHAST and color codes indicate the corresponding functions of the genes.

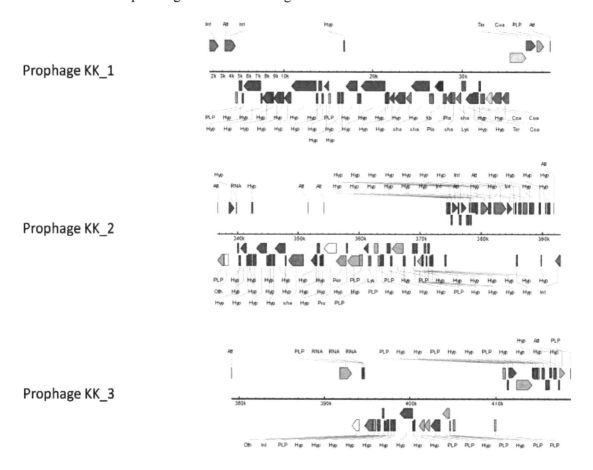

Identified CDS types:

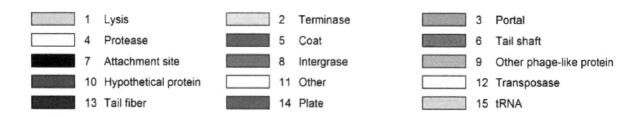

1	Lysis		2	Terminase		3	Portal
4	Protease		5	Coat		6	Tail shaft
7	Attachment site		8	Intergrase		9	Other phage-like protein
10	Hypothetical protein		11	Other		12	Transposase
13	Tail fiber		14	Plate		15	tRNA

A region of 6 genes, named KK_11, was present in all the KK strains in between PA3768 and PA3769 (*guaA*), of which 3 genes had homologs (PA14_15620 to PA14_15650) in RGP36 of PACS2 or PA14 strains [25].

Finally, the KK strains all displayed a 38 gene locus (region KK_12, 57.2 kb) located between the PA2077 and PA2078 genes of PAO1, encoding proteins involved in mercuric resistance (with *merE*, *merD*, *merA*, *merP*, *merR* and *merT* homologs [28]), corresponding to an RND multi-drug efflux pump and a regulator of EAL family.

All phage regions were confirmed by mapping reads and therefore we could confirm that when stated these regions are missing.

2.2.1.2. Minor Genomic Changes between KK Strains

Regarding additional genomic DNA differences between KK strains and PAO1, more discrete remodeling events were noticed. For instance, in KK strains a gene encoding a putative acetyltransferase was found inserted downstream the *pdxY* (PA5516) gene compared to PAO1. Similarly, an additional gene encoding an asparagine synthetase was identified downstream the *rfaE* (PA4996) gene of PAO1, in all the KK strains just as in *P. aeruginosa* M18. The gene encoding AlgP, the prokaryotic transcriptional positive regulator required for transcription of key alginate biosynthetic gene *algD*, contained in all the KK strains an extra 12-bp repeated sequence corresponding to a KPAA additional module as compared to PAO1. However, although the repetitive structure of the *algP* gene appears to participate in the processes underlying the metastable character of mucoidy in *P. aeruginosa*, variations in the number of the 12-bp repeats found did not appear to influence the mucoid status of the examined strains [29].

On the other side, several specific regions of PAO1 were not identified in the KK strains. As mentioned previously, this was the case of region KK_2 and of three ORF (PA3486-PA3488) including *pldA* and *vgrA1* genes which encodes a phospholipase D and an effector of the HSI-I T6SS, respectively. These later genes are present on a 7 kb mobile genetic element acquired horizontally, perhaps from an eukaryotic organism, of which *pldA* has been demonstrated to contribute to the ability of *P. aeruginosa* PAO1 to persist in a chronic pulmonary infection model in rats [30]. The region PA3497-PA3514 of PAO1 corresponding to RGP34 was absent from the KK strains as it is from strains PA14, PACS2, PA2192 and C3719 [25].

2.2.1.3. Genetic Changes Related to Evolution of Phenotypic Traits of KK Strains over Time in CF Patient

Quorum Sensing and Alginate. We previously demonstrated that KK1 strain produces a phosphate limitation-like secretome very different from the PAO1 one, in particular lacking the elastase LasB [12]. We thus examined what could explain this particular secretory phenotype. Interestingly, this strain lacks the PA1430-1433 genes encoding the LasR-LasI quorum sensing cell-cell communication system that controls expression of many exoproducts in *P. aeruginosa* [31], the RsaL negative regulator of LasR-LasI system [32] and a protein of unknown function (Figure 5). Interestingly, KK14 and KK72 strains have this locus. Moreover, LasR of KK72 strain displays a K218R substitution (Figure 8A) in the C-terminal part of this LuxR type regulator forming an HTH domain contacting DNA [33]. The impact of this amino-acid substitution in the α9 helix critical for DNA recognition [34] and for binding of the LasR transcriptional activator in KK72 strain requires further examination. These genetic changes seem to correlate well with the global analysis of proteolytic activity of these strains (Figure 1E), although in depth analysis has to be performed. This suggests that the absence of this particular region could represent a fitness advantage for *P. aeruginosa* onset of infection in the KK environment.

Figure 5. KK strain regions of genome plasticity (RGPs) varying between KK strains using WallGene facility. KK1 genome was chosen as the reference genome. The following color codes are used for genes in WallGene: (1) genes of the reference organism with a homologous gene in at least one of the non-reference genomes have an attributed color (except black, grey, or white) at random; (2) genes of the reference genome with no homology at all are black; (3) genes of non-reference genomes with exactly one homology in the reference genome are the same color as the homologous gene; (4) genes of non-reference genome with more than one homology in the reference genome are white; (5) genes of non-reference genomes with no homology in the reference genome are dark grey. If homology links are displayed, those genes are hidden.

KK1 and KK72 strains display a non mucoid phenotype, while KK14 strain exhibits a mucoid phenotype (Figure 1A). Examination of sequence of the *mucA* gene in KK strains identified a deletion of one G base in a stretch of 5G specific to KK14 strain already identified as a hot spot of mutation in *mucA* gene and leading to a frameshift [35]. The non mucoid phenotype of KK72 is associated with a wild type *mucA* gene. Transcriptomic data obtained from these three strains further confirmed the derepression of the *alg* biosynthetic genes in KK14 as compared to KK1 and KK72 strains (data not shown). Additionally, examination of variants showed that *algD* gene encoding a periplasmic epimerase which converts ß-D-mannuronic acid into α-L-guluronic acids at the polymer level of the alginate biosynthetis machinery [36] exhibits a SNP R401H in KK14 as compared to KK1 and KK72 strains. Whether this SNP contributes to KK14 mucoidy conversion remains to be elucidated.

GacS/GacA regulatory pathway and related phenotypes. We further examined KK genomes for the central GacS/GacA regulatory pathway controlling sRNA Rsm levels, since it has been demonstrated to be impaired in several clinical strains [5,37,38]. High expression of *rsmY* and *rsmZ* leads to massive biofilm formation and T6SS production and to repression of T3SS expression, while an impaired biofilm formation and no T6SS production and an induction of T3SS expression is associated with low or null levels of RsmY and RsmZ [39]. In *P. aeruginosa*, transcription of these two sRNAs is under a complex and sophisticated regulatory network involving the GacS/GacA two-component system (TCS) but also other TCS pathways including (i) the two histidine kinases (HK) LadS and RetS which triggers and represses expression of both *rsm* genes by interfering with the GacS/GacA TCS activity, respectively [40–42]; (ii) the GacS-structurally related PA1611 hybrid HK interacting with RetS in *P.*

aeruginosa in a very similar manner than GacS and RetS do [43]; (iii) the HptB regulatory pathway which also intersects with the GacS/GacA TCS and induces only the expression of *rsmY* gene [39] and their associated HK PA2824 (SagS) [44] and PA1975 and iv/ the TCS BfiS/BfiR [45]. We thus checked if partners of the complex and sophisticated regulatory networking controlling Rsm production display or not mutations in KK strains. No mutation in LadS, GadS, GacA, RetS, PA1611 or PA1975, the regulator of PA1611, or in HptB was identified although these proteins are sharing polymorphism in all KK strains as compared to PAO1. No SNP was identified in promoter sequences of these genes or in *rsm* promoters between the three KK strains. Thus, this regulatory pathway remains functional during the period of isolation of KK strains, a feature interesting since LadS or GacS have been found to be susceptible to mutations in PA14 [38] or in the CF CHA [5,37] strains. TCS are not the only players involved in controlling *rsm* expression. Intracellular level of cyclic di-GMP has been described to control *rsm* expression [46] and an elevated intracellular concentration of cyclic di-GMP leads to an increased production of RsmY and RsmZ. This intracellular level of cyclic di-GMP is oppositely controlled by phosphodiesterases (PDE) and diguanylate cyclases (DGC) and any modification of the expression level of these proteins could thus lead to modification of *rsm* expression. Interestingly, KK14 strain does not produce and secrete T6SS components while forming biofilm and KK72 produces and secretes T6SS components while not forming biofilm, thus in these two strains, T6SS production is not following the same Rsm-dependent regulation than biofilm. This Rsm-independent regulation of T6SS has to be confirmed. As AlgU is exerting a negative effect on HSI-I genes (Tart *et al.*, 2005), this could explain at least the KK14 defective T6SS production.

KK72 strain exhibits a deregulated T3SS production and secretion (effective in non-induced and induced conditions, Figure 1E) that is coupled to an increased ExsA amount. Beside high levels of free RsmA that positively regulates *exsA* expression [47], additional levels of regulation might be implied, T3SS expression and activity being finely tuned (for review [48,49]). No particular mutation was found specific to this KK72 strain in key regulatory T3SS genes such as *vfr* and *exsC* and *exsE*. Examination of the promoters and genes of the transcriptional activator ExsA and its repressor ExsD was made indicating that ExsD accumulates mutations in KK14 and KK72 as compared to KK1 strain such as P126A and G235V; whether these mutations participate in hyper production of T3SS in KK72 strain remains to be studied. Additionally, the negative T3SS producing KK14 strain exhibits a unique S232R mutation in ExsA, whether it contributes to its DNA binding activity remains to be elucidated. ExsA expression, the master regulator of T3SS gene expression, has been demonstrated to be reduced in *mucA* mutants through either a Vfr-independent mechanism involving the RsmAYZ regulatory system and the TCS AlgZ/AlgR [47] or a Vfr-dependent mechanism [50] possibly on the promoter of the regulatory operon *exsCEBA* [51]. Whether it contributes to absence of T3SS expression in the mucoid KK14 strain has to be elucidated as well.

Figure 6. Prophages identified in ST395 strains. The identification has been performed using PHAST software; each arrow represents a gene predicted by PHAST and color codes indicate the corresponding functions of the genes.

Figure 6

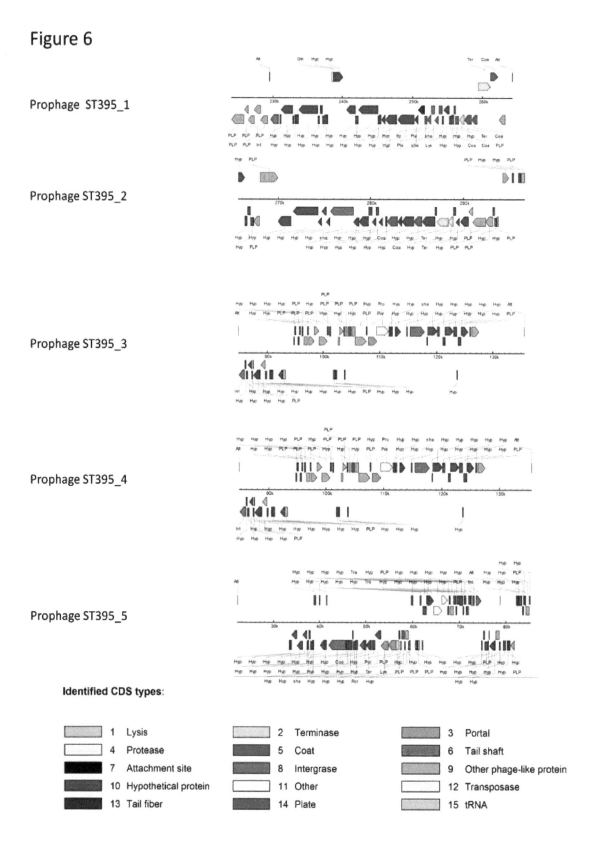

2.2.2. ST395 Strain Microevolution and Phenotypic Consequences

As proposed previously, an even short-term habitat differentiation can cause major phenotypic diversification driven by single genomic variation events and uptake of phage DNA (Bezuidt, 2013). Rearrangements observed in ST395 strains (Table 4 and Figures 6, 7 and S2) are good illustrations of this feature in a non CF clinical context.

Table 4. Regions of genome plasticity of the sequenced *P. aeruginosa* ST395 strains.

	Location in PAO1 genome	Phagic origin	ST395E	ST395P
Region ST395_1&2	PA5149.1	no	+ (26.483 kb)	+ (12.871 kb)
Region ST395_1&2 Prophage ST395_1	PA5160.1	yes ΦCTX	+ (40.4 kb)	+ (22.7 kb)
Region ST395_3 Prophage ST395_2	PA2603.1	yes Φ297	+ (31 kb)	-
Region ST395_4 Prophage ST395_3	PA4138-PA4139	yes F10	+ (42,196kb)	?
Region ST395_5 Prophage ST395_4	PA2794-PA2795	yes F116	-	+ (70.9 kb)
Region ST395_6	PA2583.1	no	+ (99.342 kb)	+ (79.699 kb)
Region ST395_7	PA0728 -PA0730	no	+ (91 kb)	+ (104.3 kb)
Region ST395_8	*phnA -phnB* genes	no	-	+ (74 kb)
Region ST395_9 Prophage ST395_5	PA3824.1	yes B3	-	+ (63.1 kb)
Region ST395_10	PA2817-PA2820	no	+ (104.5 kb)	+ (7.46 kb)
Region ST395_11	PA0976.1	no	+ PAPI-1 like	+ PAPI-1 like
Region ST395_12	PA2730-PA2736.1	no	+ (25.6 kb)	+ (57.25 kb)
Region ST395_13	PA4231-PA4232	no	+ (19.6 kb)	+ (19.6 kb)
Region ST395_14	PA3835-PA3836	no	+ (PAGI-9) (7.192 kb)	+ (PAGI-9) (7.192 kb)

2.2.2.1. Major Genomic Changes between ST395 Strains

The ST395_1 region was identified in place of the tRNA-Phe PA5149.1 of PAO1 strain, the location of the previously described RGP62 [25]. However, none of the genes of ST395 strains display homologies with those of PACS2 strain. This region varies in size from 26,483 bp in ST395E and 12,871 bp in ST395P (Figure 7), respectively due to the absence of the last four genes in ST395P.

Figure 7. ST395 strain RGPs varying between ST395 strains using Wallgene facility. ST395P was chosen as the reference genome. The same color codes presented for Figure 5 are used.

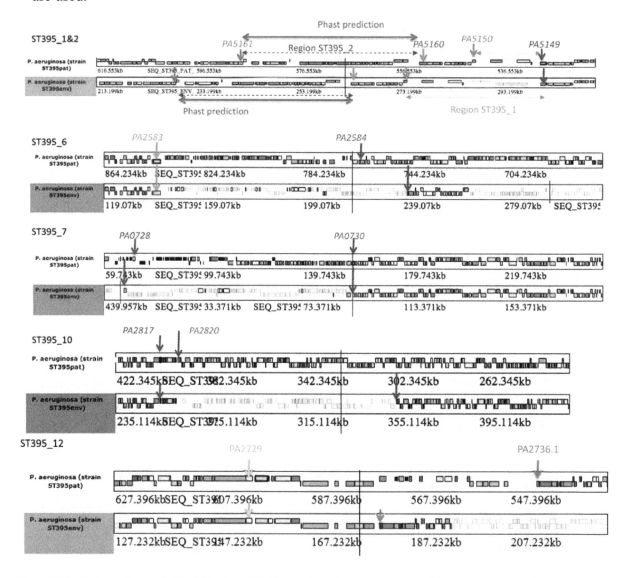

The ST395_2 region of 40.4 kb in ST395 strains (prophage ST395_1 corresponding to 49 ORF, (Figures 6 and 7), with a GC% of 63.7 and 65.2 for ST395E and ST395P, respectively) was identified in both ST395 strains and present in between PA5160 and PA5161 (*rmlD*) of PAO1 strain in place of the tRNA-Thr PA5160.1.

The ST395_3 region of 50 kb (prophage ST395_2 corresponding to 68 ORF with a GC% of 62.7) was specifically identified in ST395E strain in place of the tRNA-Ser PA2603.1. PHAST predicts an incomplete prophage which displays homology with the phage Φ297 (Figure 6). This region ST395_3 is probably incomplete since present at the ends of two contigs.

The ST395_4 region of 50.8kb (prophage ST395_3 corresponding to 60 ORF with a GC% of 62.8) was identified ST395E strain in a region which was not previously identified as a RGP [25]. Its existence in ST395P could not be ascertained since both bording genes were present at the ends of two contigs. This prophage (Figure 6) is homologous to prophage 2 identified in LESB58 strain of which 32 genes are homologous to the sequenced bacteriophage F10 [52].

The ST395_5 region (prophage ST395_4 corresponding to 70 ORF with a GC% of 63) of 70.9 kb was specifically identified in ST395P strain between PA2794 and PA2795 genes of PAO1 strain. This region is an intact prophage which displays homology with the bacteriophage F116 (Figure 6).

The region ST395_6 was identified in both ST395 strains in place of the tRNA-Gly PA2583.1 of PAO1 strain with a respective size of 99,342 and 79,699 bp in ST395E and ST395P strains (Figure 7). In ST395E it represents part of RGP29 of strain 2192 lacking the Dit Island genes encoding proteins of abietane diterpenoids metabolism [25], while in ST395P, this region is organized as the RGP27 of PACS2 [25]. Thus, whereas both ST395 display additional regions in this genome location, it appears that these two regions are not well conserved between the two ST395 strains, resequencing this region with NGS long reads technology could thus be decisive.

The region ST395_7 inserted in between PA0728 and PA0730 from PAO1 strain, described as the RGP5 [25], is in ST395E an homologous region of 91kb (PSTAB_1168-PSTAB_1251) identified in *Pseudomonas stutzeri,* strain ATCC 17588 (LMG 11199) [53]. In ST395P strain, bording genes of this DNA region of 104.3kb are homologous to PA7_5324 and PA7_5328 and the inserted region derives from the *P. aeruginosa* NCGM2.S1 strain and thus differs widely as compared to the corresponding region in ST395E strain (Figure 7). For example, ST395P strain has an *int1*-like gene (99.9% of identity), a trace of an integron but no complete cassette gene could be identified. There is a questionable prophage (11 ORF) related to the Pf1 prophage in this region for ST395P but no homologous phage was found using PHAST for ST395E.

The region ST395_8 of 67.15kb was specifically identified in ST395P strain inserted in between *phnA* and *phnB* genes of PAO1 strain. This region is part of the RGP29 (PA2G_02071-PA2G_02148) identified in strain 2192 of *P. aeruginosa* [25].

The region ST395_9 of 63.1 kb was also specifically identified in ST395P strain (prophage ST395_5 corresponding to 85 ORF with a GC% of 63.2) inserted in place of the tRNA-Leu (PA3824.1) of PAO1 strain, however the other bording gene is unavailable due to the end of the corresponding contig (Figure 6). The region exhibits high homologies with the region of 39016 strain of *P. aeruginosa* (PA39016_000840119-PA39016_000840070) derived from Phage pseudoB3.

Additionally, these ST395 strains were characterized by several other major genomic rearrangements. For example, the region between PA2817 and PA2820 in PAO1 strain containing the gene encoding the aminoglycoside response regulator (Arr) [27] is varying in between the two ST395 strains (ST395_10) and compared to PAO1 strain (Figure 7). In ST395E, this region is 104 kb long whereas in S395P this region is only 7.46 kb long, suggesting that most of this region was lost in ST395P. Genes present in this region in ST395P strain are also present in ST395E strain. In ST395E, additional region resembles the RGP29 inserted locus of PAGC2 strain but lacking the Dit Island genes encoding proteins of abietane diterpenoids metabolism [25].

The ICE PAPI-1 identified in PA14 strain was found in both strains (ST395_11) but instead of being inserted in the PA4514.1-4541.3 tRNA region as in PA14 strain [54], this ICE is inserted in place of the tRNA-Lys PA0976.1 in both ST395 strains, the place where the ICE PAPI-2 is inserted in PA14, this latter region being identical to PAO1. Whether this ICE PAPI-1 is complete requires extended PCR since genes of the end of this PAPI-1-like element are present at the ends of sequenced contigs in both strains.

The region ST395_12 is located in place of PA2730-2736.1 of PAO1 strain. This region of 25.6 kb and 57.25kb in ST395E and ST395P (Figure 7), respectively is containing genes common to both strains but STP395P contains additional genes encoding an integrase, a protein involved in DNA repair (RadC like) and a protein homologous of ThiJ from *E. coli* belonging to the DJ-1 superfamily [55].

The region ST395_13 present in both ST395 strains of 19.6 kb is located in between PA4231 (*pchA*) gene and PA4232 (*ssb*) gene of PAO1. It contains a majority of genes encoding integrase family proteins with high homologies with those identified in *P. putida* GB-1 strain.

Glycosylation locus involved in A-band and B-band lipopolysaccharide synthesis [56] is absent in draft genomes of ST395 strains.

All phage regions were confirmed by mapping reads and therefore we could confirm that when stated these regions are missing.

2.2.2.2. Minor Genomic Changes between ST395 Strains

More discrete remodeling events were noticed in ST395 strains. For example, the region upstream the *cupA* locus, which contains the *cgrABC* genes controlling *cupA* gene expression [57,58], exhibits in ST395P a probable frameshift in *cgrA* gene. Whether this disturbs *cgr*-dependent *cupA* regulation in this strain requires functional studies.

The PA2152 gene encoding a protein with maltose alpha-D-glucosyltransferase activity probably involved in trehalose biosynthesis in PAO1 strain [59] exhibits premature stop codons in both ST395 strains, possibly suggesting that this pathway is altered in ST395 strains.

ST395 strains possess additional genes such as a gene encoding an asparagine synthetase recovered only in LESB58 and M18 *P.aeruginosa* strains in between *rfaE* [60] and PA4995 genes of PAO1 strains, a gene in between PA2790 and P2791 genes of PAO1 recovered in LESB58 and B136-33 *P. aeruginosa* strains whose corresponding putative product contains a right handed beta helix region that shares some similarity with pectate lyases. The PA3164 gene which in PAO1 strain seems to be a pseudogene due to frameshift is probably encoding a functional 3-phoshoshikimate 1-carboxyvinyltransferase prephenate dehydrogenase in both ST395 strains. Other discrete variations were identified in particular in *algP* gene from ST395 strains, the gene which encodes a regulator involved in regulation of mucoidy in *P. aeruginosa* [29]. None of the open reading frame of these strains was matching with the *algP* wild type version, probably highlighting a defect in mucoidy conversion in ST395 strains. Another example comes from the PA2690 gene in PAO1 which encodes a probable transposase which is absent from the ST395 strain genomes.

Interestingly, ST395 strains possess as B136-33, 2192 and RP73 and PSE9 [61] strains of *P. aeruginosa* an additional gene (ST395_14) present in between PA3835 and PA3836 genes of PAO1 strain. This gene forms the PAGI-9 island of 7.192 kb identified in PSE9 strain [61]. Thus strains ST395 possess the PAGI-9 island formed of the *rhs* gene and could probably contribute to virulence of these strains in acute pneumonia in the context of ventilator-associated pneumonia in ICU [62].

The ST395 strains are thus highly differing in their prophage regions but also major differences are observed between their RGP, suggesting that environmental constraints have highly shaped genome backbones in between the two times of isolation, although intermediate sampling could help in identifying whether changing habitat may have caused these rearrangements.

2.2.2.3. Genetic Changes Related to ST395P Multi-Drug Resistance towards Antibiotics as Compared to ST395E

Genes or regions known to be implicated in resistance to ß-lactams, aminoglycosides and fluoroquinolones were investigated in detail [63,64] (Table 5).

Table 5. Genetic events in target genes controlling acquired resistance in ST395 strains.

	ST395E	**ST395P**
Resistance to ß lactams		
AmpC derepression		
AmpD, AmpDh2, AmpDh3	A134V, wt, R66C	T139M and A134V, wt, R66C
OprD	wt	c703t SNP introducing a premature stop codon
MexAB-OprM overproduction		
MexR	wt	H107P
NalC	G71E	G71E
NalD	wt	wt
ArmR	wt	wt
MexXY-OprM overproduction	See Resistance to aminoglycosides	See Resistance to aminoglycosides
MexCD-OprJ overproduction		
NfxB	wt	wt
Resistance to aminoglycosides		
Aminoglycoside modifying enzymes		
APH(3')-IIb	wt	wt
MexXY-OprM overproduction		
MexZ (*agrZ* mutant)	wt	del nt452-459 of *mexZ* gene
RplA (*agrW1* mutant)	wt	wt
Fmt (*agrW1* mutant)	wt	wt
FolD (*agrW1* mutant)	wt	wt
ArmZ (*agrW1* mutant)	wt	wt
rplU-rpmA promoter (*agrW1* mutant)	wt	Insertion of 2g at -186nt before the start codon of the *rplU* gene
ParRS (*agrW2* mutant)	ParR wt, ParS wt	ParR wt, ParS V216A
PA2572-PA2573	wt,R206G Q210K S217A N236D	wt,R206G Q210K S217A N236D
Resistance to fluoroquinolones		
DNA gyrase and topoisomerase		
GyrA	925 aa (PA01 923 aa)	925 aa T83I
ParC	wt	S87L
GyrB	wt	wt
ParE	V200M	V200M
MexAB-OprM overproduction	See Resistance to ß lactams	See Resistance to ß lactams
MexXY-OprM overproduction	See Resistance to aminoglycosides	See Resistance to aminoglycosides
MexCD-OprJ overproduction	See Resistance to ß lactams	See Resistance to ß lactams
MexEF-OprN overproduction	MexT wt, MexS wt	MexT R48C, MexS T19P

Resistance to ß-lactams. In *P. aeruginosa,* resistance to ß-lactams may be due to overproduction of intrinsic ß-lactamase AmpC, acquisition of various secondary *β*-lactamases through horizontal gene transfer, decrease in the outer membrane permeability (loss of porins) [65] and/or overproduction of active efflux systems, mainly MexAB-OprM and MexXY-OprM [66].

While no acquired ß-lactamase gene could be detected in ST395P, the strain turned out to harbor a mutation in the *ampD* gene leading to a T139M substitution in amidase AmpD, compared with its wild-type susceptible counterpart ST395E. Inactivation of this enzyme which plays an important role in the recycling of muropeptides during the remodeling of peptidoglycan is a well known cause of AmpC upregulation in *P. aeruginosa* and of pan-resistance to ß-lactams except carbapenems [67]. Interestingly, we found that the decreased susceptibility of ST395P to carbapenems (imipenem and meropenem) was related to a C703T substitution introducing a premature stop codon in *oprD*, the gene which encodes the major uptake pathway of carbapenems in *P. aeruginosa*, namely porin OprD [68]. While no clear evidence was obtained of mutations upregulating efflux pumps in ST395P except for MexXY(OprM) (see below) and a H107P substitution in MexR that could explain the *mexAB-oprM* overexpression, although this substitution located in the α5 helix (Figure 8B) of the protein [69] has not been described as critical for MexR oligomerization or DNA binding [70], both the overproduction of intrinsic ß-lactamase and the loss of porin OprD are sufficient to account for the resistance phenotype displayed by this isolate.

Figure 8. (A) Modelization of the C-terminal end of the LasR activator of QS. LasR from KK14 and KK72 differed by an amino-acid substitution K218R (K for KK14, and R for KK72 strains) present in the α9 helix important for recognition of DNA before binding. **(B)** Modelization of the dimer of the MexR variant of the transcriptional repressor of the MexAB-OprM efflux pump in strain ST395P. Each monomer is colored differently (green and blue), both harboring amino acid substitution (in red) in α5 helix (H107P) which is probably not critical for MexR oligomerization or DNA binding.

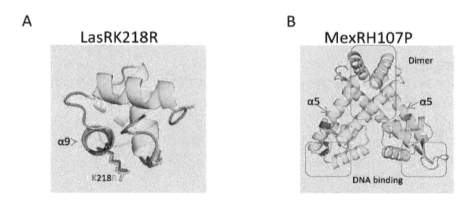

Resistance to aminoglycosides. High aminoglycoside resistance in *P. aeruginosa* is due to horizontally acquired aminoglycoside-modifying enzymes (AME). Beyond the AME named APH(3')-IIb, contributing to intrinsic kanamycin resistance, none additional AME encoding gene was identified in the ST395 strains. This result was not surprising by itself in view of the low resistance levels to aminoglycosides (gentamicin, tobramycin and amikacin) displayed by ST395P. Strongly supporting that the efflux system MexXY-OprM is upregulated in this isolate and plays a role in its resistance phenotype, we found a deletion (nt 452–459) in the *mexZ* gene that encodes the TetR-like repressor (MexZ) of operon *mexXY* [71]. Comparatively, ST395E harbored an intact, wild-type gene *mexZ*. Recently, mutational inactivation of MexZ has been reported as the main cause of low-level efflux-based resistance to aminoglycosides in clinical strains of *P. aeruginosa* [72]. It should be noted here that MexXY-OprM is the only pump able to extrude these antibiotics in this organism. Potential other mutations contributing to overexpression of operon *mexXY* in ST395P have been revealed by genome sequencing, the role of which remains to be confirmed (Table 5).

Resistance to fluoroquinolones. Accounting for the elevated resistance of ST395P to fluoroquinolones, a T83I mutation could be identified in the QRDR (Quinolone Resistance Determining Region) of the A subunit (GyrA) of the main target enzyme DNA gyrase [73]. Another prevalent mutation (S87L) responsible for high fluoroquinolone resistance in *P. aeruginosa* was characterized in the C subunit (ParC) of the secondary target enzyme, topoisomerase IV. Beside these mutations that strongly affect the interaction of fluoroquinolones with their cellular targets, upregulation of the MeXY(OprM) system was also expected to contribute to some extend to the resistance phenotype of ST395P to these agents.

In final, our whole genome sequencing experiments revealed that ST395P has become multiresistant through a series of mutations activating intrinsic mechanisms that involve drug hydrolysis (ß-lactamase AmpC), membrane impermeability (loss of porin OprD), and drug efflux (overproduction of MexXY(OprM)). This evolution from the environmental isolate ST395E was not dependent upon lateral gene transfer (summarized in Table 5).

3. Experimental Section

3.1. Origin of Strains

The CF KK strains were sequentially isolated in a CF patient followed at the CF clinic Hannover who died after the isolation of isolate KK72. The ICU ST395 strains were isolated at the Besançon Hospital, ST395E in a sink of an ICU department and ST395P has been isolated in a patient hospitalized in the same ICU unit and under ventilated assistance.

3.2. Genome Sequencing and Bioinformatics

Genomic DNA was sequenced on Illumina Hiseq 2000 system (Beijing Genomics Institute, BGI, China). Mean genome coverage varied between 121 to 140 X. The paired-end reads were assembled *de novo* using SOAPdenovo 1.05. The resulting number of contigs varied between 55 to 125 with an average length from 70,000 to 127,000 bases. Genome sizes and sequencing data are indicated for each strain in Tables 1 and 2.

Annotation of the assembled contig sequences was performed with the Genostar Suite software. The Genostar Suite, together with the reference MicroB database, is an integrated bioinformatics interactive software application dedicated to microbial genome analysis and comparison. MicroB integrates and updates data from several databases, *i.e.*, NCBI Reference Sequence, UniProtKB, ENZYME, Gene Ontology and KEGG. GenoAnnot module was used to annotate the 5 genomes. A variant of the PRIAM algorithm [74] was used to predict the enzymatic activities of the proteins. The five annotated genomes were integrated in MicroB database. The genomic comparative analyses were performed using Genostar Suite and WallGene and datasets from the present study are available in a free access [24].

WallGene is an interactive web application developed by Genostar (Montbonnot, France) in collaboration with the Pasteur Institute (Paris, France) [75], to facilitate large-scale comparative analysis by computing homologies and visualizing syntenies between a set of genomes, The WallGene visualization tools include several types of views, each with a different purpose from a biological perspective. Six views are currently available: (1) the Wall designed to explore homologies and syntenies in a linear way by focusing on genes of interest; (2) the Line Plot and Dot Plot tools allowing comparison 2-by-2 of the general organization of assembled genomes, and explore some biological events such as conservation, inversion, and duplication; (3) the Core Genome exploring common and specific genes of selected genomes; (4) the Circular View showing the overall organization and homologies of organisms in a set of circular graphs; (5) the Gene List view to retrieve genes and homologies according to gene name or function in tabular form. A user guide is available on the web page [24].

Datasets can be calculated with as reference genome any assembled genome of *P. aeruginosa*, or with a reference genome of choice that could be a neo-sequenced and annotated genome to compare directly with clonal derivatives. In the present example, we did both (PAO1 *versus* KK strains and KK1 *versus* KK14 and KK72, and PAO1 *versus* ST395 strains and ST395P *versus* ST395E) using the same parameters (see comparison between Figure 5 and Figure S1 on one hand and Figure 7 and Figure S2 on the other hand). Unidirectional blastP best hits were computed using the following parameters: 80% coverage, 40% identity and 10^{-5} e-value.

PHAST [76] was used to identify, annotate and graphically display prophage sequences within bacterial genomes. Additionally, any absent phage region from a given genome was further checked to be absent using further mapping of crude reads of this genome against the assembled genomes of strains containing it.

3.3. Phenotypic Studies

3.3.1. Antibiograms

MHA plates were inoculated with calibrated suspensions of ST395 strains as recommended by the CLSI.

3.3.2. Motilities

Swarming and twitching behaviors were determined for strains grown on M8 medium supplemented with 0.5% agar for 48 h at 30 °C and on LB medium supplemented with 1.5% agar for 48 h at 37 °C, respectively [77]. All plates were inoculated with bacteria from overnight cultures on LB agar using sterile toothpicks.

3.3.3. Biofilm

Subcultures of overnight LB cultures were prepared in minimal growth medium M63 prepared at an initial optical density (OD) at 600 nm of 0.10 and inoculated in 96 well microplates in six replicates per strain or in glass tubes. Plates or glass tubes were incubated 24 h at 30 °C. Bacterial biofilm formation was evaluated by crystal violet staining, extraction by ethanol treatment and sonication and measurement of OD at 570 nm with a TECAN device.

3.3.4. Transcriptional Activities

The miniCTX-*rsmY-lacZ* and miniCTX-*rsmZ-lacZ* vectors [41] were introduced in the different *P. aeruginosa* strains and site specific recombination at the *attB* site generated chromosomal *rsmY-lacZ*, *rsmZ-lacZ* fusions. The FRT cassette-excision step was performed, resulting in the generation of strains without tetracycline resistance.

3.3.5. T2SS

Proteolytic activity mainly due to T2SS substrates in *P. aeruginosa* ([78] was tested on TSA plates supplemented with 1.5% milk and after 48 h at 37 °C. 9 spots were done for each strain, proteolytic halo was measured and mean and standard deviation were calculated and submitted to appropriate t-test comparison.

3.3.6. T3SS

T3SS-dependent cytotoxicity was evaluated on J774 cells by measuring LDH release using Cytotoxicity Detection kit (Roch) after 1, 2 and 3 h of contact with bacteria at a MOI of 10 [79]. Induction of T3SS *in vitro* was obtained by adding 5 mM EGTA and 20 mM $MgCl_2$ to bacterial cultures at OD_{600nm} of 0.1. When the cells reached OD_{600nm} 1.0, supernatants were collected and analyzed by immunoblot using anti-PcrV, anti-PopB and anti-ExoS antibodies. Cells were 5-fold concentrated and analysed for PcrV, PopB, ExoS synthesis (WC) and secretion (SN). Cytosolic fractions from 50-fold concentrated cells (Cytos) were also subjected to immunoblot analysis with anti-ExsA and anti-ExsD polyclonal antibodies [79,80].

3.3.7. T6SS

Production and secretion of the Hcp1 of the HSI-1 T6SS were assessed as described [81] with cells grown up to OD_{600nm} of 2.0. Extracellular proteins and whole cell lysates were 50-fold and 5-fold concentrated, respectively. 5 μL of each samples were subjected to SDS-PAGE and immunoblotted with polyclonal antibodies anti-Hcp1 [81].

3.3.8. Modelling

Modelling of LasRK218R and of MexRH107P was performed using PyMol.

4. Conclusions

Through this study, we identified common genomic features of *P. aeruginosa* strains from two different medical contexts. Among these, it is important to note the key role of prophages in shaping *P. aeruginosa* genomes, the Arr region which is systematically different in all strains from the one from PAO1 genome (with extra-pieces of DNA ranging from 7,460 to 122,566 bp), and whatever is derived from CF (chronic evolution) and ICU (fast evolution) infections. Of note is the systematic absence in our set of strains of the glycosylation locus involved in A-band and B-band LPS synthesis. Something notably different between CF and ICU strains is that whereas RGP are highly conserved in CF strains, they could have reduced size. In ICU-derived strains we identified RGP present at the same location, which, however, differed from one to another (ST396_6 and ST395_7). This could probably reflect the variability of environmental constraints which is probably much higher in hospital than in a CF lung environment. Furthermore, genome examination of CF strains allowed us to put RGP into three categories which are: (1) RGP which are present in early or mid-term colonization but absent in late clones (regions KK_1 and KK_3); (2) RGP which are continuously present over the period of sampling in KK strains (regions KK_4, KK_5, KK_7, KK_8, KK_9, KK_10, KK_11 and KK12); and (3) RGP which could be considered as "fitness regions", whose loss or maintenance could improve clonal fitness at one stage of the disease (regions KK_6, the PA1430-1433 region and the case of *mucA* gene). This latter category illustrates the fact that the clones studied here probably represent the ones with the most adequate fitness regarding the CF airway environment at that stage. Several clones with less appropriate fitness could coexist but were not picked up. It has been reported that high phenotypic diversity was apparent in the *P. aeruginosa* populations from each chronically infected CF patient [82]. Contemporary isolates from a single sputum sample can differ at the SNP, indel, and accessory genome levels and the cross-sectional genomic variation among coeval pairs of *P. aeruginosa* CF isolates can be comparable to the variation previously reported to differentiate between paired longitudinally sampled isolates [9]. Additionally, in a panel of 135 concurrent *P. aeruginosa* isolates from eight different adult CF patients (9 to 20 isolates per patient) for various QS-controlled phenotypes, most patients contained complex mixtures of QS-proficient and -deficient isolates [83]. All these evidences support the fact that there is likely to be a "cloud" of variation and K14 and KK72 that just represent one isolate from amongst the diversity. We thus essentially observed a final reduction of genome size of CF strains along the disease. Regarding ICU strains studied here, as mentioned above regarding the differences observed between their RGP, this could suggest that environmental constraints have highly shaped genome backbones in a very short period (between the two times of isolation), although intermediate sampling could help in identifying whether changing habitat may have caused these rearrangements. We finally observed an increase in their genome size, while switching from a sensitive to a resistant strain to antibiotics.

We thus unraveled diversity of genomes in between clonal derivatives and the potential key role of prophages in shaping bacterial genomes in these two clinical contexts. It is very tempting to speculate that both types of environments (CF or VAP (ventilator-associated pneumonia) in ICU) are selective pressure conditions that result in the changes observed in these *P. aeruginosa* strains. The examination of these genomes at the different levels (contigs, locus, gene) questions the reliability of genotyping methods used to classify strains in a clonal lineage. The availability of genome sequencing facilities would probably help in redefining the clonal notion.

From our dataset, we would like to go further in depth into the relationship between genetic or genomic events that we observed and phenotypic traits of our strains. This is illustrated for example for KK strains by the Rsm-independent T6SS regulation in KK14 and KK72 strains which can probably be attributed to AlgU in KK14 or to an unknown mechanism in KK72; the role of KK_8 region in antifungal defense in CF airways; the absence of the KK_2 region in CF strains, a region described as essential for increased ability to persist in a chronic pulmonary animal model; the contribution of K218R in LasR in KK72 strain to the absence of proteolytic activity of this strain and the role of G235V mutation in ExsD in deregulated T3SS in KK72 strain or of S232R mutation in ExsA in T3SS defective phenotype of KK14. For ST395 strains, it is of interest to test how the single or multiple punctual mutations identified in AmpD, OprD, MexR, MexZ, *rplU-rpmA* promoter, ParS, ParC, MexT and MexS observed in the ST395P strain act in synergy to shape the resistant phenotype of this strain, because most of these mutations have not been described yet. It would be also very interesting to study whether the RGP ST395_14 region could contribute to the success of this clone in the VAP context.

Thus, possible sequencing application and easy access to draft genomes would probably contribute towards a virulence and antibiotic resistance survey in clinical contexts in the near future.

Acknowledgments

SdB's work has been supported by the GDR3171, ANR grant ERA-NET ADHRES 27481 and FUI ANTIPYO. The authors are very grateful to Michel Ragno for western blot skills.

Author Contributions

S.de.B designed the experiments and wrote the paper. C.L.-M. and S.de.B. performed the bioinformatic analyses. C.B., D.R., G.M., I.A., SE. and K.J. made the phenotypic characterization of the different isolates. C.B., I.A., S.E., F.R., K.J., P.P. helped improving the manuscript.

References

1. Dark, M.J. Whole-genome sequencing in bacteriology: State of the art. *Infec. Drug Resist.* **2013**, *6*, 115–123.
2. Marvig, R.L.; Jochumsen, N.; Johansen, H.K.; Hoiby, N.; Molin, S.; Sommer, M.O.; Jelsbak, L.; Folkesson, A. Draft genome sequences of Pseudomonas aeruginosa B3 strains isolated from a cystic fibrosis patient undergoing antibiotic chemotherapy. *Genome Announc.* **2013**, *1*, e00804-13.
3. Marvig, R.L.; Johansen, H.K.; Molin, S.; Jelsbak, L. Genome analysis of a transmissible lineage of Pseudomonas aeruginosa reveals pathoadaptive mutations and distinct evolutionary paths of hypermutators. *PLoS Genet.* **2013**, *9*, e1003741.

4. Jeukens, J.; Boyle, B.; Bianconi, I.; Kukavica-Ibrulj, I.; Tummler, B.; Bragonzi, A.; Levesque, R.C. Complete genome sequence of persistent cystic fibrosis isolate Pseudomonas aeruginosa strain rp73. *Genome Announc.* **2013**, *1*, e00568-13.

5. Bezuidt, O.K.; Klockgether, J.; Elsen, S.; Attree, I.; Davenport, C.F.; Tummler, B. Intraclonal genome diversity of Pseudomonas aeruginosa clones CHA and TB. *BMC Genom.* **2013**, *14*, 416.

6. Klockgether, J.; Miethke, N.; Kubesch, P.; Bohn, Y.S.; Brockhausen, I.; Cramer, N.; Eberl, L.; Greipel, J.; Herrmann, C.; Herrmann, S.; *et al.* Intraclonal diversity of the pseudomonas aeruginosa cystic fibrosis airway isolates TBCF10839 and TBCF121838: Distinct signatures of transcriptome, proteome, metabolome, adherence and pathogenicity despite an almost identical genome sequence. *Environ. Microbiol.* **2013**, *15*, 191–210.

7. Naughton, S.; Parker, D.; Seemann, T.; Thomas, T.; Turnbull, L.; Rose, B.; Bye, P.; Cordwell, S.; Whitchurch, C.; Manos, J. Pseudomonas aeruginosa AES-1 exhibits increased virulence gene expression during chronic infection of cystic fibrosis lung. *PloS One* **2011**, *6*, e24526.

8. Cramer, N.; Klockgether, J.; Wrasman, K.; Schmidt, M.; Davenport, C.F.; Tummler, B. Microevolution of the major common pseudomonas aeruginosa clones C and PA14 in cystic fibrosis lungs. *Environ. Microbiol.* **2011**, *13*, 1690–1704.

9. Chung, J.C.; Becq, J.; Fraser, L.; Schulz-Trieglaff, O.; Bond, N.J.; Foweraker, J.; Bruce, K.D.; Smith, G.P.; Welch, M. Genomic variation among contemporary Pseudomonas aeruginosa isolates from chronically infected cystic fibrosis patients. *J. Bacteriol.* **2012**, *194*, 4857–4866.

10. Xiong, J.; Alexander, D.C.; Ma, J.H.; Deraspe, M.; Low, D.E.; Jamieson, F.B.; Roy, P.H. Complete sequence of pOZ176, a 500-kilobase IncP-2 plasmid encoding IMP-9-mediated carbapenem resistance, from outbreak isolate Pseudomonas aeruginosa 96. *Antimicrob. Agents. Ch.* **2013**, *57*, 3775–3782.

11. Ciornei, C.D.; Novikov, A.; Beloin, C.; Fitting, C.; Caroff, M.; Ghigo, J.M.; Cavaillon, J.M.; Adib-Conquy, M. Biofilm-forming Pseudomonas aeruginosa bacteria undergo lipopolysaccharide structural modifications and induce enhanced inflammatory cytokine response in human monocytes. *Innate Immun.* **2010**, *16*, 288–301.

12. Bastonero, S.; Le Priol, Y.; Armand, M.; Bernard, C.S.; Reynaud-Gaubert, M.; Olive, D.; Parzy, D.; de Bentzmann, S.; Capo, C.; Mege, J.L. New microbicidal functions of tracheal glands: Defective anti-infectious response to Pseudomonas aeruginosa in cystic fibrosis. *PloS One* **2009**, *4*, e5357.

13. Mougous, J.D.; Cuff, M.E.; Raunser, S.; Shen, A.; Zhou, M.; Gifford, C.A.; Goodman, A.L.; Joachimiak, G.; Ordonez, C.L.; Lory, S.; *et al.* A virulence locus of Pseudomonas aeruginosa encodes a protein secretion apparatus. *Science* **2006**, *312*, 1526–1530.

14. Yahr, T.L.; Frank, D.W. Transcriptional organization of the trans-regulatory locus which controls exoenzyme s synthesis in Pseudomonas aeruginosa. *J. Bacteriol.* **1994**, *176*, 3832–3838.

15. McCaw, M.L.; Lykken, G.L.; Singh, P.K.; Yahr, T.L. ExsD is a negative regulator of the Pseudomonas aeruginosa type III secretion regulon. *Mol. Microbiol.* **2002**, *46*, 1123–1133.

16. Chatterjee, S.; Chaudhury, S.; McShan, A.C.; Kaur, K.; De Guzman, R.N. Structure and biophysics of type III secretion in bacteria. *Biochemistry* **2013**, *52*, 2508–2517.

17. Hauser, A.R. The type III secretion system of Pseudomonas aeruginosa: Infection by injection. *Nature reviews. Microbiology* **2009**, *7*, 654–665.

18. Engel, J.; Balachandran, P. Role of Pseudomonas aeruginosa type III effectors in disease. *Curr. Opin. Microbiol.* **2009**, *12*, 61–66.

19. Cisz, M.; Lee, P.C.; Rietsch, A. ExoS controls the cell contact-mediated switch to effector secretion in Pseudomonas aeruginosa. *J. Bacteriol.* **2008**, *190*, 2726–2738.

20. Lapouge, K.; Schubert, M.; Allain, F.H.; Haas, D. Gac/Rsm signal transduction pathway of gamma-proteobacteria: From RNA recognition to regulation of social behaviour. *Mol. Microbiol.* **2008**, *67*, 241–253.

21. Brencic, A.; McFarland, K.A.; McManus, H.R.; Castang, S.; Mogno, I.; Dove, S.L.; Lory, S. The GacS/GacA signal transduction system of Pseudomonas aeruginosa acts exclusively through its control over the transcription of the RsmY and RsmZ regulatory small RNAs. *Mol. Microbiol.* **2009**, *73*, 434–445.

22. Cholley, P.; Thouverez, M.; Hocquet, D.; van der Mee-Marquet, N.; Talon, D.; Bertrand, X. Most Multidrug-Resistant *Pseudomonas aeruginosa* Isolates from Hospitals in Eastern France Belong to a Few Clonal Types. *J. Clin. Microbiol.* **2011**, *49*, 2578–2583.

23. Magiorakos, A.P.; Srinivasan, A.; Carey, R.B.; Carmeli, Y.; Falagas, M.E.; Giske, C.G.; Harbarth, S.; Hindler, J.F.; Kahlmeter, G.; Olsson-Liljequist, B., *et al.* Multidrug-resistant, extensively drug-resistant and pandrug-resistant bacteria: An international expert proposal for interim standard definitions for acquired resistance. *Clin. Microbiol. Infec.* **2012**, *18*, 268–281.

24. Wallgene. Available online: https://www.wallgene.com/WallGene/papers (accessed on 4 April 2014).

25. Mathee, K.; Narasimhan, G.; Valdes, C.; Qiu, X.; Matewish, J.M.; Koehrsen, M.; Rokas, A.; Yandava, C.N.; Engels, R.; Zeng, E.; *et al.* Dynamics of Pseudomonas aeruginosa genome evolution. *Proc. Natl. Acad. Sci. USA* **2008**, *105*, 3100–3105.

26. Nowak-Thompson, B.; Chaney, N.; Wing, J.S.; Gould, S.J.; Loper, J.E. Characterization of the pyoluteorin biosynthetic gene cluster of Pseudomonas fluorescens Pf-5. *J. Bacteriol.* **1999**, *181*, 2166–2174.

27. Hoffman, L.R.; D'Argenio, D.A.; MacCoss, M.J.; Zhang, Z.; Jones, R.A.; Miller, S.I. Aminoglycoside antibiotics induce bacterial biofilm formation. *Nature* **2005**, *436*, 1171–1175.

28. Brown, N.L.; Shih, Y.C.; Leang, C.; Glendinning, K.J.; Hobman, J.L.; Wilson, J.R. Mercury transport and resistance. *Biochem. Soc. Trans.* **2002**, *30*, 715–718.

29. Deretic, V.; Konyecsni, W.M. A procaryotic regulatory factor with a histone H1-like carboxy-terminal domain: Clonal variation of repeats within *algP*, a gene involved in regulation of mucoidy in Pseudomonas aeruginosa. *J. Bacteriol.* **1990**, *172*, 5544–5554.

30. Wilderman, P.J.; Vasil, A.I.; Johnson, Z.; Vasil, M.L. Genetic and biochemical analyses of a eukaryotic-like phospholipase D of Pseudomonas aeruginosa suggest horizontal acquisition and a role for persistence in a chronic pulmonary infection model. *Mol. Microbiol.* **2001**, *39*, 291–303.

31. Passador, L.; Cook, J.M.; Gambello, M.J.; Rust, L.; Iglewski, B.H. Expression of Pseudomonas aeruginosa virulence genes requires cell-to-cell communication. *Science* **1993**, *260*, 1127–1130.

32. de Kievit, T.; Seed, P.C.; Nezezon, J.; Passador, L.; Iglewski, B.H. RsaL, a novel repressor of virulence gene expression in pseudomonas aeruginosa. *J. Bacteriol.* **1999**, *181*, 2175–2184.

33. Fukushima, J.; Ishiwata, T.; Kurata, M.; You, Z.; Okuda, K. Intracellular receptor-type transcription factor, lasr, contains a highly conserved amphipathic region which precedes the putative helix-turn-helix DNA binding motif. *Nucleic Acids Res.* **1994**, *22*, 3706–3707.

34. Vannini, A.; Volpari, C.; Gargioli, C.; Muraglia, E.; Cortese, R.; De Francesco, R.; Neddermann, P.; Marco, S.D. The crystal structure of the quorum sensing protein TraR bound to its autoinducer and target DNA. *EMBO J.* **2002**, *21*, 4393–4401.

35. Martin, D.W.; Schurr, M.J.; Mudd, M.H.; Govan, J.R.; Holloway, B.W.; Deretic, V. Mechanism of conversion to mucoidy in Pseudomonas aeruginosa infecting cystic fibrosis patients. *Proc. Natl. Acad. Sci. USA* **1993**, *90*, 8377–8381.

36. Rehman, Z.U.; Wang, Y.; Moradali, M.F.; Hay, I.D.; Rehm, B.H. Insights into the assembly of the alginate biosynthesis machinery in Pseudomonas aeruginosa. *Appl. Environ. Microbiol.* **2013**, *79*, 3264–3272.

37. Sall, K.M.; Casabona, G.; Bordi, C.; Huber, P.; de Bentzmann, S.; Attrée, I.; Elsen, S. A gacS deletion in Pseudomonas aeruginosa cystic fibrosis isolate CHA shapes its virulence. *PloS One* **2014**, in press.

38. Mikkelsen, H.; McMullan, R.; Filloux, A. The Pseudomonas aeruginosa reference strain PA14 displays increased virulence due to a mutation in LadS. *PloS One* **2011**, *6*, e29113.

39. Bordi, C.; Lamy, M.C.; Ventre, I.; Termine, E.; Hachani, A.; Fillet, S.; Roche, B.; Bleves, S.; Mejean, V.; Lazdunski, A.; *et al.* Regulatory RNAs and the HptB/RetS signalling pathways fine-tune Pseudomonas aeruginosa pathogenesis. *Mol. Microbiol.* **2010**, *76*, 1427–1443.

40. Goodman, A.L.; Merighi, M.; Hyodo, M.; Ventre, I.; Filloux, A.; Lory, S. Direct interaction between sensor kinase proteins mediates acute and chronic disease phenotypes in a bacterial pathogen. *Genes Dev.* **2009**, *23*, 249–259.

41. Roux, L.; Filloux, A.; Sivaneson, M.; de Bentzmann, S.; Bordi, C. The LadS hybrid histidine kinase triggers Pseudomonas aeruginosa chronic infection by forming a multicomponent signal transduction system with the GacS/GacA two component system. *Env. Microbiol.* **2014**, in press.

42. Ventre, I.; Goodman, A.L.; Vallet-Gely, I.; Vasseur, P.; Soscia, C.; Molin, S.; Bleves, S.; Lazdunski, A.; Lory, S.; Filloux, A. Multiple sensors control reciprocal expression of Pseudomonas aeruginosa regulatory RNA and virulence genes. *Proc. Natl. Acad. Sci. USA* **2006**, *103*, 171–176.

43. Kong, W.; Chen, L.; Zhao, J.; Shen, T.; Surette, M.G.; Shen, L.; Duan, K. Hybrid sensor kinase PA1611 in Pseudomonas aeruginosa regulates transitions between acute and chronic infection through direct interaction with rets. *Mol. Microbiol.* **2013**, *88*, 784–797.

44. Petrova, O.E.; Sauer, K. SagS contributes to the motile-sessile switch and acts in concert with BfiSR to enable Pseudomonas aeruginosa biofilm formation. *J. Bacteriol.* **2011**, *193*, 6614–6628.

45. Petrova, O.E.; Sauer, K. The novel two-component regulatory system BfiSR regulates biofilm development by controlling the small RNA Rsmz through CafA. *J. Bacteriol.* **2010**, *192*, 5275–5288.

46. Moscoso, J.A.; Mikkelsen, H.; Heeb, S.; Williams, P.; Filloux, A. The Pseudomonas aeruginosa sensor RetS switches type III and type VI secretion via c-di-GMP signalling. *Environ. Microbiol.* **2011**, *13*, 3128–3138.

47. Intile, P.J.; Diaz, M.R.; Urbanowski, M.L.; Wolfgang, M.C.; Yahr, T.L. The AlgZR Two-Component System Recalibrates the RsmAYZ Posttranscriptional Regulatory System To Inhibit Expression of the Pseudomonas aeruginosa Type III Secretion System. *J. Bacteriol.* **2014**, *196*, 357–366.

48. Yahr, T.L.; Wolfgang, M.C. Transcriptional regulation of the Pseudomonas aeruginosa type III secretion system. *Mol. Microbiol.* **2006**, *62*, 631–640.

49. Coggan, K.A.; Wolfgang, M.C. Global regulatory pathways and cross-talk control Pseudomonas aeruginosa environmental lifestyle and virulence phenotype. *Curr. Issues Mol. Biol.* **2012**, *14*, 47–70.

50. Jones, A.K.; Fulcher, N.B.; Balzer, G.J.; Urbanowski, M.L.; Pritchett, C.L.; Schurr, M.J.; Yahr, T.L.; Wolfgang, M.C. Activation of the pseudomonas aeruginosa algu regulon through muca mutation inhibits cyclic amp/vfr signaling. *J. Bacteriol.* **2010**, *192*, 5709–5717.

51. Lykken, G.L.; Chen, G.; Brutinel, E.D.; Chen, L.; Yahr, T.L. Characterization of ExsC and ExsD self-association and heterocomplex formation. *J. Bacteriol.* **2006**, *188*, 6832–6840.

52. Winstanley, C.; Langille, M.G.; Fothergill, J.L.; Kukavica-Ibrulj, I.; Paradis-Bleau, C.; Sanschagrin, F.; Thomson, N.R.; Winsor, G.L.; Quail, M.A.; Lennard, N.; *et al.* Newly introduced genomic prophage islands are critical determinants of in vivo competitiveness in the liverpool epidemic strain of Pseudomonas aeruginosa. *Genome Res.* **2009**, *19*, 12–23.

53. Chen, M.; Yan, Y.; Zhang, W.; Lu, W.; Wang, J.; Ping, S.; Lin, M. Complete genome sequence of the type strain pseudomonas stutzeri cgmcc 1.1803. *J. Bacteriol.* **2011**, *193*, 6095.

54. He, J.; Baldini, R.L.; Deziel, E.; Saucier, M.; Zhang, Q.; Liberati, N.T.; Lee, D.; Urbach, J.; Goodman, H.M.; Rahme, L.G. The broad host range pathogen Pseudomonas aeruginosa strain pa14 carries two pathogenicity islands harboring plant and animal virulence genes. *Proc. Natl. Acad. Sci. USA* **2004**, *101*, 2530–2535.

55. Wilson, M.A.; Ringe, D.; Petsko, G.A. The atomic resolution crystal structure of the YajL (ThiJ) protein from Escherichia coli: A close prokaryotic homologue of the parkinsonism-associated protein DJ-1. *J. Mol. Biol.* **2005**, *353*, 678–691.

56. Rocchetta, H.L.; Burrows, L.L.; Pacan, J.C.; Lam, J.S. Three rhamnosyltransferases responsible for assembly of the A-band D-rhamnan polysaccharide in Pseudomonas aeruginosa: A fourth transferase, WbpL, is required for the initiation of both A-band and B-band lipopolysaccharide synthesis. *Mol. Microbiol.* **1998**, *28*, 1103–1119.

57. McManus, H.R.; Dove, S.L. The CgrA and CgrC proteins form a complex that positively regulates cupA fimbrial gene expression in Pseudomonas aeruginosa. *J. Bacteriol.* **2011**, *193*, 6152–6161.

58. Vallet-Gely, I.; Sharp, J.S.; Dove, S.L. Local and global regulators linking anaerobiosis to cupA fimbrial gene expression in Pseudomonas aeruginosa. *J. Bacteriol.* **2007**, *189*, 8667–8676.

59. Tsusaki, K.; Nishimoto, T.; Nakada, T.; Kubota, M.; Chaen, H.; Sugimoto, T.; Kurimoto, M. Cloning and sequencing of trehalose synthase gene from Pimelobacter sp. R48. *BBA* **1996**, *1290*, 1–3.

60. Valvano, M.A.; Marolda, C.L.; Bittner, M.; Glaskin-Clay, M.; Simon, T.L.; Klena, J.D. The rfaE gene from Escherichia coli encodes a bifunctional protein involved in biosynthesis of the lipopolysaccharide core precursor ADP-L-glycero-D-manno-heptose. *J. Bacteriol.* **2000**, *182*, 488–497.

61. Battle, S.E.; Rello, J.; Hauser, A.R. Genomic islands of Pseudomonas aeruginosa. *FEMS Microbiol. Lett.* **2009**, *290*, 70–78.

62. Kung, V.L.; Khare, S.; Stehlik, C.; Bacon, E.M.; Hughes, A.J.; Hauser, A.R. An rhs gene of Pseudomonas aeruginosa encodes a virulence protein that activates the inflammasome. *Proc. Natl. Acad. Sci. USA* **2012**, *109*, 1275–1280.

63. Mérens, A.; Delacour, H.; Plésiat, P.; Cavallo, J.D.; Jeannot, K. Pseudomonas aeruginosa et résistance aux antibiotiques. *Revue Francophone Des Laboratoires* **2011**, 29–62.

64. Poole, K. Multidrug efflux pumps and antimicrobial resistance in Pseudomonas aeruginosa and related organisms. *J. Mol. Microbiol. biotechnol.* **2001**, *3*, 255–264.

65. Li, H.; Luo, Y.F.; Williams, B.J.; Blackwell, T.S.; Xie, C.M. Structure and function of oprd protein in Pseudomonas aeruginosa: From antibiotic resistance to novel therapies. *IJMM* **2012**, *302*, 63–68.

66. Lister, P.D.; Wolter, D.J.; Hanson, N.D. Antibacterial-resistant Pseudomonas aeruginosa: Clinical impact and complex regulation of chromosomally encoded resistance mechanisms. *Clin. Microbiol. Rev.* **2009**, *22*, 582–610.

67. Juan, C.; Macia, M.D.; Gutierrez, O.; Vidal, C.; Perez, J.L.; Oliver, A. Molecular mechanisms of beta-lactam resistance mediated by AmpC hyperproduction in Pseudomonas aeruginosa clinical strains. *Antimicrob. Agents Chemother.* **2005**, *49*, 4733–4738.

68. Fukuoka, T.; Ohya, S.; Narita, T.; Katsuta, M.; Iijima, M.; Masuda, N.; Yasuda, H.; Trias, J.; Nikaido, H. Activity of the carbapenem panipenem and role of the OprD (D2) protein in its diffusion through the Pseudomonas aeruginosa outer membrane. *Antimicrob. Agents Chemother.* **1993**, *37*, 322–327.

69. Lim, D.; Poole, K.; Strynadka, N.C. Crystal structure of the MexR repressor of the mexRAB-oprM multidrug efflux operon of pseudomonas aeruginosa. *J. Biol. Chem.* **2002**, *277*, 29253–29259.

70. Andresen, C.; Jalal, S.; Aili, D.; Wang, Y.; Islam, S.; Jarl, A.; Liedberg, B.; Wretlind, B.; Martensson, L.G.; Sunnerhagen, M. Critical biophysical properties in the pseudomonas aeruginosa efflux gene regulator mexr are targeted by mutations conferring multidrug resistance. *Protein Sci.* **2010**, *19*, 680–692.

71. Matsuo, Y.; Eda, S.; Gotoh, N.; Yoshihara, E.; Nakae, T. MexZ-mediated regulation of mexXY multidrug efflux pump expression in Pseudomonas aeruginosa by binding on the mexZ-mexX intergenic DNA. *FEMS Microbiol. Lett.* **2004**, *238*, 23–28.

72. Guenard, S.; Muller, C.; Monlezun, L.; Benas, P.; Broutin, I.; Jeannot, K.; Plesiat, P. Multiple mutations lead to MexXY-OprM-dependent aminoglycoside resistance in clinical strains of pseudomonas aeruginosa. *Antimicrob. Agents Chemother.* **2014**, *58*, 221–228.

73. Piddock, L.J. Mechanisms of fluoroquinolone resistance: An update 1994–1998. *Drugs* **1999**, *58* (Suppl. 2), 11–18.

74. Claudel-Renard, C.; Chevalet, C.; Faraut, T.; Kahn, D. Enzyme-specific profiles for genome annotation: PRIAM. *Nucleic Acids Res.* **2003**, *31*, 6633–6639.

75. Lechat, P.; Souche, E.; Moszer, I. Syntview - an interactive multi-view genome browser for next-generation comparative microorganism genomics. *BMC bioinformatics* **2013**, *14*, 277.

76. Phast. Available online: http://phast.wishartlab.com (accessed on 4 April 2014).

77. Rashid, M.H.; Rao, N.N.; Kornberg, A. Inorganic polyphosphate is required for motility of bacterial pathogens. *J. Bacteriol.* **2000**, *182*, 225–227.

78. Michel, G.P.; Durand, E.; Filloux, A. XphA/XqhA, a novel GspCD subunit for type II secretion in Pseudomonas aeruginosa. *J. Bacteriol.* **2007**, *189*, 3776–3783.

79. Goure, J.; Pastor, A.; Faudry, E.; Chabert, J.; Dessen, A.; Attree, I. The V antigen of Pseudomonas aeruginosa is required for assembly of the functional PopB/PopD translocation pore in host cell membranes. *Infect. Immun.* **2004**, *72*, 4741–4750.

80. Thibault, J.; Faudry, E.; Ebel, C.; Attree, I.; Elsen, S. Anti-activator ExsD forms a 1:1 complex with ExsA to inhibit transcription of type III secretion operons. *J. Biol. Chem.* **2009**, *284*, 15762–15770.

81. Casabona, M.G.; Silverman, J.M.; Sall, K.M.; Boyer, F.; Coute, Y.; Poirel, J.; Grunwald, D.; Mougous, J.D.; Elsen, S.; Attree, I. An ABC transporter and an outer membrane lipoprotein participate in posttranslational activation of type VI secretion in Pseudomonas aeruginosa. *Environ. Microbiol.* **2013**, *15*, 471–486.

82. Ashish, A.; Paterson, S.; Mowat, E.; Fothergill, J.L.; Walshaw, M.J.; Winstanley, C. Extensive diversification is a common feature of Pseudomonas aeruginosa populations during respiratory infections in cystic fibrosis. *J. Cystic Fibrosis* **2013**, *12*, 790–793.

83. Wilder, C.N.; Allada, G.; Schuster, M. Instantaneous within-patient diversity of Pseudomonas aeruginosa quorum-sensing populations from cystic fibrosis lung infections. *Infect. immun.* **2009**, *77*, 5631–5639.

3

Antimicrobial and Antibiofilm Activity of Chitosan on the Oral Pathogen *Candida albicans*

Eduardo Costa, Sara Silva [†]**, Freni Tavaria** [†] **and Manuela Pintado** *

Universidade Católica Portuguesa/Porto, Rua Arquiteto Lobão Vital, Apartado 2511, 4202-401 Porto, Portugal; E-Mails: emcosta@porto.ucp.pt (E.C.); snsilva@porto.ucp.pt (S.S.); ftavaria@porto.ucp.pt (F.T.)

[†] These authors contributed equally to this work.

* Author to whom correspondence should be addressed; E-Mail: mpintado@porto.ucp.pt;

External Editor: Gianfranco Donelli

Abstract: Oral candidiasis is particularly evident, not only in cancer patients receiving chemotherapy, but also in elderly people with xerostomy. In general, *Candida* is an opportunistic pathogen, causing infections in immunocompromised people and, in some cases, when the natural microbiota is altered. Chitosan, a natural derivative of chitin, is a polysaccharide that has been proven to possess a broad spectrum of antimicrobial activity that encompasses action against fungi, yeast and bacteria. While recent studies have revealed a significant antibiofilm activity upon several microorganisms, including *C. albicans*, little is known regarding the impact of chitosan upon the adhesive process or mature biofilms. With that in mind, the purpose of this work was to evaluate, *in vitro*, the capability of chitosan to inhibit *C. albicans* growth and biofilm formation. The results obtained showed that chitosan is capable of inhibiting *C. albicans* planktonic growth (HMW, 1 mg/mL; LMW, 3 mg/mL). Regarding biofilm growth, chitosan inhibited *C. albicans* adhesion (*ca.* 95%), biofilm formation (percentages above 90%) and reduced mature biofilms by *ca.* 65% and dual species biofilms (*C. albicans* and *S. mutans*) by *ca.* 70%. These results display the potential of this molecule to be used as an effective anti-*Candida* agent capable of acting upon *C. albicans* infections.

Keywords: candidiasis; *Candida albicans*; chitosan; biofilm; antibiofilm

---

1. Introduction

Since the 1970s, there has been an increase in candidiasis incidence, mostly due to the use of plastic permanent catheters, antibiotics and immunosuppressive drugs [1]. These *Candida*-derived infections may occur in the skin, mucous membranes (such as the mouth and vagina) and in the viscera, with the main etiological agent being *Candida albicans* [1,2]. Among the various human fungal pathogens, *C. albicans* accounts for the majority of systemic infections in immunocompromised patients, with overall mortality rates ranging from 29% to 76% [2–6]. This opportunistic fungi causes great problems, as it is resistant to most antimicrobial compounds, namely amphotericin-B, which is considered the standard for the treatment of systemic mycoses. Despite still being considered the drug of choice against *C. albicans*, these antifungal agents are being increasingly reported as inefficient with numerous cases of resistances, particularly to fluconazole, being observed [1–4]. This problem has led to the search for alternative drugs and compounds to be used in the treatment and management of *C. albicans* infections.

Chitin is the primary structural component of the shells of crustaceans, arthropods and the fungal cell wall and is obtained mainly as a byproduct of the fishing industry. Partial deacetylation of chitin leads to chitosan, a polysaccharide composed of units of glucosamine (2-amino-2-deoxy-D-glucose) and *N*-acetyl glucosamine (2-acetamido-2-deoxy-D–glucose) linked by β(1→4) bonds. Chitosan is the only natural polysaccharide that presents a cationic character due to its amino groups, which, at low pH, are protonated and can interact with negatively-charged compounds, such as proteins, anionic polysaccharides (e.g., alginates, carraghenates, pectins), fatty acids, bile acids and phospholipids [7]. This behavior, along with its biocompatibility, biodegradability and lack of toxicity, has led to the usage of chitosan in diverse fields, such as technology, food, cosmetics, medicine, biotechnology, agriculture and the paper industry [8,9]. However, chitosan possesses some limitations, namely its insolubility in water, high viscosity and tendency to coagulate proteins at high pH [10–12].

Chitosan's antimicrobial activity is well established against a variety of microorganisms, including fungi [10,13–15]. When considering chitosan antifungal activity, several authors have already shown that it is active upon yeasts, molds and dermatophytes [16–19]. While the antifungal activity of chitosan upon *C. albicans* is well established, the same cannot be said regarding the effect of chitosan upon *C. albicans* biofilm formation. Early reports [20–22] suggest that chitosan may be active upon *C. albicans* biofilms; however, the real effect of chitosan upon the different steps of *C. albicans* biofilms has not yet been fully explored. As such, the aim of this work was to fully assess chitosan's potential as a means to prevent *C. albicans*-derived infections through the control of its growth, adhesion and biofilm formation.

2. Results and Discussion

2.1. MIC Determination

The MIC values, obtained by broth microdilution, for chitosan activity upon *C. albicans* were relatively low. In fact, HMW chitosan presented a MIC value of 1 mg/mL and LMW chitosan a MIC value of 3 mg/mL. The antifungal activity of chitosan upon *C. albicans* is well established, with several authors [16–19] presenting various MIC values for different chitosans against this yeast. Tayel, Moussa, El-Tras, Knittel, Opwis and Schollmeyer [2] previously reported a MIC of 1.25 mg/mL (32 kDa, deacetylation degree (DD) 86%). Qin *et al.* [23] reported an even lower MIC of 0.8 mg/mL (2.91 kDa, DD 86.4%), and Şenel *et al.* [24] reported a MIC of 10 mg/mL (1,000 kDa, DD 80%). Comparing these results with the ones obtained, it is possible to see that for LMW chitosan, the MIC value obtained was slightly superior to those previously reported [2,23], with this differences being probably due to the higher DD used in those assays. On the other hand, for HMW chitosan, the values here obtained were significantly lower than those reported by Şenel, İkinci, Kaş, Yousefi-Rad, Sargon and Hıncal [24]. From here, the ½ and the ¼ of the MIC were calculated to be used in the biofilm assays, as previously described by Cerca *et al.* [25].

2.2. Adherence to Coated Surfaces

The effect of chitosan upon *C. albicans* adhesion to surfaces can be seen in Figure 1. The results obtained showed that both MW and the times tested were capable of producing adhesion inhibition percentages above 90%. In fact, the lowest inhibition percentage was obtained for LMW chitosan after only 30 s of exposure. When considering the differences between 30 s and 90 s of exposure, there were no significant statistical differences ($p > 0.05$) found, either for HMW or LMW chitosan. On the other hand, when considering the impact of the MW and the exposure time, some differences are ascertainable; 90 s of exposure for HMW presented statistically significant ($p < 0.05$) higher inhibition values than both LMW assays; LMW, at 30 s of exposure, presented a significantly lower ($p < 0.05$) inhibition value than the one registered in both HMW assays. These results are in line with those previously reported by Carlson, Taffs, Davison and Stewart [20], who showed that chitosan reduced *C. albicans* adhesion up to 99%.

2.3. Microtiter-Plate Test

When considering the impact of chitosan upon *C. albicans* biofilm formation (Figure 2), here analyzed indirectly through biomass production, one can see that, as with the previous assay, the highest inhibition percentage (66.94%) was obtained for HMW chitosan (0.5 mg/mL) and the lowest inhibition percentage (37.97%) was obtained for LMW chitosan (0.75 mg/mL). When comparing the results obtained for the ½ and ¼ of the MIC of both MWs, no statistically significant ($p > 0.05$) differences were found when considering the effect of the MW upon chitosan's activity. On the other hand, when considering the effect of the MW in conjunction with the concentration, one can see clear differences in behavior (Figure 2). In fact, 0.5 mg/mL of HMW chitosan presented significantly higher ($p < 0.05$) inhibition values than the remaining assays, while no significant ($p > 0.05$) differences were found between the ¼ of the MIC for HMW (0.25 mg/mL) and ½ of the MIC for LMW (1.5 mg/mL). On the other hand, 0.75 mg/mL of LMW chitosan presented statistically significant ($p < 0.05$) lower inhibition percentages than the remaining assays. These results are in line with those registered by Martinez, Mihu, Tar, Cordero, Han, Friedman, Friedman and Nosanchuk [22], who reported that chitosan was capable of reducing *C. albicans* biofilm formation by a 2.5 factor, and by those of Cobrado *et al.* [26] and of Cobrado *et al.* [27], who showed that chitosan was capable of reducing *C. albicans* biomass production up to 90%.

Figure 1. Inhibitory effect of chitosan upon *C. albicans* adhesion. Values obtained given as the percentage of adhesion inhibition. Different letters represent the statistically significant differences found ($p < 0.05$). All assays performed in triplicate. HMW, high molecular weight; LMW, low molecular weight.

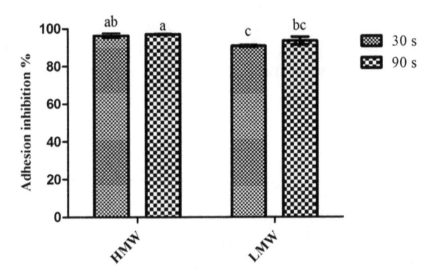

Figure 2. Effect of sub-MIC concentrations of chitosan (½ and ¼ of the MICs; values in mg/mL) upon *C. albicans* biofilm formation. Values obtained are given as the percentage of biofilm formation inhibition. Different letters represent the statistically significant differences found ($p < 0.05$). All assays were performed in triplicate.

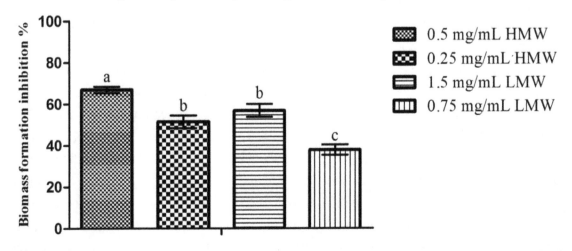

2.4. Mature Biofilms Assays

Regarding the effect of chitosan upon *C. albicans* mature biofilms, the results obtained can be seen in Figure 3. Once again, the highest inhibition percentage was obtained for HMW chitosan (51.77% for 0.25 mg/mL), and the lowest inhibition was registered for LMW chitosan (45.37% for 1.5 mg/mL). Statistical analysis of the results showed that when considering the effect of the MW, there were statistically significant differences ($p < 0.05$) between HMW chitosan at 0.25 mg/mL and both LMW concentrations tested. Simultaneously, when considering the effect of the MW in conjunction with concentration (Figure 3), differences were also observed with 0.25 mg/mL HMW chitosan, presenting significantly ($p < 0.05$) higher inhibition values than the assays that utilized LMW chitosan. Between the remaining assays, no statistically significant ($p > 0.05$) differences were found.

Figure 3. Effect of sub-MIC concentrations of chitosan (½ and ¼ of the MICs; values in mg/mL) upon *C. albicans* mature biofilms. Results are presented as biofilm reduction percentages. Different letters represent the statistically significant differences found ($p < 0.05$). All assays performed in triplicate.

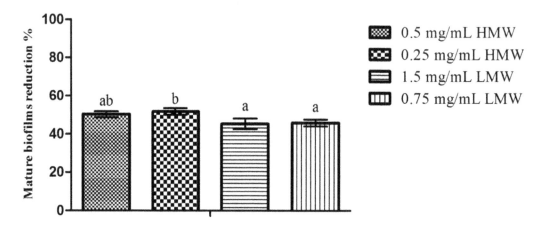

2.5. Dual-Species Biofilms

Results obtained regarding the activity of chitosan upon *C. albicans* mature biofilms can be observed in Figure 4. Contrary to the pattern observed in previous assays, LMW chitosan presented the highest biofilm inhibition percentage (66.77% for 0.75 mg/mL) and HMW chitosan the lowest (55.10% for 0.25 mg/mL). Statistical analysis of the results showed that the only statistically significant difference observed was for 0.25 mg/mL of HMW chitosan, which presented an inhibition value significantly lower than the inhibition values obtained in the remaining test conditions. When considering the differences in chitosan's activity between single species *C. albicans* biofilm and dual species *C. albicans* and *S. mutans* biofilms (Figure 5), the statistical analysis shows that there are statistically significant differences ($p < 0.05$) in LMW chitosan's activity between a single and a dual species population. On a closer look, LMW chitosan presents a statistically significant ($p < 0.05$) increase in activity between single species and dual species biofilms. This translates as an increase of biomass production inhibition of *ca.* 10%, for 1.5 mg/mL, and of *ca.* 31%, for 0.75 mg/mL of chitosan, for LMW chitosan between populations.

Despite the lack of previous results regarding the effect of chitosan upon *C. albicans* mature and dual species biofilms, the inhibitions here registered are quite interesting, especially when considering that

C. albicans biofilms produce an exopolymeric matrix that serves as a diffusion barrier to antimicrobials and that, under these conditions, *Candida* cells overexpress efflux pumps to enhance antifungal resistance [28]. This mechanism may be the reason why HMW chitosan possessed higher activity than LMW upon mature biofilms, as it is known that the latter must enter the cells in order to be active [15]. In the dual species biofilms, one cannot underestimate the importance of *S. mutans*, as it is known to be crucial to *C. albicans* colonization of the oral cavity, mainly due to providing adhesion sites and producing lactate that can be used as a carbon source by yeasts. This symbiosis has been well established in several studies, which have shown that there is a strong coadherence between these microorganisms [29]. Considering that, both *S. mutans* and *C. albicans*, have been described as being more sensitive to HMW chitosan [16–19,30], it is somewhat surprising that LMW chitosan presented higher inhibition percentages than HMW chitosan for the dual species biofilms. It is possible that an unknown mechanism, possibly located at the adhesins level, as hypothesized by Azcurra *et al.* [31], or at the cell to cell communication level, where the larger HMW molecules are incapable of acting, is responsible for the higher activity registered for LMW chitosan.

Figure 4. Effect of sub-MIC concentrations of chitosan (½ and ¼ of the MICs; values in mg/mL) upon biofilms formed by *C. albicans* and *S. mutans*. Results presented as the percentage of biofilm formation inhibition. Different letters represent the statistically significant differences found ($p < 0.05$). All assays performed in triplicate.

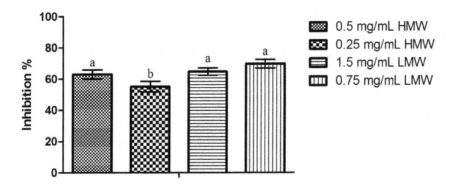

Figure 5. Comparison of the effect of sub-MIC concentrations of chitosan upon *C. albicans* single species and dual species biofilms. Results presented as the percentage of biofilm formation inhibition. Different letters represent the statistically significant differences found ($p < 0.05$). All assays performed in triplicate.

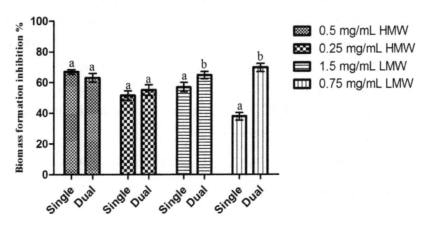

3. Experimental Section

3.1. Sources of Chitosan and Microorganisms

High and low molecular weight chitosan were obtained from Sigma-Aldrich (St. Louis, MO, USA). High molecular weight chitosan was characterized by a DD > 75% and a MW of 624 kDa. Low molecular weight chitosan was characterized by a DD between 75% and 85% and a MW of 107 kDa. Chitosan solutions were prepared in 1% (v/v) solution of glacial acetic acid 99% (Panreac, Barcelona, Spain). Chitosan was added to 1% acetic acid to the desired concentration. Afterwards, the solution was stirred overnight at 50 °C to promote complete dissolution of chitosan. The pH was adjusted with NaOH (Merck, Darmstad, Germany) to a final value of 5.6–5.8, and solutions were stored at refrigerated temperature.

Candida albicans used in this study was obtained from the culture collection of the Göteburg University (CCUG) (Sweden) (CCUG 49242). Inocula were prepared in yeast malt broth (YMB) (Difco, Franklin Lakes, NJ, USA) and incubated at 37 °C for 24 h. Viable counts were performed in yeast malt agar (YMA) (Difco, Franklin Lakes, NJ, USA).

3.2. Determination of Minimal Inhibitory Concentration

Determination of the MIC was performed as described by Costa, Silva, Pina, Tavaria and Pintado [10]. Briefly, an inoculum of 0.5 in the MacFarland scale (1.5×10^8 CFU/mL) of *C. albicans* was prepared from overnight cultures and inoculated in YMB with chitosan concentrations ranging from 0.1 mg/mL to 7 mg/mL. Two controls were simultaneously assessed: one with 0.1 mg/mL chitosan, but without inoculum, and another where chitosan was replaced by sterile water and with added inoculum. The MIC was determined by observing the lowest concentration of chitosan that inhibited microbial growth. All assays were performed in triplicate.

3.3. Adherence

The effect of chitosan on *C. albicans* adhesion to surfaces was performed as described by Costa, Silva, Tavaria and Pintado [30], tested using 24-well microplates. Briefly, 1 cm aluminum disks were dipped for 30 or 90 s in a well containing either 1% (v/v) HMW or LMW chitosan. Following that, the disks were rinsed with sterile water and submerged in a well containing inoculum for 60 s, after which disks were placed into wells containing the appropriate medium and incubated for 24 h at 37 °C. Two controls were simultaneously assessed. In the first one, disks were dipped in sterile water and then inoculated and incubated. In the second one, disks were dipped in the test solutions and, after rinsing in sterile water, were then incubated without inoculum. After 24 h, the disks were recovered, and after serial dilutions, viable counts were assessed by the drop method, as described by Miles *et al.* [32], in YMA. Plates were then incubated at 37 °C for 24 h under aerobic conditions. Results were given as inhibition percentages using the following formula:

$$\% I = 100 - (\log CFU \text{ sample}/\log CFU \text{ control}) \times 100$$

All assays were performed in duplicate.

3.4. Microtiter-Plate Test

Biofilm quantification was carried out by adapting the protocol of Stepanovic *et al.* [33]. Briefly, in a flat bottom, 96-well microplate, wells were filled with 200 µL of test solutions with chitosan added at sub-MIC concentrations (½ and ¼ of the MIC) and inoculated at 1% (v/v). The plate was then incubated at 37 °C for 24 h in aerobiosis. All assays were performed in triplicate in the appropriate media supplemented with 5% sucrose.

To visualize adhesion, the contents of each well were discarded and then washed 3 times with sterile deionized water in order to remove non-adherent cells. The remaining attached microorganisms were fixed with 200 µL of ethanol (Panreac, Barcelona, Spain) for 15 min. Ethanol was discarded, and the wells were air dried. After that, 200 µL of crystal violet solution were added to the wells for 5 min, the excess stain removed by rinsing the plate under tap water followed by air drying. Adherence was quantified by measuring the OD at 630 nm using a microplate reader (FLUOstar, OPTIMA, BGM Labtech).

Optical density values from wells with liquid media, chitosan and no inoculum were used as negative controls, while OD from wells with liquid media, deionized water and inoculum were used as positive controls. Additionally, a control with 1% (v/v) acetic acid for each microorganism was used.

Results for this test were given as the percentage of biofilm formation inhibition applying the following formula:

$$\% \text{ biofilm formation inhibition} = 100 - (OD_{assay}/OD_{control}) \times 100$$

3.5. Mature Biofilms Assay

The assessment of chitosan's effect on mature biofilms was performed through adaptation of the microplate protocol described by Stepanovic, Vukovic, Dakic, Savic and Svabic-Vlahovic [33]. Briefly, in a flat bottom 96-well microplate, wells were filled with 200 µL of medium, inoculated at 1% (v/v) and incubated 48 h at 37 °C. After 48 h, the medium was carefully aspirated, and the wells were rinsed with phosphate buffer. Following that, 200 µL of medium, with chitosan at sub-MIC concentrations, was added and incubated at 37 °C for 24 h.

To visualize biofilms, the contents of each well were discarded and the wells washed 3 times with sterile deionized water in order to remove non-adherent cells. The remaining attached microorganisms were fixed with 200 µL of ethanol (Panreac, Barcelona, Spain) for 15 min. Ethanol was then discarded and the wells air dried. After that, 200 µL of crystal violet solution (Merck, Darmstadt, Germany) were added to the wells for 5 min. Excess stain was removed by rinsing the plate under tap water followed by air drying of the plate.

Adherence was quantified by measuring the OD at 660 nm using a microplate reader.

All experiments were done in triplicate for each microorganism. OD values from wells only with YMB were used as negative controls. A positive control with media and sterile deionized water was used. Additionally a control with 1% (v/v) acetic acid for each microorganism was used.

Results for this test were given as the reduction of the present biofilm, applying the following formula:

$$\text{Mature biofilm inhibition percentage} = 100 - (OD_{assay}/OD_{control}) \times 100$$

3.6. Dual-Species Biofilms

Quantification of the effect of chitosan upon biofilms formed by two different microorganisms was performed as previously described by Costa, Silva, Tavaria and Pintado [30]. Briefly, a test solution, with chitosan at sub-MIC concentrations, was inoculated with *C. albicans* and *Streptococcus mutans* (CCUG 45091) (1:1) to achieve a 2% (v/v) inoculum concentration. Impact upon biofilm formation was evaluated using the biofilm microtiter plate assay as described above. Results were obtained as referred above, and all assays were done in triplicate.

3.7. Statistical Treatment

The statistical differences in the methods were evaluated using PASW Statistics v. 21.0.0.0 (New York, NY, USA). The normality of the results' distribution was evaluated through Shapiro–Wilk's test. The differences were assessed using the one-way ANOVA test associated with Scheffe's test (for normal distributions). The differences were considered significant at a 0.05 significance level.

4. Conclusions

In conclusion, chitosan showed remarkable potential as a possible anti-candidiasis agent, as it was active upon *C. albicans* in the planktonic state and, more importantly, upon its sessile growth, with significant activity upon the several phases—adhesion, formation, mature and co-aggregation—of biofilm establishment and growth.

Acknowledgments

The author hereby gratefully acknowledges the Agency of Innovation (Agência de Inovação, ADI, Portugal) and Quadro de Referência Estratégico Nacional (QREN, Portugal), which, through the project "QUITORAL—Desenvolvimento de novas formulações de quitosanos com aplicação em medicina oral" (QREN-ADI 3474) and the National Funds from FCT (Fundação para a Ciência e a Tecnologia) through project PEst-OE/EQB/LA0016/2013, provided funding for the realization of this work.

Author Contributions

Eduardo Costa was responsible for the experimental planning and execution, data processing and writing of the article; Sara Silva was responsible for the experimental execution, data processing, statistical analysis and writing of the article; Freni Tavaria was responsible for the experimental planning, data validation, article proofing and validation; Manuela Pintado was responsible for the experimental planning and article proofing and validation.

References

1. Seyfarth, F.; Schliemann, S.; Elsner, P.; Hipler, U.C. Antifungal effect of high- and low-molecular-weight chitosan hydrochloride, carboxymethyl chitosan, chitosan oligosaccharide and *N*-acetyl-D-glucosamine against candida albicans, candida krusei and candida glabrata. *Int. J. Pharm.* **2008**, *353*, 139–148.

2. Tayel, A.A.; Moussa, S.; El-Tras, W.F.; Knittel, D.; Opwis, K.; Schollmeyer, E. Anticandidal action of fungal chitosan against candida albicans. *Int. J. Biol. Macromol.* **2010**, *47*, 454–457.

3. Sgherri, C.; Porta, A.; Castellano, S.; Pinzino, C.; Quartacci, M.F.; Calucci, L. Effects of azole treatments on the physical properties of *Candida albicans* plasma membrane: A spin probe epr study. *Biochim. Biophys. Acta (BBA)–Biomembr.* **2014**, *1838*, 465–473.

4. Wisplinghoff, H.; Ebbers, J.; Geurtz, L.; Stefanik, D.; Major, Y.; Edmond, M.B.; Wenzel, R.P.; Seifert, H. Nosocomial bloodstream infections due to *Candida* spp. In the USA: Species distribution, clinical features and antifungal susceptibilities. *Int. J. Antimicrob. Agent* **2014**, *43*, 78–81.

5. Lortholary, O.; Renaudat, C.; Sitbon, K.; Madec, Y.; Denoeud-Ndam, L.; Wolff, M.; Fontanet, A.; Bretagne, S.; Dromer, F. Worrisome trends in incidence and mortality of candidemia in intensive care units (Paris area, 2002–2010). *Intensive Care Med.* **2014**, *40*, 1303–1312.

6. Bassetti, M.; Merelli, M.; Righi, E.; Diaz-Martin, A.; Rosello, E.M.; Luzzati, R.; Parra, A.; Trecarichi, E.M.; Sanguinetti, M.; Posteraro, B.; *et al.* Epidemiology, species distribution, antifungal susceptibility, and outcome of candidemia across five sites in Italy and Spain. *J. Clin. Microbiol.* **2013**, *51*, 4167–4172.

7. Ramos, V.M.; Rodrıguez, N.M.; Rodriguez, M.S.; Heras, A.; Agulló, E. Modified chitosan carrying phosphonic and alkyl groups. *Carbohydrate Polymers* **2003**, *51*, 425–429.

8. Kim, S.-K.; Rajapakse, N. Enzymatic production and biological activities of chitosan oligosaccharides (COS): A review. *Carbohydr. Polym.* **2005**, *62*, 357–368.

9. Kittur, F.S.; Kumar, A.B.V.; Gowda, L.R.; Tharanathan, R.N. Chitosanolysis by a pectinase isozyme of *Aspergillus niger*—A non-specific activity. *Carbohydr. Polym.* **2003**, *53*, 191–196.

10. Costa, E.M.; Silva, S.; Pina, C.; Tavaria, F.K.; Pintado, M.M. Evaluation and insights into chitosan antimicrobial activity against anaerobic oral pathogens. *Anaerobe* **2012**, *18*, 305–309.

11. Kumar, M.N.V.R. A review of chitin and chitosan applications. *React. Funct. Polym.* **2000**, *46*, 1–27.

12. Rabea, E.I.; Badawy, M.E.; Stevens, C.V.; Smagghe, G.; Steurbaut, W. Chitosan as antimicrobial agent: Applications and mode of action. *Biomacromolecules* **2003**, *4*, 1457–1465.

13. Upadhyaya, L.; Singh, J.; Agarwal, V.; Tewari, R.P. Biomedical applications of carboxymethyl chitosans. *Carbohydr. Polym.* **2013**, *91*, 452–466.

14. Leceta, I.; Guerrero, P.; Ibarburu, I.; Dueñas, M.T.; de la Caba, K. Characterization and antimicrobial analysis of chitosan-based films. *J. Food Eng.* **2013**, *116*, 889–899.

15. Raafat, D.; Sahl, H.G. Chitosan and its antimicrobial potential—A critical literature survey. *Microb. Biotechnol.* **2009**, *2*, 186–201.

16. Muzzarelli, R.; Tarsi, R.; Filippini, O.; Giovanetti, E.; Biagini, G.; Varaldo, P.E. Antimicrobial properties of *N*-carboxybutyl chitosan. *Antimicrob. Agents Chemother.* **1990**, *34*, 2019–2023.

17. Gil, G.; del Monaco, S.; Cerrutti, P.; Galvagno, M. Selective antimicrobial activity of chitosan on beer spoilage bacteria and brewing yeasts. *Biotechnol. Lett.* **2004**, *26*, 569–574.

18. Guo, Z.; Chen, R.; Xing, R.; Liu, S.; Yu, H.; Wang, P.; Li, C.; Li, P. Novel derivatives of chitosan and their antifungal activities *in vitro*. *Carbohydr. Res.* **2006**, *341*, 351–354.

19. Zakrzewska, A.; Boorsma, A.; Brul, S.; Hellingwerf, K.J.; Klis, F.M. Transcriptional response of *Saccharomyces cerevisiae* to the plasma membrane-perturbing compound chitosan. *Eukaryot. Cell* **2005**, *4*, 703–715.

20. Carlson, R.P.; Taffs, R.; Davison, W.M.; Stewart, P.S. Anti-biofilm properties of chitosan-coated surfaces. *J. Biomater. Sci. Poly. Ed.* **2008**, *19*, 1035–1046.

21. Schinabeck, M.K.; Long, L.A.; Hossain, M.A.; Chandra, J.; Mukherjee, P.K.; Mohamed, S.; Ghannoum, M.A. Rabbit model of *Candida albicans* biofilm infection: Liposomal amphotericin B antifungal lock therapy. *Antimicrob. Agents Chemother.* **2004**, *48*, 1727–1732.

22. Martinez, L.R.; Mihu, M.R.; Tar, M.; Cordero, R.J.B.; Han, G.; Friedman, A.J.; Friedman, J.M.; Nosanchuk, J.D. Demonstration of antibiofilm and antifungal efficacy of chitosan against candidal biofilms, using an *in vivo* central venous catheter model. *J. Infect. Dis.* **2010**, *201*, 1436–1440.

23. Qin, C.; Li, H.; Xiao, Q.; Liu, Y.; Zhu, J.; Du, Y. Water-solubility of chitosan and its antimicrobial activity. *Carbohydr. Polym.* **2006**, *63*, 367–374.

24. Şenel, S.; İkinci, G.; Kaş, S.; Yousefi-Rad, A.; Sargon, M.F.; Hıncal, A.A. Chitosan films and hydrogels of chlorhexidine gluconate for oral mucosal delivery. *Int. J. Pharm.* **2000**, *193*, 197–203.

25. Cerca, N.; Martins, S.; Pier, G.B.; Oliveira, R.; Azeredo, J. The relationship between inhibition of bacterial adhesion to a solid surface by sub-mics of antibiotics and subsequent development of a biofilm. *Res. Microbiol.* **2005**, *156*, 650–655.

26. Cobrado, L.; Azevedo, M.M.; Silva-Dias, A.; Ramos, J.P.; Pina-Vaz, C.; Rodrigues, A.G. Cerium, chitosan and hamamelitannin as novel biofilm inhibitors? *J. Antimicrob. Chemother.* **2012**, *67*, 1159–1162.

27. Cobrado, L.; Silva-Dias, A.; Azevedo, M.M.; Pina-Vaz, C.; Rodrigues, A.G. *In vivo* antibiofilm effect of cerium, chitosan and hamamelitannin against usual agents of catheter-related bloodstream infections. *J. Antimicrob. Chemother.* **2013**, *68*, 126–130.

28. Cuéllar-Cruz, M.; Vega-González, A.; Mendoza-Novelo, B.; López-Romero, E.; Ruiz-Baca, E.; Quintanar-Escorza, M.A.; Villagómez-Castro, J.C. The effect of biomaterials and antifungals on biofilm formation by *Candida* species: A review. *Eur. J. Clin. Microbiol. Infect. Dis.* **2012**, *31*, 2513–2527.

29. Metwalli, K.H.; Khan, S.A.; Krom, B.P.; Jabra-Rizk, M.A. *Streptococcus mutans*, *Candida albicans*, and the human mouth: A sticky situation. *PLoS Pathog.* **2013**, *9*, e1003616.

30. Costa, E.M.; Silva, S.; Tavaria, F.K.; Pintado, M.M. Study of the effects of chitosan upon streptococcus mutans adherence and biofilm formation. *Anaerobe* **2013**, *20*, 27–31.

31. Azcurra, A.I.; Barembaum, S.R.; Bojanich, M.A.; Calamari, S.E.; Aguilar, J.; Battellino, L.J.; Dorronsoro, S.T. Effect of the high molecular weight chitosan and sodium alginate on *Candida albicans* hydrophobicity and adhesion to cells. *Med. Oral Patol. Oral Cir. Bucal* **2006**, *11*, E120–E125.

32. Miles, A.A.; Misra, S.S.; Irwin, J.O. The estimation of the bactericidal power of the blood. *J. Hyg–Camb.* **1938**, *38*, 732–749.

33. Stepanovic, S.; Vukovic, D.; Dakic, I.; Savic, B.; Svabic-Vlahovic, M. A modified microtiter-plate test for quantification of staphylococcal biofilm formation. *J. Microbiol. Meth.* **2000**, *40*, 175–179.

4

Iron and *Acinetobacter baumannii* Biofilm Formation

Valentina Gentile, Emanuela Frangipani, Carlo Bonchi, Fabrizia Minandri, Federica Runci and Paolo Visca *

Department of Sciences, Roma Tre University, Viale Marconi 446, 00146 Rome, Italy;
E-Mails: valentina.gentile@uniroma3.it (V.G.); emanuela.frangipani@uniroma3.it (E.F.);
carlo.bonchi@uniroma3.it (C.B.); fabrizia.minandri@uniroma3.it (F.M.);
federica.run@gmail.com (F.R.)

* Author to whom correspondence should be addressed; E-Mail: paolo.visca@uniroma3.it;

Abstract: *Acinetobacter baumannii* is an emerging nosocomial pathogen, responsible for infection outbreaks worldwide. The pathogenicity of this bacterium is mainly due to its multidrug-resistance and ability to form biofilm on abiotic surfaces, which facilitate long-term persistence in the hospital setting. Given the crucial role of iron in *A. baumannii* nutrition and pathogenicity, iron metabolism has been considered as a possible target for chelation-based antibacterial chemotherapy. In this study, we investigated the effect of iron restriction on *A. baumannii* growth and biofilm formation using different iron chelators and culture conditions. We report substantial inter-strain variability and growth medium-dependence for biofilm formation by *A. baumannii* isolates from veterinary and clinical sources. Neither planktonic nor biofilm growth of *A. baumannii* was affected by exogenous chelators. Biofilm formation was either stimulated by iron or not responsive to iron in the majority of isolates tested, indicating that iron starvation is not sensed as an overall biofilm-inducing stimulus by *A. baumannii*. The impressive iron withholding capacity of this bacterium should be taken into account for future development of chelation-based antimicrobial and anti-biofilm therapies.

Keywords: *Acinetobacter baumannii*; biofilm; chelator; deferasirox; deferiprone; deferoxamine; dipyridyl; iron; transferrin

1. Introduction

Acinetobacter baumannii has emerged worldwide as a leading cause of hospital-acquired infections, especially among severely ill patients in intensive care units (ICUs) [1]. Although *A. baumannii* was initially regarded to as a low-grade pathogen, evidence has been accumulated suggesting that *A. baumannii* infections are associated with increased mortality in critically ill patients [2]. *A. baumannii* causes a broad range of nosocomial infections, including ventilator-associated pneumonia, urinary tract infections, wound infection, bacteremia, endocarditis, meningitis [3], and has recently been associated with very severe community-acquired infections, especially among individuals with predisposing factors in Southern Asia and other tropical regions [4]. *A. baumannii* can also be isolated from veterinary sources, and show common characteristics with strains described in human infection [5].

Tendency to the epidemic spread, resistance to antibiotics and persistence in the hospital setting are hallmarks of *A. baumannii* infection [3]. Successful strains of multidrug-resistant (MDR) *A. baumannii* are notorious for their ability to rapidly spread among hospitalized patients, overcome geographical borders, and become epidemic worldwide [6]. Epidemiologic and population genetics studies indicate that the majority of *A. baumannii* infections are caused by strains belonging to three international clonal lineages (ICLs) [1,3,6]. *A. baumannii* strains belonging to the most widespread ICLs are invariably characterized by an MDR phenotype, which is progressively evolving towards pandrug resistance, thereby challenging the current antimicrobial armamentarium [7,8]. This poses the urgent need for the development of novel treatment strategies to combat infections caused by MDR *A. baumannii* [9].

The capacity of MDR clinical isolates of *A. baumannii* to resist to desiccation and to form biofilms are regarded as crucial factors contributing to the clinical success and persistence of this species in healthcare facilities. *A. baumannii* can survive for up to months on the dry surface of inanimate objects [10,11], enabling transmission of infection for long times under both epidemic and endemic situations [12]. A number of reports have demonstrated that *A. baumannii* can form biofilms on several biotic and abiotic surfaces, providing the bacteria with protection against antibiotic/antiseptic treatment(s) and the host immune defenses *in vivo* (reviewed in [13,14]). Biofilm formation is crucial for several *A. baumannii* infections, since these are often associated with indwelling medical devices, e.g., vascular and urinary catheters, cerebrospinal fluid shunts, and endotracheal tubes [15]. While it is apparent that the capacity to form biofilms is a general phenotypic trait of *A. baumannii*, remarkable differences in the amount of biofilm formed by different strains have been reported, even if belonging to the same clonal lineage or epidemiological cluster [12,15–18]. A number of environmental factors can influence biofilm formation, including the presence of metal cations [16,19]. Among these, iron represents an essential nutrient for infecting bacteria, and a key determinant in host-pathogen interactions. This is because bacteria must counteract an iron-poor environment during infection, due to iron sequestration by iron carrier and storage proteins of the host and adaptive hypoferremia during infection [20]. *A. baumannii* has evolved an impressive capacity to acquire iron from the host, due to the production of multiple siderophores for Fe(III) transport, combined with uptake specificities for heme and Fe(II) [21,22].

Given the crucial role of iron in *A. baumannii*-host interactions [22–24], attention has recently been given to non-antibiotic approaches that target iron metabolism to achieve antibacterial activity, including chelation therapy and use of iron mimetics (reviewed in [9]). Interestingly, it was noted that: (*i*) high concentrations of deferiprone (DFP, (Sigma Aldrich, St. Louis, MO, USA)), a compound used for chelation therapy in humans, inhibited to some extent logarithmic growth of *A. baumannii* ATCC 17978 in a chemically defined medium [25]; (*ii*) gallium, an iron-mimetic drug, suppressed the growth of MDR *A. baumannii* strains both *in vitro* and *in vivo*, acting through disruption of bacterial iron metabolism [25–27]; (*iii*) mutants impaired in production of the acinetobactin siderophore show reduced fitness *in vivo* [23]. On the other hand, it was also reported that biofilm formation on plastic by the type strain *A. baumannii* ATCC 19606^T was stimulated under conditions of iron scarcity imposed by the addition of the chelator 2,2′-dipyridyl (DIP) [19]. Therefore, the effect of iron availability on both planktonic and biofilm mode of *A. baumannii* growth deserves more in-depth investigation.

In this report, strains and optimal growth conditions for the generation *A. baumannii* biofilms were preliminarily established. Then, the role of iron in *A. baumannii* biofilm formation was investigated. Lastly, the activity of a new therapeutic iron chelator was assessed in search for inhibitory drugs that could be repurposed as adjuvant antimicrobials in the treatment of biofilm-based *A. baumannii* infections.

2. Results and Discussion

2.1. Definition of Culture Conditions for A. baumannii *Biofilm Formation*

Biofilm formation is a multifactorial phenotype [13,14], and in *A. baumannii* it can be modulated by iron availability, carbon sources, growth temperature, and different expression levels of adhesive and cell-aggregating factors [13,14,16,18,19,28]. Therefore, as a preliminary step to the investigation of the effect of iron on *A. baumannii* biofilm formation, we determined the growth response of the reference strain *A. baumannii* ATCC 17978 [25,29] to iron restriction imposed by different chelators in M9 minimal medium [30] containing 20 mM sodium succinate as the carbon source [26]. In line with previous observations [25], *A. baumannii* ATCC 17978 showed an impressive ability to multiply under conditions of iron deficiency, as those imposed by the addition of up to 128 μM human apo-transferrin (h-TF (Sigma Aldrich)), trisodium citrate (CIT (Sigma Aldrich)), desferrioxamine (DFO (Ciba Geigy, Origgio, Italy)), deferasirox (DFX (Novartis, Basel, Switzerland)) and DFP (Figure 1).

None of the tested chelators reduced *A. baumannii* ATCC 17978 growth yields at 48 h, even when 100 μM DIP (a chelator of the intracellular Fe(II) pool) was added to further reduce iron availability. As expected, growth in M9 was stimulated by *ca.* 25% in the presence of 100 μM FeCl$_3$. A similar resistance to exogenously supplied chelators in M9 was also observed for strains AYE [31] and ACICU [32], representatives for ICL-I and ICL-II, respectively (data not shown). These data can be explained by the presence in *A. baumannii* of very efficient iron uptake systems [11,21], capable of counteracting the iron withholding capacity of exogenously added chelators. The observation that DFX, DFO, and DFP do not stimulate bacterial growth in the presence of DIP (a chelator of the intracellular Fe(II) pool) suggests that these chelators are unlikely to serve as an iron source for *A. baumannii*.

Figure 1. Effect of different iron chelators on planktonic growth of *A. baumannii* ATCC 17978. Bacteria were grown for 48 h at 37 °C in 96-wells microtiter plates containing 100 μL M9 supplemented with the indicated iron chelator at different concentrations: 32 μM (light grey bars), 128 μM (dark grey bars) or 128 μM chelator + 100 μM DIP (black bars). Growth was measured as OD_{600} and expressed as percentage relative to the untreated control (*i.e.*, OD_{600} in M9). The average of the OD_{600} in control M9 was 0.318 ± 0.008 and represents 100% of growth (white bar). Relative growth in M9 supplemented with 100 μM $FeCl_3$ is reported (striped bar). Data represent the average of three independent experiments ± standard deviation. h-TF, tranferrin; CIT, citrate; DFX, deferasirox; DFO, desferrioxamine; DFP, deferiprone.

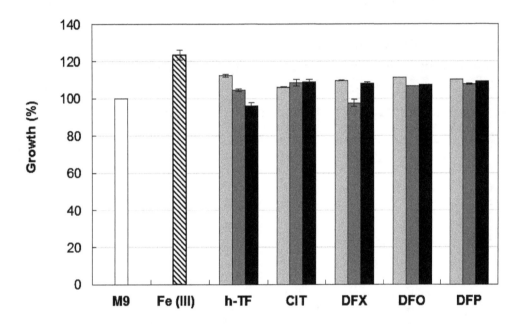

Next, the inter-strain variability and the growth medium-dependence of biofilm formation was investigated. Five well-characterized *A. baumannii* strains (AYE, representative for ICL-I [31]; ACICU, representative for ICL-II [32]; 50C, ICL-II pandrug resistant isolate [33]; RUH5875, prototypic strain for ICL-III [34]; ATCC 17978 [29]] were grown in three iron-poor media [M9, M9 supplemented with 100 μM DIP, and Chelex-100-treated Tryptic Soy Broth dialysate, TSBD [35]) in order to determine both growth and biofilm levels at 24 and 48 h. Quantitative estimation of the bacterial biomass in biofilms was assessed in 96-well polystyrene microtiter plates (BD Falcon, Milano, Italy), using the crystal-violet (CV) staining method [36]. There was a wide range of variation in growth and biofilm levels between *A. baumannii*, depending on strains and culture media, though for some strains moderate correlation was observed between growth yields and biofilm levels (Figure 2).

Remarkably, all strains produced more abundant biofilm in TSBD than in the other iron-poor media, and biofilm levels in strain ACICU were significantly higher ($p < 0.05$ in the student's *t*-test) than all the other strains tested (Figure 2). These findings corroborate the notion that biofilm levels in *A. baumannii* can vary even between closely related isolates (e.g., strains ACICU and 50C belonging to the same genetic cluster according to ref. [33]), and that different media have a profound impact on biofilm yields [15–18].

To rule out the possibility that differences in biofilm levels between TSBD and M9 or M9 plus DIP were due to different iron content of these media, an iron biosensor consisting of the Fur-controlled *basA* promoter fused to the reporter *lacZ* gene [26] was used as a probe to determine the intracellular iron level in *A. baumannii* ATCC17978. Since the Fur repressor protein acts as an iron sensor, the activity of the Fur-controlled *basA* promoter provides an indirect estimate of the intracellular iron levels of bacteria grown in the different media. The β–galactosidase (LacZ) expression was higher in TSBD than in M9 or M9 plus DIP (Figure 3), and it was invariably repressed by iron, indicating that TSBD is sensed by *A. baumannii* as an iron-poor medium.

Figure 2. Growth and biofilm formation by selected *A. baumannii* strains in different iron-poor media. Bacterial cells were inoculated at OD_{600} of 0.01 in 100 μL of the different growth media, dispensed in a 96-wells microtiter plate, and grown at 37 °C without shaking for 24 and 48 h. Growth (circles) was measured spectrophotometrically (OD_{600}) and biofilm formation (bars) was evaluated using the CV staining assay [36]. Dark grey, TSBD; light grey M9; white M9 supplemented with 100 μM DIP. Data represent the average of three independent experiments ± standard deviation.

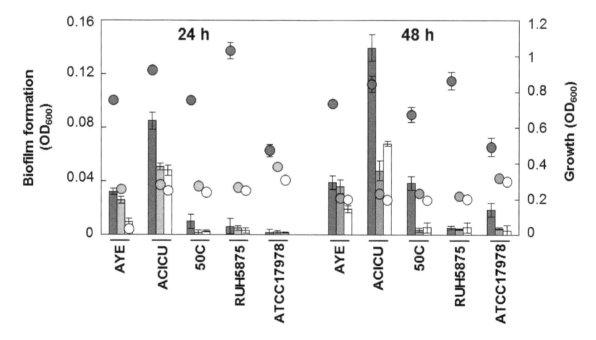

To visualize differences in biofilm structure among the five representative *A. baumannii* strains, biofilm formation on glass slides was monitored during seven days growth in TSBD by means of confocal microscopy, according to a previously described procedure [37] (Figure 4). High biofilm levels with formation of large cellular aggregates were observed for *A. baumannii* ACICU, and to a much lesser extent for the other strains (Figure 4A). Interestingly, *A. baumannii* biofilm cells were found to be embedded in a blue fluorescent material upon staining with calcofluor white (Figure 4B). In line with previous findings [18,29], this observation denotes the presence of exopolysaccharides in the matrix of *A. baumannii* biofilms, whose levels appear to be consistent with to the amount of biofilm formed in 96-well polystyrene microtiter plates (Figure 2).

Based on the above results, TSBD was considered as suitable iron-depleted medium that would allow robust biofilm formation and an easier evaluation of the effect of iron on this process. This is because the high biofilm levels achieved by *A. baumannii* in TSBD would facilitate the detection of biofilm variations in response to iron levels. Moreover, the high peptide content and balanced formula of TSBD (35, see also [38]) make it more similar to a biological fluid than the M9 mineral salt medium.

Figure 3. Regulatory mechanism and activity of the *basA::lacZ* iron biosensor in the reference *A. baumannii* strain ATCC 17978. (A) Schematic of the regulatory mechanism the *basA::lacZ* iron-regulated transcriptional fusion carried by plasmid pMP220::P$_{basA}$ [26]. Under iron proficient conditions (left), the Fur repressor protein binds the P$_{basA}$ promoter and inhibits β–galactosidase (LacZ) expression; under iron deficient conditions Fur repression is relieved and the LacZ enzyme is expressed. (B) Activity of the *basA::lacZ* iron-regulated fusion in *A. baumannii* ATCC 17978 grown for 24 and 48 h in different media, as indicated, in the absence (white bars) or presence (black bars) of 100 μM FeCl$_3$. Data are the means (±standard deviations (SD)) of triplicate experiments.

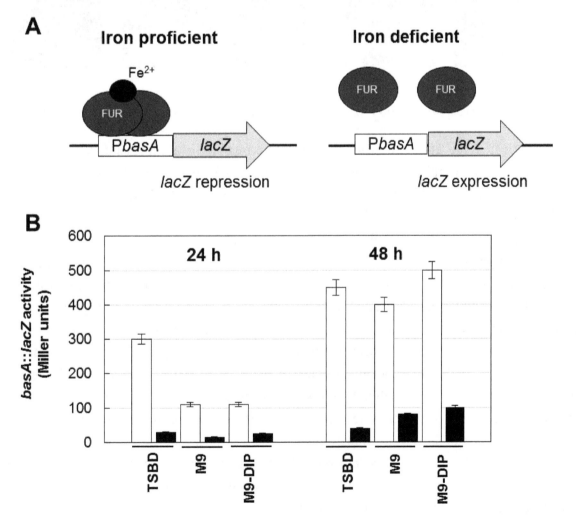

Figure 4. Seven-days biofilm of selected *A. baumannii* strains grown in TSBD. (**A**) Confocal microscope images (x-y plane and side view) of *A. baumannii* biofilms stained with acridine orange, a fluorescent dye which labels double-stranded nucleic acids (prevalently DNA) in green, and single-stranded nucleic acids (prevalently RNA) in red. (**B**) *A. baumannii* biofilms stained with the calcofluor white for exopolysaccharide labelling [19,28], and analyzed by fluorescence microscopy. Scale bar: 50 µm.

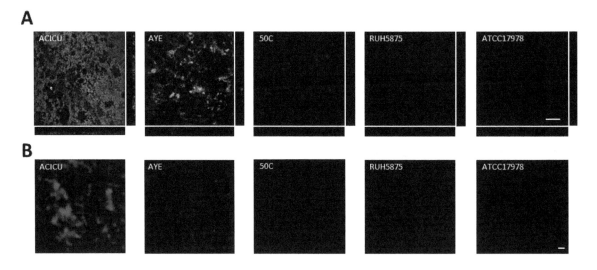

2.2. Effect of Iron Levels on Biofilm Formation by a Collection of Diverse A. baumannii Isolates

We investigated the effect of iron on biofilm formation in a representative collection of 54 *A. baumannii* strains (Table S1 in Supplementary Material), including 27 isolates from veterinary sources (67% MDR) and 27 isolates from clinical sources (96% MDR). Isolates were selected so to maximize diversity, as inferred by Random Amplified Polymorphic DNA fingerprints with primer DAF4 ([21,33]; data not shown), and represent the most widespread ICLs and some emerging lineages (Table S1 in Supplementary Material). High growth yields were observed for almost all isolates in TSBD (median OD_{600} = 0.716), which were significantly increased by the addition of 100 µM $FeCl_3$ (median OD_{600} = 1.031), consistent with iron being a nutritionally-limiting factor in TSBD (Figure 5A). Remarkably, biofilm formation was more abundant in $FeCl_3$-supplemented TSBD (median OD_{600} = 0.102) than in TSBD (median OD_{600} = 0.071) (Figure 5B). After having excluded from the analysis 4 biofilm non-producing isolates (namely, 4297, 196-1, 82D, RUH5875, see Table S1), the normalization of biofilm formation by growth yields resulted in minor differences between the two growth conditions (median values were 0.104 and 0.098 for the iron-limited and iron-rich condition, Figure 5C). This result is due to somehow opposite responses of *A. baumannii* isolates to iron starvation (*i.e.*, TSBD *vs.* $FeCl_3$-supplemented TSBD); in 21 isolates (42%) biofilm production was significantly enhanced by iron deficiency, in 12 (24%) it was significantly reduced, and in 17 (34%) iron had no effect on biofilm formation (significance in the Student's *t*-test was set at $p < 0.05$). Although stimulation of biofilm formation in response to iron-limited growth was observed for a minority (42%) of *A. baumannii* isolates, this may have relevant medical implications, since transition of these isolates from planktonic to biofilm-growing cells could be favored *in vivo*, where infecting bacteria are normally challenged with iron shortage. However, this behavior cannot be generalized, since biofilm production was either unchanged or even inhibited by iron deficiency in the majority (66%) of the isolates.

2.3. Effect of Deferasirox on A. baumannii Biofilm Formation

We showed that planktonic *A. baumannii* has an impressive ability to grow in the presence of exogenously added therapeutic chelators DFP, DFO, and DFX (Figure 1), and previous data indicate only modest inhibition of *A. baumannii* growth at high DFP concentrations (*ca.* 200 µM, ref. [25]). To gain further insight into the effect of iron withholding on *A. baumannii* biofilm formation, we examined the effect of DFX, a newly developed orally active Fe(III) chelator, on our collection of 50 biofilm-producing isolates. DFX is a synthetic compound with high affinity and specificity for Fe(III) ($\log\beta_2$ = 36.9 according to ref. [39]), and is unlikely to serve as an iron carrier to *A. baumannii* based on growth assays (Figure 1). It was successfully used in combination therapy against murine staphylococcemia [40], and in treatment of invasive fungal infections [41].

Here, biofilm formation was tested in a DFX concentration range 4–128 µM, in order to match the DFX plasma levels achievable during treatment of iron overload in humans [42]. Notably, biofilm formation by most of the isolates was not significantly affected by DFX up to 128 µM, either in TSBD or in TSBD plus 100 µM $FeCl_3$ (Figure 6A).

Figure 5. Growth and biofilm formation in a representative collection of 54 *A. baumannii* strains from clinical and veterinary sources. (**A**) Growth of 54 *A. baumanni* strains for 48 h in 96-wells microtiter plates containing 100 µL TSBD supplemented (black circles) or not (white circles) with 100 µM $FeCl_3$, as indicated. (**B**) Absolute values of biofilm formation by the same isolates shown in panel A, evaluated by the CV staining assay (OD_{600}). Grey circles (B) represent the values for strains that in either or both conditions yielded negative biofilm values, and were excluded from calculations in panel C. (**C**) Relative values of biofilm formation (Biofilm formation (OD_{600})/Growth (OD_{600})) for a subset of 50 biofilm-producing isolates. The line bar represents the median value for each group. Values for each strain are the average of three independent experiments.

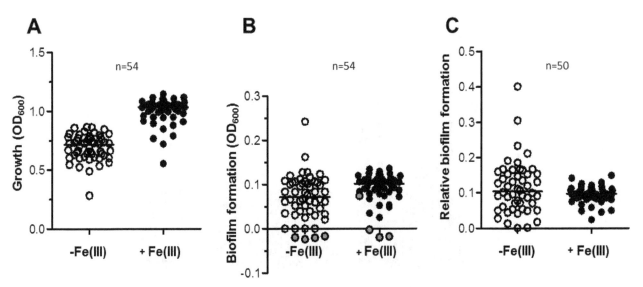

Figure 6. Effect of DFX on *A. baumannii* biofilm formation. (**A**) *A. baumannii* strains were grown statically for 48 h in microtiter plates containing 100 μL TSBD supplemented with DFX at indicated concentrations, or 128 μM DFX plus 100 μM $FeCl_3$. Biofilm formation (OD_{600} in the CV staining assay) was normalized by the growth yield (OD_{600} of the culture) and expressed as percentage relative to the DFX-untreated control (TSBD). Boxes represent medians, second and third interquartiles; whiskers represent range of 50 isolates tested. (**B**) Relative biofilm levels produced by individual isolates in presence of 128 μM DFX, expressed as % of the untreated control in TSBD. With reference to Figure 5C, the bar filling denotes: isolates in which biofilm production was significantly enhanced by iron deficiency (white, 21 isolates), or significantly reduced (black, 12 isolates), or in which iron had no effect on biofilm formation (grey, 17 isolates). In both panels data represent the average of three independent experiments.

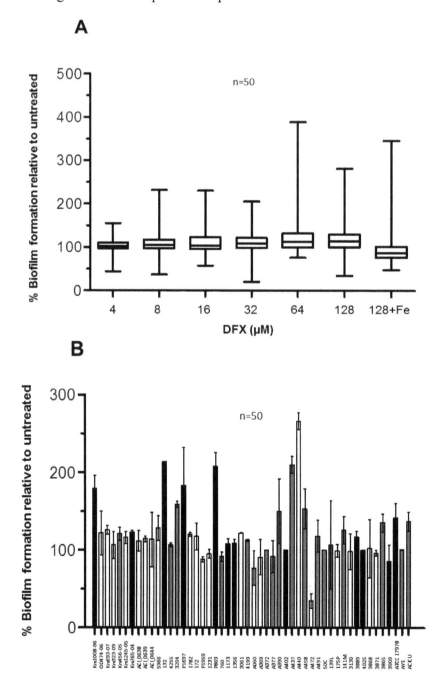

No obvious correlation could be observed between the biofilm response to iron starvation in TSBD (see Figure 5 and associated text) and in the presence of 128 μM DFX (Figure 6B). The observation that a minority of isolates (*i.e.*, Km1008-06, 132, P1697, P869, A472, and ATCC17978) showed opposite responses to iron starvation induced by TSBD with and without iron (Figure 5), compared with TSBD and TSBD plus DFX (Figure 6B), suggests that either DFX exerts iron chelation-independent effects, or that the iron deficiency threshold that determines the biofilm response in *A. baumannii* can vary for these isolates. Apart from this, the ability to generate biofilms is scarcely influenced by the presence of DFX for most *A. baumannii* isolates, indicating that, at least *in vitro*, this therapeutic chelator is incapable of overcoming the iron withholding capacity of *A. baumannii* biofilms.

3. Experimental Section

3.1. Bacterial Strains and Growth Media

Relevant characteristics of the 54 *A. baumannii* strains used in this study are provided in Table S1 in the Supplementary Material. The collection includes representative strains for ICLs I, II, and III, namely AYE (ICL-I) [43], ACICU (ICL-II) [32], and RUH 5875 (ICL-III). Strain ATCC 17978 is a well-characterized clinical isolate dated 1950s and showing moderate antibiotic resistance [29]. Strain 50C is a pandrug resistant clinical isolate [33,44]. Other clinical and veterinary isolates were provided as part of the collections from various European laboratories [5,21,45–48]. Iron-poor culture media used in this study were the M9 minimal medium [30] supplemented with 20 mM sodium succinate as the carbon source, and TSBD, a Chelex 100-treated Trypticase Soy Broth dialysate [35]. When required, media were supplemented with either 100 μM DIP or 100 μM $FeCl_3$.

3.2. Chemicals

The chemicals used in this study were deferiprone (DFP, (Sigma Aldrich)), tri-sodium citrate [CIT, (Sigma Aldrich), desferrioxamine (DFO, (Ciba Geigy)); human apo-transferrin (h-TF, iron content ≤ 0.005%, (Sigma Aldrich)), and deferasirox (DFX, (Novartis)).

3.3. Growth Inhibitory Activity of Iron-Chelators

The activity of the iron chelators on bacterial growth was tested in 96-well microtiter plates (BD Falcon) containing increasing concentrations (4–128 μM) of iron chelators. Plates were inoculated at OD_{600} of 0.01 in a 100 μL final volume of M9 supplemented or not with 100 μM DIP at the highest iron-chelator concentration tested, or 100 μM $FeCl_3$, and incubated at 37 °C for 48 h with moderate shaking (100 r.p.m.). Spectrophotometric readings were performed in a Wallac 1420 Victor3V multilabel plate reader (Perkin Elmer, Milano, Italy).

3.4. Biofilm Formation

Biofilm formation was measured according to the microtiter plate assay [36]. Briefly, bacterial cells were inoculated at OD_{600} of 0.01 in 100 μL of medium and grown at 37 °C for up to 48 h in 96-wells microtiter plates without shaking. Planktonic cells were removed and the attached cells were gently washed three times with sterile PBS, air dried, and stained with 150 μL of 0.1% CV water solution for 20 min. The wells were gently washed four times with distilled water, and the surface-associated dye was eluted in 200 μL of 95% ethanol. The OD_{600} of the eluate was measured in a Wallac 1420 Victor3V multilabel plate reader (Perkin Elmer).

3.5. Biofilm Inhibition

To investigate the effect of DFX on biofilm formation, fifty biofilm-producing *A. baumannii* strains were inoculated (OD_{600} of 0.01) into 96-well microtiter plates containing 100 μL TSBD supplemented with increasing DFX concentrations (4 to 128 μM) or 128 μM DFX plus 100 μM $FeCl_3$ The assay was performed as described above.

3.6. Microscopy Analysis

For microscopic visualization of *A. baumannii* biofilms, strains were grown in an 8-well chamber slide as previously described [37]. Briefly, bacteria were inoculated at OD_{600} of 0.01 in 200 μL of TSBD and incubated at 37 °C for 48 h to allow the adhesion of the bacterial cells on the glass surface. To maintain bacterial viability, the medium was changed every 24 h until the seventh day. To visualize biofilms structure, *A. baumannii* biofilms were stained with the acridine orange (0.1% water solution), a fluorescent dye, which labels double-stranded nucleic acids (prevalently DNA) in green, and single-stranded nucleic acids (prevalently RNA) in red, and examined using Leica TCS SP5 confocal microscope. For detection of matrix exopolysaccharides, samples were stained with calcofluor white (Fluka) and analyzed with an epifluorescence microscope. The Image J software [49] was used for image analysis.

3.7. β-Galactosidase Activity Assay

The *basA* promoter was cloned upstream of the *lacZ* reporter gene in plasmid pMP220::P*basA* (carrying the tetracycline-resistance (Tc^R) determinant) as previously described [26]. For reporter gene activity measurements, *A. baumannii* ATCC 17978 (Tc^S) was transformed with P*basA::lacZ* (Tc^R) and grown for 16 h at 37 °C in M9 medium supplemented with 10 μg/mL Tc. Cultures were then appropriately diluted in TSBD, M9 and M9 supplemented with 100 μM DIP, with or without 100 μM $FeCl_3$ to reach an initial cell concentration corresponding to $OD_{600} \sim 0.01$ and incubated at 37 °C with vigorous shaking. The β-galactosidase (LacZ) activity expressed by *A. baumannii* ATCC 17978 (pMP220::P*basA*) after 24 and 48 h growth was determined spectrophotometrically on toluene/SDS-permeabilized cells using *o*-nitrophenyl-β-D-galactopyranoside as the substrate, and expressed in Miller units [50].

$$\text{Miller units} = 1{,}000 \times [OD_{420} - (1.75 \times OD_{550})] / \text{Volume (ml)} \times \text{Time (min)} \times OD_{600}$$

4. Conclusions

The formation and maturation of *A. baumannii* biofilms depend on the complex interplay of many environmental and cell-associated factors [13,14]. In this study, attention has been focused on the role of iron, since this metal is essential for bacterial nutrition and virulence [22–24], and plays a central role in host defense from bacterial infection [20]. In agreement with a previous study [25], we showed that planktonic *A. baumannii* cells can overcome iron restriction imposed by a variety of exogenous chelators, likely due to the presence in this species of multiple iron scavenging systems [21,22]. Then, we observed relevant differences in biofilm levels depending on *A. baumannii* strain and growth medium, and established suitable conditions for testing the effect of iron on biofilm formation. The two most relevant findings of these experiments were: (*i*) the strong influence of medium composition on biofilm yields; (*ii*) the high variability in biofilm levels produced by *A. baumannii* strains of clinical and veterinary origin, irrespective of their genetic relatedness or epidemic potential; (*iii*) the strain-dependent response of *A. baumannii* biofilms to iron scarcity. Since biofilm formation was either stimulated by iron or not responsive to this metal in the majority of strains tested, we conclude that iron starvation is not sensed as an overall biofilm-inducing stimulus by *A. baumannii*. Consistent with these findings, a recently developed clinical chelator, endowed with extremely high affinity for iron, showed no significant anti-biofilm activity in *A. baumannii*. Thus, while iron metabolism continues to represent a promising target for *A. baumannii* inhibition, the impressive iron withholding capacity of this bacterium should be taken into account for future development of chelation-based antimicrobial and anti-biofilm therapies.

Acknowledgments

This work was supported by a grant from the Italian Ministry of University and Research-PRIN 2012 (prot. 2012WJSX8K) to Paolo Visca. The Authors wish to thank Novartis Pharma AG (Basel, Switzerland) for the generous gift of deferasirox, and the many European laboratories that provided *A. baumannii* strains.

Author Contributions

Conceived and designed the experiments: Emanuela Frangipani, Paolo Visca. Supervised the laboratory work: Emanuela Frangipani, Paolo Visca. Performed the experimental work: Valentina Gentile, Carlo Bonchi, Federica Runci, Fabrizia Minandri. Wrote the manuscript: Paolo Visca.

References

1. Antunes, L.C.; Visca, P.; Towner, K.J. *Acinetobacter baumannii*: Evolution of a global pathogen. *Pathog. Dis.* **2014**, *71*, 292–301.
2. Falagas, M.E.; Bliziotis, I.A.; Siempos, I.I. Attributable mortality of *Acinetobacter baumannii* infections in critically ill patients: A systematic review of matched cohort and case-control studies. *Crit. Care* **2006**, *10*, R48.

3. Dijkshoorn, L.; Nemec, A.; Seifert, H. An increasing threat in hospitals: Multidrug-resistant *Acinetobacter baumannii*. *Nat. Rev. Microbiol.* **2007**, *5*, 939–951.

4. Eveillard, M.; Kempf, M.; Belmonte, O.; Pailhoriès, H.; Joly-Guillou, M.L. Reservoirs of *Acinetobacter baumannii* outside the hospital and potential involvement in emerging human community-acquired infections. *Int. J. Infect. Dis.* **2013**, *17*, e802–e805.

5. Endimiani, A.; Hujer, K.M.; Hujer, A.M.; Bertschy, I.; Rossano, A.; Koch, C.; Gerber, V.; Francey, T.; Bonomo, R.A.; Perreten, V. *Acinetobacter baumannii* isolates from pets and horses in Switzerland: Molecular characterization and clinical data. *J. Antimicrob. Chemother.* **2011**, *66*, 2248–2254.

6. Zarrilli, R.; Pournaras, S.; Giannouli, M.; Tsakris, A. Global evolution of multidrug-resistant *Acinetobacter baumannii* clonal lineages. *Int. J. Antimicrob. Agents* **2013**, *41*, 11–19.

7. Durante-Mangoni, E.; Zarrilli R. Global spread of drug-resistant *Acinetobacter baumannii*: Molecular epidemiology and management of antimicrobial resistance. *Future Microbiol.* **2011**, *6*, 407–422.

8. Neonakis, I.K.; Spandidos, D.A.; Petinaki, E. Confronting multidrug-resistant *Acinetobacter baumannii*: A review. *Int. J. Antimicrob. Agents* **2011**, *37*, 102–109.

9. García-Quintanilla, M.; Pulido, M.R.; López-Rojas, R.; Pachón, J.; McConnell, M.J. Emerging therapies for multidrug resistant *Acinetobacter baumannii*. *Trends Microbiol.* **2013**, *21*, 157–163.

10. Jawad, A.; Seifert, H.; Snelling, A.M.; Heritage, J.; Hawkey, P.M. Survival of *Acinetobacter baumannii* on dry surfaces: Comparison of outbreak and sporadic isolates. *J. Clin. Microbiol.* **1998**, *36*, 1938–1941.

11. Antunes, L.C.; Imperi, F.; Carattoli, A.; Visca, P. Deciphering the multifactorial nature of *Acinetobacter baumannii* pathogenicity. *PLoS One* **2011**, *6*, e22674.

12. Giannouli, M.; Antunes, L.C.; Marchetti, V.; Triassi, M.; Visca, P.; Zarrilli, R. Virulence-related traits of epidemic *Acinetobacter baumannii* strains belonging to the international clonal lineages I-III and to the emerging genotypes ST25 and ST78. *BMC Infect. Dis.* **2013**, *13*, 282.

13. Gaddy, J.A.; Actis, L.A. Regulation of *Acinetobacter baumannii* biofilm formation. *Future Microbiol.* **2009**, *4*, 273–278.

14. Longo, F.; Vuotto, C.; Donelli, G. Biofilm formation in *Acinetobacter baumannii*. *New Microbiol.* **2014**, *37*, 119–127.

15. Rodríguez-Baño, J.; Martí, S.; Soto, S.; Fernández-Cuenca, F.; Cisneros, J.M.; Pachón, J.; Pascual, A.; Martínez-Martínez, L.; McQueary, C.; Actis, L.A.; *et al.* Spanish Group for the Study of Nosocomial Infections (GEIH). Biofilm formation in *Acinetobacter baumannii*: Associated features and clinical implications. *Clin. Microbiol. Infect.* **2008**, *14*, 276–278.

16. Lee, H.W.; Koh, Y.M.; Kim, J.; Lee, J.C.; Lee, Y.C.; Seol, S.Y.; Cho, D.T.; Kim, J. Capacity of multidrug-resistant clinical isolates of *Acinetobacter baumannii* to form biofilm and adhere to epithelial cell surfaces. *Clin. Microbiol. Infect.* **2008**, *14*, 49–54.

17. Wroblewska, M.M.; Sawicka-Grzelak, A.; Marchel, H.; Luczak, M.; Sivan, A. Biofilm production by clinical strains of *Acinetobacter baumannii* isolated from patients hospitalized in two tertiary care hospitals. *FEMS Immunol. Med. Microbiol.* **2008**, *53*, 140–144.

18. McQueary, C.N.; Actis, L.A. *Acinetobacter baumannii* biofilms: Variations among strains and correlations with other cell properties. *J. Microbiol.* **2011**, *49*, 243–250.

19. Tomaras, A.P.; Dorsey, C.W.; Edelmann, R.E.; Actis, L.A. Attachment to and biofilm formation on abiotic surfaces by *Acinetobacter baumannii*: Involvement of a novel chaperone-usher pili assembly system. *Microbiology* **2003**, *149*, 3473–3484.

20. Weinberg, E.D. Iron availability and infection. *Biochim. Biophys. Acta* **2009**, *1790*, 600–605.

21. Antunes, L.C.; Imperi, F.; Towner, K.J.; Visca, P. Genome-assisted identification of putative iron-utilization genes in *Acinetobacter baumannii* and their distribution among a genotypically diverse collection of clinical isolates. *Res. Microbiol.* **2011**, *162*, 279–284.

22. Zimbler, D.L.; Penwell, W.F.; Gaddy, J.A.; Menke, S.M.; Tomaras, A.P.; Connerly, P.L.; Actis, L.A. Iron acquisition functions expressed by the human pathogen *Acinetobacter baumannii*. *Biometals* **2009**, *22*, 23–32.

23. Gaddy, J.A.; Arivett, B.A.; McConnell, M.J.; López-Rojas, R.; Pachón, J.; Actis, L.A. Role of acinetobactin-mediated iron acquisition functions in the interaction of *Acinetobacter baumannii* strain ATCC 19606^{T} with human lung epithelial cells, *Galleria mellonella* caterpillars, and mice. *Infect. Immun.* **2012**, *80*, 1015–1024.

24. Mortensen, B.L.; Skaar, E.P. The contribution of nutrient metal acquisition and metabolism to *Acinetobacter baumannii* survival within the host. *Front. Cell. Infect. Microbiol.* **2013**, *3*, 95.

25. De Léséleuc, L.; Harris, G.; KuoLee, R.; Chen, W. *In vitro* and *in vivo* biological activities of iron chelators and gallium nitrate against *Acinetobacter baumannii*. *Antimicrob. Agents Chemother.* **2012**, *56*, 5397–5400.

26. Antunes, L.C.; Imperi, F.; Minandri, F.; Visca, P. *In vitro* and *in vivo* antimicrobial activities of gallium nitrate against multidrug-resistant *Acinetobacter baumannii*. *Antimicrob. Agents Chemother.* **2012**, *56*, 5961–5970.

27. Minandri, F.; Bonchi, C.; Frangipani, E.; Imperi, F.; Visca, P. Promises and failures of gallium as an antibacterial agent. *Future Microbiol.* **2014**, *9*, 379–397.

28. Nucleo, E.; Steffanoni, L.; Fugazza, G.; Migliavacca, R.; Giacobone, E.; Navarra, A.; Pagani, L.; Landini, P. Growth in glucose-based medium and exposure to subinhibitory concentrations of imipenem induce biofilm formation in a multidrug-resistant clinical isolate of *Acinetobacter baumannii*. *BMC Microbiol.* **2009**, *9*, 270.

29. Smith, M.G.; Gianoulis, T.A.; Pukatzki, S.; Mekalanos, J.J.; Ornston, L.N.; Gerstein, M.; Snyder, M. New insights into *Acinetobacter baumannii* pathogenesis revealed by high-density pyrosequencing and transposon mutagenesis. *Genes Dev.* **2007**, *21*, 601–614.

30. Guterman, S.K. Colicin B: Mode of action and inhibition by enterochelin. *J. Bacteriol.* **1973**, *114*, 1217–1224.

31. Fournier, P.E.; Vallenet, D.; Barbe, V.; Audic, S.; Ogata, H.; Poirel, L.; Richet, H.; Robert, C.; Mangenot, S.; Abergel, C.; *et al.* Comparative genomics of multidrug resistance in *Acinetobacter baumannii*. *PLoS Genet.* **2006**, *2*, e7.

32. Iacono, M.; Villa, L.; Fortini, D.; Bordoni, R.; Imperi, F.; Bonnal, R.J.; Sicheritz-Ponten, T.; de Bellis, G.; Visca, P.; Cassone, A.; *et al.* Whole-genome pyrosequencing of an epidemic multidrug-resistant *Acinetobacter baumannii* strain belonging to the European clone II group. *Antimicrob. Agents Chemother.* **2008**, *52*, 2616–2625.

33. D'Arezzo, S.; Principe, L.; Capone, A.; Petrosillo, N.; Petrucca, A.; Visca, P. Changing carbapenemase gene pattern in an epidemic multidrug-resistant *Acinetobacter baumannii* lineage causing multiple outbreaks in central Italy. *J. Antimicrob. Chemother.* **2011**, *66*, 54–61.

34. Van Dessel, H.; Dijkshoorn, L.; van der Reijden, T.; Bakker, N.; Paauw, A.; van den Broek, P.; Verhoef, J.; Brisse, S. Identification of a new geographically widespread multiresistant *Acinetobacter baumannii* clone from European hospitals. *Res. Microbiol.* **2004**, *155*, 105–112.

35. Ohman, D.; Sadoff, J.; Iglewski, B. Toxin A-deficient mutants of *Pseudomonas aeruginosa* PA103: Isolation and characterization. *Infect. Immun.* **1980**, *28*, 899–908.

36. O'Toole, G.; Kaplan, H.B.; Kolter, R. Biofilm formation as microbial development. *Annu. Rev. Microbiol.* **2000**, *54*, 49–79.

37. Jurcisek, J.A.; Dickson, A.C.; Bruggeman, M.E.; Bakaletz, L.O. *In vitro* biofilm formation in an 8-well chamber slide. *J. Vis. Exp.* **2011**, *47*, doi:10.3791/2481.

38. Sigma-Aldrich. Available online: www.sigmaaldrich.com (accessed on 14 August 2014).

39. Hider, R.; Xiaole, K.; Lucker, T.; Conlon, K.; Harland, R. SPD602 is a selective iron chelator which is able to mobilise the non-transferrin-bound iron pool. *Blood* **2013**, *122*, 1673.

40. Luo, G.; Spellberg, B.; Gebremariam, T.; Lee, H.; Xiong, Y.Q.; French, S.W.; Bayer, A.; Ibrahim, A.S. Combination therapy with iron chelation and vancomycin in treating murine staphylococcemia. *Eur. J. Clin. Microbiol. Infect. Dis.* **2014**, *33*, 845–851.

41. Lewis, R.E.; Pongas, G.N.; Albert, N.; Ben-Ami, R.; Walsh, T.J.; Kontoyiannis, D.P. Activity of deferasirox in *Mucorales*: Influences of species and exogenous iron. *Antimicrob. Agents. Chemother.* **2011**, *55*, 411–413.

42. Nisbet-Brown, E.; Olivieri, N.F.; Giardina, P.J.; Grady, R.W.; Neufeld, E.J.; Séchaud, R.; Krebs-Brown, A.J.; Anderson, J.R.; Alberti, D.; Sizer, K.C.; *et al.* Effectiveness and safety of ICL670 in iron-loaded patients with thalassaemia: A randomised, double-blind, placebo-controlled, dose-escalation trial. *Lancet* **2003**, *361*, 1597–1602.

43. Vallenet, D.; Nordmann, P.; Barbe, V.; Poirel, L.; Mangenot, S.; Bataille, E.; Dossat, C.; Gas, S.; Kreimeyer, A.; Lenoble, P.; *et al.* Comparative analysis of Acinetobacters: Three genomes for three lifestyles. *PLoS One* **2008**, *19*, e1805.

44. D'Andrea, M.M.; Giani, T.; D'Arezzo, S.; Capone, A.; Petrosillo, N.; Visca, P.; Luzzaro, F.; Rossolini, G.M. Characterization of pABVA01, a plasmid encoding the OXA-24 carbapenemase from Italian isolates of *Acinetobacter baumannii. Antimicrob. Agents Chemother.* **2009**, *53*, 3528–3533.

45. Vaneechoutte, M.; Devriese, L.A.; Dijkshoorn, L.; Lamote, B.; Deprez, P.; Verschraegen, G.; Haesebrouck, F. *Acinetobacter baumannii*-infected vascular catheters collected from horses in an equine clinic. *J. Clin. Microbiol.* **2000**, *38*, 4280–4281.

46. Zordan, S.; Prenger-Berninghoff, E.; Weiss, R.; van der Reijden, T.; van den Broek, P.; Baljer, G.; Dijkshoorn, L. Multidrug-resistant *Acinetobacter baumannii* in veterinary clinics, Germany. *Emerg. Infect. Dis.* **2011**, *17*, 1751–1754.

47. MacKenzie, F.M.; Struelens, M.J.; Towner, K.J.; Gould, I.M.; ARPAC Steering Group; ARPAC Consensus Conference Participants. Report of the Consensus Conference on Antibiotic Resistance; Prevention and Control (ARPAC). *Clin. Microbiol. Infect.* **2005**, *11*, 938–954.

48. Towner, K.J.; Levi, K.; Vlassiadi, M.; on behalf of the ARPAC Steering Group. Genetic diversity of carbapenem-resistant isolates of *Acinetobacter baumannii* in Europe. *Clin. Microbiol. Infect.* **2008**, *14*, 161–167.

49. ImageJ. Available online: http://rsbweb.nih.gov/ij/ (accessed on 14 August 2014).

50. Miller, J.H. *Experiments in Molecular Genetics*; Cold Spring Harbor Laboratory: Cold Spring Harbor, NY, USA, 1972; pp. 252–255.

5

Evolution of Antimicrobial Peptides to Self-Assembled Peptides for Biomaterial Applications

Alice P. McCloskey, Brendan F. Gilmore and Garry Laverty *

Biomaterials, Biofilm and Infection Control Research Group, School of Pharmacy,
Queen's University Belfast, Medical Biology Centre, 97 Lisburn Road, Belfast BT9 7BL, N. Ireland;
E-Mails: amccloskey16@qub.ac.uk (A.P.M.); b.gilmore@qub.ac.uk (B.F.G.)

* Author to whom correspondence should be addressed; E-Mail: garry.laverty@qub.ac.uk;

External Editor: Dr. Gianfranco Donelli

Abstract: Biomaterial-related infections are a persistent burden on patient health, recovery, mortality and healthcare budgets. Self-assembled antimicrobial peptides have evolved from the area of antimicrobial peptides. Peptides serve as important weapons in nature, and increasingly medicine, for combating microbial infection and biofilms. Self-assembled peptides harness a "bottom-up" approach, whereby the primary peptide sequence may be modified with natural and unnatural amino acids to produce an inherently antimicrobial hydrogel. Gelation may be tailored to occur in the presence of physiological and infective indicators (e.g. pH, enzymes) and therefore allow local, targeted antimicrobial therapy at the site of infection. Peptides demonstrate inherent biocompatibility, antimicrobial activity, biodegradability and numerous functional groups. They are therefore prime candidates for the production of polymeric molecules that have the potential to be conjugated to biomaterials with precision. Non-native chemistries and functional groups are easily incorporated into the peptide backbone allowing peptide hydrogels to be tailored to specific functional requirements. This article reviews an area of increasing interest, namely self-assembled peptides and their potential therapeutic applications as innovative hydrogels and biomaterials in the prevention of biofilm-related infection.

Keywords: antimicrobial; bacteria; biofilm; biomaterial; infection; peptide; self-assembly

1. Introduction

Biomaterials have an increasingly important role in patient care. Approximately five million medical devices and implants are used in the US each year [1]. They are beneficial not only as temporary interventions but also as permanent features to replace or facilitate normal bodily functions. There is a diverse array of such materials available including: intravascular and urinary catheters, heart valve prostheses, artificial hip joints, dental implants, and intraocular lenses [2]. Their use is particularly prominent in modern medicine as population demographics demonstrate an increasing trend toward an ageing population, in tandem with increased life expectancy and improved healthcare [3].

Grainger and colleagues researched the contribution medical devices have to improving patients' quality of life [4]. They concluded that 50% of patients with aortic heart valve disease could potentially die within three years of diagnosis. Valve replacements resulted in an increase in ten year survival to approximately 70% of patients. Despite this improvement, 60% of these patients were shown to have device-associated complications thus affecting patient quality of life. Implantation of a medical device is an invasive surgical procedure that may result in irritation, wounding and infection of the surgical site. A macrophage-mediated collection of immune responses, collectively referred to as the host or foreign body response, is triggered leading to compromised device function and scarring of surrounding tissue [5]. Anderson and colleagues provide a comprehensive outline of the sequence of events following surgical implantation [6]. The initial response follows the normal wound-healing cascade of: injury, blood-material interactions, provisional matrix formation, acute inflammation, chronic inflammation, granulation tissue development, foreign body reaction, and fibrosis. The resulting host or foreign body response to a device is estimated to affect approximately 5% of patients and can have a significant impact on patient recovery and long-term health. Surgical trauma can result in a compromised immune response leading to unchallenged accumulation and adherence of pathogens at the site of implantation, resulting in biofilm formation. Biomaterials provide an optimal surface for biofilm formation [1,7]. The long-term effects are considerable. Economically, biomaterial associated infections have costly implications on health-care budgets. Bacterial accumulation and the subsequent formation of a biofilm contributes to an infectious profile 10–1000 times more resistant to standard therapeutic regimens, leading to compromised implant function and/or failure [8]. Symptomatic infection often occurs within 2 weeks of implantation [4,6,7,9].

Biofilms are phenotypically heterogeneous, sessile microbial communities that form at biotic and abiotic sites. They may be composed of a single or multiple species (poly-microbial) of bacteria and fungi [10–12]. Biofilm formation can be divided into three significant stages: (1) initial non-specific, reversible primary adhesion; (2) specific irreversible adhesion (coating of the device, transport of cells to the interface, adhesion of cells; accumulation at the surface involving biomolecular processes including quorum sensing, up-regulation of virulence factors and secretion of extracellular polymers; (3) biofilm detachment/dispersal and recolonization of alternative sites. Following implantation the surface chemistry of a biomaterial is modified by the laying down of a host-derived conditioning film. Primary adhesion is dependent on two key factors—hydrophilicity and charge at the cell-device interface. Primary adhesion is a non-specific process mediated by hydrophobic and van der Waal's interactions between the microbial cell and the generally hydrophobic surface, as is the case for silicone [1,10,11]. Binding sites such as fibrinogen, fibronectin, vitronectin, binding autolysin, albumin and extracellular matrix binding protein become exposed on the biomaterial surface. Microbial adhesins, for example teichoic acid expressed in *Staphylococcus epidermidis*, specifically recognize binding sites and mediate adherence to the surface via covalent attachment.

The potential for microbial spoilage is not confined to hydrophobic surfaces. More hydrophilic materials, for example Teflon®, also suffer from microbial contamination due to mechanical rather than chemical factors [13]. MacKintosh and co-workers investigated how the modification of poly(ethylene terephthalate) surface chemistry affected bacterial-biomaterial interaction, attachment and subsequent biofilm formation of *Staphylococcus epidermidis* [14]. They demonstrated that hydrophobic interactions do influence the adhesion of bacteria to the material surface. Of greater significance is the presence of serum proteins within the conditioning film. These tend to have a greater effect on adhesion and biofilm formation *in vivo*. Similar research performed by the Gottenbos group suggested that biofilm formation is a complex relationship involving not only the biomaterial surface properties and the ability of the bacteria to bind to a given surface, but also the availability of nutrients at the site of adherence [15].

Accumulation on a surface occurs when bacterial cells multiply and form multi-layered cell clusters resulting in a complex three dimensional architecture- the classic biofilm [16]. The biofilm is maintained through specific quorum sensing pathways. Quorum sensing is a communicatory and regulatory process controlling the up- and down-regulation of genes that govern virulence and adhesion factors, relative to environmental conditions and population density. It is an essential process for biofilm survival ensuring that biofilms act as a mutualistic community rather than individual cells [17]. As the microbial population increases the supply of nutrients and oxygen become limited within the confines of the biofilm. Therefore biofilm bacteria generally grow more slowly than planktonic bacteria due to a reduced rate of respiration/metabolism. The protective environment, provided by the polymeric exopolysaccharide matrix, means that bacteria are much more resistant to the host's immune response and therapeutic antimicrobials than their planktonic counterparts [1,18,19]. Biofilm mediated infections are thus extremely difficult to treat and the extent and rate of eradication is largely determined by the most resistant phenotype within the biofilm. Chemotherapeutic failure often results in surgical removal of the biomaterial, particularly those involving *Staphylococcus aureus* and *Candida* species [7]. Removal, combined with potential chemotherapeutic failure, is not an ideal scenario as concerns grow regarding increased antimicrobial resistance, and the relative lack of new antimicrobials in development [20–22].

Typical biofilm related medical device infections include: Catheter associated urinary tract infections; peristomal skin infections following insertion of percutaneous endoscopic gastrostomy feeding tubes; and pneumonia or tracheobronchitis with tracheostomy devices. The most commonly implicated pathogens are: staphylococci, enterococci, *Escherichia coli*, *Proteus mirabilis*, *Pseudomonas*, and *Candida* [19,23,24]. The prognosis for such infections depend on the patient's initial health, which in many cases is poor due to age and co-morbidities, and the duration of implantation. Medical implants are commonly required in immunocompromised patients. Therefore, insertion of an implant and the resulting trauma further compromises the immune response increasing patient recovery time and morbidity.

Numerous strategies to reduce biomaterial-associated infections have been developed but few have translated to clinical practice [9]. Hospital stays can be up to two and a half times longer than for uninfected patients, with a total of 3.6 million extra days being spent in hospital per year in England. Nosocomial infections cost the health sector in England almost £1 billion per year [25]. In the United States medical device related infections contribute to over 50,000 deaths per year [4]. As for the majority of disease states prevention is the key aim. Poor hygiene practice within the healthcare setting has been shown to increase the risk of infection. Simple measures such as correct hand washing technique, by both staff and patients, can have a dramatic decrease in infections [26]. There is an increasing demand globally for medical devices to replace normal physiological function. Therefore managing and preventing implant associated infections is a huge challenge [1]. These problems have to be addressed on a global-scale and require the development of biomaterials that are both biocompatible and anti-infective. This review examines the current strategies employed to reduce the occurrence of biofilm mediated device related infections and investigates the potential of future innovative strategies, namely peptide based biomaterials.

2. Current Research Based Strategies for the Prevention of Medical Device Related Infection

Biomaterials cover a diverse range of pharmaceutical applications from drug delivery to tissue engineering [27]. Every device is prone to infection. Surfaces are particularly vulnerable to biofilm formation. Therefore antimicrobial coatings are a plausible solution for the development of devices with anti-infective properties. Implantation of medical devices may be classified as temporary or permanent/long-term. Temporary devices, for example contact lenses, are not fully integrated into the host tissue. Other internally-based devices, for example heart valves, tend to be more permanent. Prevention of temporary device-related infections can be managed with non-adhesive, antimicrobial impregnated or releasing coatings, which kill bacteria that come into contact with the device [9]. Permanent device coatings must be multi-functioning, facilitating incorporation of the device into the host tissue whilst simultaneously preventing microbial adhesion over an extended period within the lifetime of the device. Examples of such coatings include those investigated by the Saldarriaga group [28]. They produced multi-component cross-linked poly(ethylene-glycol) based polymers and demonstrated that the degree of hydration and steric hindrance contributed to the efficacy of these multi-functioning coatings. Hydrogel coatings display great promise as they can incorporate and/or release antimicrobial agents. They allow for improved tissue integration and a reduction in biofilm formation [29]. Hydrogels comprise a group of insoluble, swellable, hydrophilic polymers. When fully swollen they are composed of a significant amount of water (up to ~99%) but also display solid-like properties which provide desirable characteristics such as increased mechanical strength. Hydrogel classification is dependent upon the nature of the crosslinks which bind the hydrogel structure, influencing its swelling ability. Chemical hydrogels are also influenced by the structure of the primary monomer chains and the density of the crosslinks within the polymer system. Hydrogel architecture is also determined by secondary non-covalent molecular interactions and entangled molecules. The presence of a porous three-dimensional network means hydrogels are ideal biomaterials as they structurally similar to the extracellular matrix and tissue. The presence of defined functional groups, for example carboxylic acids, allow for the production of bioactive biomaterials that respond to environmental, chemical and physical stimuli. These so-called 'smart' polymer systems display significant potential as future drug delivery and biomaterial platforms [30–32].

Current research has seen an increased focus on the antimicrobial properties of silver. Hydrogel/silver coated urinary catheters have been investigated and promising results obtained. A reduction in the primary bacterial adherence was observed in comparison to a standard silicone catheter indicating that hydrogel/silver coatings have the potential to delay the onset of catheter associated infections [33]. Synergistic combinations of antibiotic(s) and/or antiseptics are also utilized clinically to reduce the incidence of infection. ARROWgard™ central venous catheters are coated by a combination of silver sulphadiazine and chlorhexidine, whilst the commercially available alternatives BioGuard Spectrum™ and Cook Spectrum® are both coated by a combination of minocycline and rifampicin [34]. Silver sulphadiazine and chlorhexidine coated catheters displayed significant activity against a range of microorganisms including *Candida albicans* and *Escherichia coli* for up to seven days [35]. Minocycline-rifampicin catheters were shown to display only bacteriostatic activity against slime producing forms of *Staphylococcus epidermidis* (ATCC 35984) and *Staphylococcus aureus* (ATCC 29213) but for an extended period of up to 21 days [36]. A range of other anti-infective biomaterials are available commercially, aiming to deliver antimicrobials locally at the device surface for the prevention of biofilm formation. Many challenges exist with this strategy. It is difficult to ensure the dose of antimicrobial delivered is uniform within the vicinity of the device surface. Areas of the implant may be exposed to sub-therapeutic concentrations of antimicrobials [37]. Sub-inhibitory concentrations of antimicrobial agents may lead to increased microbial resistance. Research by Rachid highlighted this effect whereby an increase in *ica* operon expression [38], linked with staphylococcal polysaccharide intercellular adhesin accumulation [39,40], occurred in response to sub-optimal levels of the antibiotic tetracycline and the semi-synthetic molecule quinuprisin- dalfopristin.

One of the major limitations regarding the delivery of antimicrobials in a biomaterial model is the effect of burst-release. Burst-release is consistent with an initial high and rapid release of the antimicrobial from the biomaterial. It is one of the major challenges of modern drug delivery. The antimicrobial reservoir depletes to sub-inhibitory levels within days allowing infection to develop unchallenged. Covalent attachment of antimicrobial, as outlined by the examples of ARROWgard™, BioGuard Spectrum™ and Cook Spectrum®, suffer from a reduction in activity due to masking of antimicrobials by the host's conditioning film [41]. A significant profile of prolonged release over weeks or an infection responsive system is more desirable [42]. A multitude of studies exist in antimicrobial drug delivery to resolve this issue. Examples include sustained release systems such as calcium-mediated delivery of the broad-spectrum antibiotic minocycline, as demonstrated by Zhang and colleagues [29]. The authors utilized layer-by-layer assembly and calcium binding to create a sustained release platform. Delivery of minocycline is due to a local change in pH in the vicinity of the device. Acidosis present in the tissues as a result of medical device induced inflammation or infection, weakens the chelation reaction between minocycline and calcium ions, resulting in subsequent release of minocycline. This so-called 'smart' approach to drug delivery shows promise for future biomedical application.

There has also been increasing interest in using peptides for biomaterial applications [43]. As antimicrobials, peptides serve as barriers to infection throughout nature as part of the innate immune response [44]. There are a multitude of examples whereby antimicrobial peptides have been synthesized to disrupt microbial biofilms [45–47]. Peptides also display a diverse array of properties making them suitable for biomaterial applications including: increased biocompatibility and minimal immunogenicity; the availability of moieties for functionalization; chemical versatility and biodegradability [48]. Peptides have also demonstrated an ability to self-assemble into supramolecular hydrogels in response to environmental stimuli for example pH, the presence of salts, heat and enzymatic cleavage [49,50]. These characteristics may allow such compounds to be utilized to form inherently antimicrobial peptide hydrogel structures in response to infection.

3. Current Approaches to Self-Assembling Biomaterials

The process of self-assembly is an important parameter for the development of novel biomaterials. It is particularly relevant with regards to nanotechnology. These principles have been adopted from nature. Ribosomes and the quaternary haemoglobin structures are examples of naturally occurring self-assembled architectures [51]. Assembly involves the spontaneous arrangement of pre-existing, disordered molecules of similar properties, to form higher ordered structures. It is mediated by non-covalent, local interactions: van der Waals forces, hydrogen bonding, π-π stacking, and electrostatic interactions [52,53]. Movement at a molecular level facilitates assembly. Environmental factors such as volume and binding influence assembly. Equilibrium between the aggregate and non-aggregate states is essential to maintain a higher ordered structure [54,55]. Self-assembly has recently attracted heavy investment from both the private and public sectors. In 2010 global public investment was estimated at approximately $8.2 billion and private sector funding slightly higher at $9.6 billion [56].

Current polymer technologies include the area of Pluronics or poloxamers. Composed of three polymers polyoxyethylene (PEO), polyoxypropylene (PPO) and polyoxyethylene (PEO), Pluronics is an area that has been extensively studied with regard to micellization and the formation of structures for drug delivery purposes. Pluronics have the ability to assemble at physiological temperatures, in a variety of solvents, and over a range of concentrations as opposed to a single critical concentration [57]. There is a great deal of interest within the drug delivery field in exploiting gels that have the ability to flow at ambient temperatures but form a gel upon exposure to physiological temperatures. These gels have great potential in terms of targeted or localized drug delivery of anticancer and antimicrobial drugs in particular [58]. Self-assembling Pluronics are examples of non-ionic and non-toxic gels [59]. F127 is an example of a Pluronic polymer whereby assembly is triggered due to temperature change. Its ability to form micelles at human body temperature means that F127 has potential in the delivery of poorly soluble, hydrophobic drugs [57]. Sustained release of drugs from Pluronics has been widely investigated. Barichello's group used F127 alone and in addition to poly-co-glycolic acid (PLGA) nanoparticles for protein delivery, using insulin as a model drug [60]. They demonstrated F127 incorporated insulin has the potential to provide a controlled release system. The short-acting, opioid analgesic fentanyl has also been delivered using gels formed by PEO-PPO-PEO. Investigations have shown to demonstrate a similar release flux to the commercially available Durogesic® patch [59]. The possibility exists that this type of delivery could be adopted for sustained delivery of antimicrobials to wounds or burns, removing the need for frequent changes of dressings. The antibiofilm activity of Pluronics has been studied due to its non-ionic surfactant-like properties [61]. Wesenberg-Ward and colleagues discovered that Pluronic F127 conditioned polystyrene reduced *Candida albicans* biofilm formation relative to untreated polystyrene controls [62]. Reduction in *Staphylococcus aureus* and *Staphylococcus epidermidis* adherence to polymethylmethacrylate and increased susceptibility to vancomycin and gentamicin was also observed in the presence of poloxamer 407 [63]. These studies highlight the potential use of Pluronics in the biomaterials field to produce surfaces that are resistant to microbial adhesion. Recent research by Leszczyńska outlined the use of Pluronic F127 topical antimicrobial in combination with the synthetic cationic antibacterial peptide Ceragenin CSA-13 [64]. In this instance, Pluronic F127 acted as the drug delivery vehicle with broad spectrum activity demonstrated against methicillin-resistant *Staphylococcus aureus* and a *Pseudomonas aeruginosa* strain isolated from cystic fibrosis patients. Pluronics have also been linked with increased wound-healing in animal models validating continuous research into their applications as effective biomaterials [65].

Related research combines innovative approaches to stimulate antimicrobial release with self-assembled hydrogel polymers. Norris and colleagues synthesized a self-assembled poly(2-hydroxyethyl methacrylate) coating containing ordered methylene chains [66]. This polymer released ciprofloxacin in response to low intensity ultrasound and displayed significantly reduced accumulation of established 24 h *Pseudomonas aeruginosa* biofilm over a three day period. Self-assembled monolayers have been created to modify the surface properties of biomaterials with the aim of reducing bacterial attachment. Recently Kruszewski *et al.* produced stainless steel, commonly employed in orthopaedic implants, modified by a self-assembled monolayer of long alkyl chains terminated with hydrophobic ($-CH_3$) or hydrophilic (oligoethylene glycol) tail groups [67]. These groups facilitated the attachment of gentamicin or vancomycin and reduced *Staphylococcus aureus* biofilm formation for up to 24 and 48 h respectively. Protein deposition by the host conditioning film remains a problem due to masking of covalently attached molecules. Studies exist for self-assembled monolayer materials that display resistance to biofilm formation and host protein adsorption. Self-assembled monolayers of alkanethiols, presenting a tri(ethylene glycol) functional group, displayed a profile of reduced protein adsorption and mammalian cell adhesion and resisted *Escherichia coli* biofilm formation [68]. The authors concluded this may be due to the ability of tri(ethylene glycol) to repel cells and inhibit bacterial cell motility, a key factor in biofilm formation. Silicon coated with a self-assembled micro-gel consisting of poly(ethylene glycol) and poly(ethylene glycol)-*co*-acrylic acid proved resistant to adhesion by *Staphylococcus epidermidis* for up to 10 h [69]. Loading the micro-gel with an antimicrobial peptide (L5) resulted in significant anti-adherent properties at the 10 h time-point due to the localized release and inhibitory action of the L5 peptide. After 10 h, colonization was observed due to depletion of the peptide reservoir.

Such approaches have been significant in advancing biofilm-resistant self-assembled polymer research. Limitations exist affecting translation into clinical practice, namely sufficient antimicrobial action over a sustained period of time. Self-assembled polymers have contributed to a multitude of innovative investigations and applications within biomedical engineering. It is now a widely accepted method of material development. The theory has been expanded to investigate the potential of peptide self-assembly and peptide-based nanomaterials. Self-assembled peptides display great promise as antimicrobial coatings. Alteration of the peptide backbone allows materials to be tailored to their application. The production of an inherently antimicrobial peptide hydrogel, which self-assembles in response to environmental or specific pathogenic stimuli, may allow for significant reduction of biofilm formation over a prolonged period.

Uses for self-assembled peptides range from medical to engineering applications. They have recently come to the fore of bioscience contributing significantly to the nanotech revolution [70]. Work by Zhang in 1993 on ionic self-complementary peptides is regarded as particularly noteworthy in terms of evolving this area [71]. Other experts of note include: Aggeli, who investigated the hierarchical structures of peptides [72]; Tirrell, who patented secondary structure forming peptide amphiphiles [27,73]; and Ghadiri, who was responsible for the development of cyclic nanopeptides [74]. To fully understand the potential of self-assembling peptides in biomaterial applications an appreciation of the chemical composition governing their hierarchical properties is required.

Peptides are ideal building blocks for the formation of nanostructures. Utilizing a "bottom up" approach, individual amino acid residues are used to build higher ordered structures [75]. The twenty naturally occurring amino acids alone allow a huge variety of potential combinations. Their structures and corresponding single letter abbreviation are detailed in Figure 1. An immense range of primary peptide sequences and higher ordered structures can be created for biomedical applications. Variation of the R-group at the alpha (α) carbon provides unique characteristics (hydrophobic, hydrophilic, aliphatic, aromatic, positive or negative charge) to each amino acid. These influence the extent to which the molecules can participate in non-covalent interactions and therefore self-assemble to form defined nanostructures. The hydrophobic: hydrophilic balance and ability of these molecules to hydrogen bond are particularly influential factors [55]. Ulijn and Smith provide detail regarding the effect of various amino acids on the process of assembly [76]. Their review refers to the relationship between an increase in methylene chains on the R-group side chain; the degree of hydrophobicity; and extent of steric hindrance in affecting assembly of monomer units. In particular, the degree of hydrophobicity is key in determining assembly. Peptide assembly is also influenced by the concentration of peptide present. Increasing the number of amino acid repeats results in the formation of higher assemblies. The number of amino acids present also affects the critical concentration of assembly. The critical concentration increases relative to a rise in the number of amino acid residues due to a shift in the entropic-enthalpic balance. For assembly to occur entropic loss must be balanced with an enthalpic gain within the system [77]. Environmental factors such as pH, temperature, light, and the presence of proteolytic enzymes influence assembly. Peptide systems commonly follow those found in nature. The greater the number of hydrophobic residues present, the lower the critical concentration for assembly to occur. Crucially the degree of charge and hydrophilicity must be optimal to ensure efficient assembly. An increase in hydrophobicity above optimal levels may result in precipitation of the peptide molecule in solution. Hydrophilic groups, including those present within the peptide bond (−NHCO), carboxylic acids (−COOH) and amines (−NH$_2$) can also contribute to assembly via hydrogen bond intermolecular interactions with surrounding solvent and neighboring peptide molecules. Charged amino acids, for example lysine, result in charge-charge electrostatic interactions. These have potential to drive or prevent assembly depending on the degree of polarity and charge density. Salt concentration is also a contributing factor, as demonstrated through work on the peptide EAK16-II by Hong and colleagues [78]. A low salt concentration resulted in a desired level of intermolecular interaction, driving assembly. Ionisation, which is strongly linked to pH and pKa, has a large influence on the self-assembly process. The natural amino acid tyrosine allows further functionalization of peptide molecules. Its R-group consists of an amphiphilic phenol grouping which allows, for example, formation of imines under relatively mild conditions (pH ~6.5) [79]. The use of microbial enzymes to facilitate self-assembly of antimicrobial peptides is covered in detail in Section 5.4. The phenol grouping of tyrosine provides an alternative functional group for conjugation of possible microbial enzyme targets, for example phosphate groupings [80].

Figure 1. The structures and single amino acid code for the twenty naturally occurring amino acids. Each amino acid shares a carboxylic acid (−COOH) and a primary amine group (−NH$_2$). The properties of the individual amino acids are governed by the nature and functionality of the R-group attached to the α-carbon. Researchers exploit the differences in individual amino acid units to develop peptide-based therapeutics. Of particular importance to antimicrobial peptides and peptide self-assembly is the hydrophobic: hydrophilic balance of the primary peptide structure.

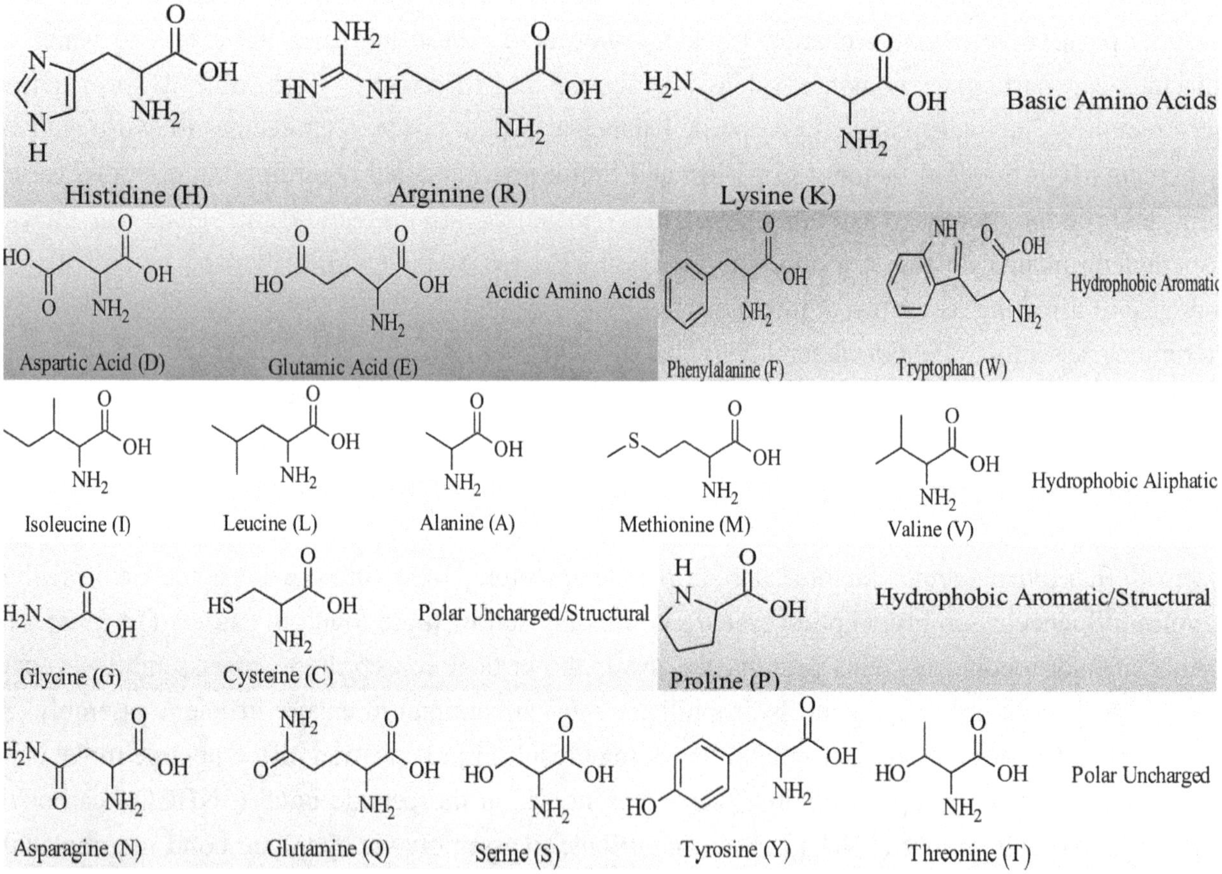

Peptide derivatives as detailed include amphiphiles and π-stacked aromatic peptides. Amphiphiles have a similar structure to membrane phospholipids, possessing a hydrophobic alkyl tail conjugated to a charged moiety. They are ideal molecules for interacting with and disrupting bacterial membranes [81]. Assembly results in a variety of higher structures, mainly rods, which possess a hydrophobic core and a hydrophilic exterior. The process of assembly is modified by altering the charge of the residues involved or by changing the position of the alkyl chain on the alternative termini (amine or carboxylic acid functional groups) [82]. Conjugated amphiphilic peptides with assembling properties for example IKVAV, have been employed in tissue engineering where the assembled nanofibrous network created scaffolds facilitating differentiation of cells into neurons [83].

Reviews such as those by Gazit and Martinez [84,85] provide more detailed information regarding π-stacked peptides. In brief, π-stacked peptides are composed of residues with aromatic groups such as phenylalanine, tryptophan, tyrosine and histidine. Burley and Petsko [86] initially investigated the aforementioned, naturally occurring aromatic amino acids, and their interactions with neighboring aromatic moieties. They highlighted the influence of a residue's environment on the availability of free energy to interact with other residues, and the contribution of this to the resulting structural stability. More recently π-π interactions particularly diphenylalanine interactions, are attracting a great deal of interest. They have a key role in β-amyloid polypeptide/ fibril formation and subsequent formation of fibrous plaques, which are implicated in disease states such as Alzheimer's [87]. π-π stacking may also be attributed to peptides that have a 9-fluorenylmethoxycarbonyl (Fmoc), naphthalene (Nap), or benzyloxycarbonyl (Cbz) group on the amine terminal (Figure 2). π-stacking occurs due to the presence of a conjugated system, allowing the aromatic π electrons within this system to overlap and interact [88]. The restricted geometries within the aromatic systems provide direction to the assembled structure, with interactions between the stacks acting as a glue and contributing to the overall rigidity of such assembled structures [84].

Figure 2. Examples of aromatic moieties utilized to provide π-π electrostatic interactions. The polycyclic aromatic hydrocarbon residues of fluorene (in 9-fluorenylmethoxycarbonyl groups), naphthalene (as in 2-naphthylacetyl) and benzene (as in 2-benzyloxycarbonyl) facilitates π-stacking due to the presence of a conjugated system of delocalized π-electrons. Such intermolecular interactions are enhanced by the presence of hydrophobic aromatic amino acid molecules, for example phenylalanine.

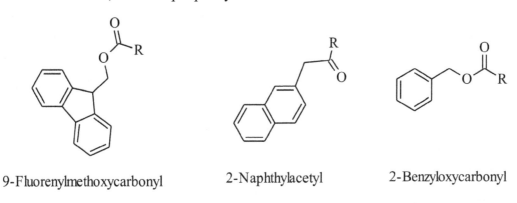

9-Fluorenylmethoxycarbonyl   2-Naphthylacetyl   2-Benzyloxycarbonyl

Although the aim of assembly is to achieve higher-ordered structures, these must be uniform, homogenous and reproducible with defined and useful properties. Peptides provide an ideal basis for such structures for many reasons. They are biocompatible and biodegradable [89]. Their synthesis is relatively uncomplicated [90]. They can assemble (forming gels) *in situ* [71]. Peptide bioactivity, such as antimicrobial potency, can also be modified according to the amino acid residues selected and structure activity relationships can often be determined with high levels of precision. Aromatic groups contribute to π-π intermolecular van der Waal's interactions. Molecules that contain such groups act as hydrogelators by supplying increased hydrophobic bulk to the molecule. Fmoc, naphthalene, and Cbz may facilitate assembly at a reduced peptide length and cost. Naphthalene is preferred due to an established safety profile as it is used in many licensed drug molecules including propranolol. The cytotoxicity of naphthalene-based peptides was previously investigated by Yang and co-workers [89]. They determined a cell survival of almost 100% when HeLa cells were exposed to 200 micromolar of naphthalene dipeptides. Supramolecular properties of these structures including electrical, mechanical and bioactivity are also determined by the process and kinetics of self-assembly. Therefore the nature of the route and rate of assembly must also be carefully considered when designing self-assembling peptide systems.

4. Antimicrobial Peptides

The chemical, physical and structural properties that govern peptide self-assembly are closely associated with factors that determine the antimicrobial potency and spectrum of activity of antimicrobial peptides. Antimicrobial peptides occur throughout nature and are involved in the innate immune response. This response is mounted a short time following exposure to an infective agent and stimulation of cells known as Toll-like receptors [91]. Unlike conventional antimicrobials, most naturally occurring antimicrobial peptides act synergistically in great numbers and at micromolar concentrations. The combined effect of this is a relatively potent antimicrobial response due to action at multiple sites, in comparison to a single target as is the case with most conventional antibiotics [92].

The amphiphilicity of antimicrobial peptides allows them to target microbial cell membranes, particularly those of bacterial cells. Bacterial membranes possess an overall negative charge, compared with neutrally charged eukaryotic membranes, due to the presence of acidic hydroxylated phospholipids. These include cardiolipin, phosphatidylglycerol and phosphatidylserine [93]. The presence of phosphate groups on membrane-bound lipopolysaccharides in Gram-negative bacteria and acidic polymers, such as teichoic acids, in Gram-positive bacteria, allow areas of dense anionic charge to develop on bacterial membranes [44]. Cationic peptides target these areas to exert their effect. Antimicrobial peptides act directly on the cell membrane by disrupting the integrity or function of the phospholipid bilayer via four recognized mechanisms: the aggregate, toroidal pore, barrel-stave and carpet models [94]. Bacterial membranes are an excellent antimicrobial target as bacteria would be required to alter the overall properties of their membrane to confer resistance characteristics, rather than modifying individual receptors. The likelihood for bacteria developing resistance is significantly decreased as antimicrobial peptides also possess intracellular targets. Peptides have been proven to inhibit ATP-dependent enzymes and disrupt processes within the cell, for example RNA and protein synthesis, DNA replication and protein folding [95–99].

Cationic peptides are the most studied form of antimicrobial peptides. Possessing a net positive charge, they are most commonly composed of 12–50 amino acids, approximately 50% of which are hydrophobic [100]. Cationic antimicrobial peptides were first derived from insect haemolymph in the 1970s. They are amphiphilic in nature enabling them to interact with the dense phospholipid exterior of bacterial cell membranes [95]. Cationic peptides have been referred to as 'nature's antibiotics,' however the term "defence proteins" may be more appropriate due to their role in modulating the innate immune response [101]. Anionic peptides are also found throughout nature and have a role in providing innate immunity in a variety of animals and plants. Typically, composed of 7–50 residues, they are also amphiphilic in nature but have an overall net negative charge due to the presence of aspartic acid residues [102,103]. Anionic peptides often require cationic co-factors, for example zinc ions, to produce an antimicrobial effect. Brogden hypothesized zinc ions may form a cationic salt bridge between anionic antimicrobial peptides and the anionic microbial cell surface [104]. These interactions facilitate movement of such peptides across the bacterial membrane, into the cell cytoplasm, allowing intracellular attack. Epithelial cells are prime locations for host defense anionic peptides, not only are they key sites for ion exchange but they are also commonly exposed to pathogenic microbes [105].

Antimicrobial activity and self-assembly of peptides are influenced by similar factors namely: charge, bulk and lipophilicity. Strøm and co-workers investigated the contribution of these factors to antimicrobial activity [106]. Their findings showed that an optimal balance exists between degree of hydrophobicity or bulk and charge governing antimicrobial potency and spectrum of activity. Modification of the peptide sequence with unnatural molecules possessing amino and/or carboxylic acid groups may be of benefit in increasing the cost-effectiveness and activity of the peptide. For example, the addition of cinnamic acid has been shown to increase antimicrobial activity by providing hydrophobic bulk to the primary peptide sequence, at a reduced cost compared with commercially available hydrophobic amino acids [107]. Hydrophobicity and antimicrobial activity can be optimized sequentially via the addition of fatty acids to the peptide motif, creating the promising antimicrobial lipopeptides [45,108]. The type and nature of amino acids employed to generate peptide motifs are also important. Utilizing unnatural amino acids, for example ornithine, may provide the peptide with stability against proteases which are unable to be recognized at a molecular level for incorporation into enzyme active sites [107]. Most amino acids in nature are present as the L-stereoisomer form. Stereoisomerism is based on the ability of molecules to rotate plane-polarized light. L-amino acids are easily recognized by host and bacterial enzymes. They are ideal substrates for proteolysis by peptide specific enzymes termed proteases. In theory this limitation can be reduced, to increase both therapeutic efficacy and retention within the host, by replacement with D-amino acids. Amino acids that are in the D-enantiomeric form do not fit in the active site of proteases and therefore cannot be broken down. D-amino acids do have limitations. They are typically expensive, and for short peptides the realistic enzyme stability they offer is debatable [109].

Lipopeptides are a form of antimicrobial peptides present in nature among bacteria and provide selective advantage against competing microbial strains. Their success is reflected in the pharmaceutical industry, with antimicrobial lipopeptides already successfully utilized clinically. These include anionic daptomycin [110], which forms micelles in the presence of calcium ions facilitating membrane interaction, and cationic polymyxins which interact with membrane-bound lipopolysaccharides inserting into bacterial membranes causing membrane disruption [111]. Cost and toxicity has rendered their use restricted to mainly topical application and second or even third line treatments for pathogens resistant to other antimicrobials. A research paper by Levine presented the findings of patients registered on the Cubicin® Outcomes Registry and Experience (CORE) 2004 database. This covered patients administered with the injectable form of daptomycin (brand name: Cubicin®) for the treatment of infective endocarditis [112]. Of those treated, 83% of *Staphylococcus aureus* infections were methicillin resistant, and 43% enterococci infections were vancomycin resistant. The findings showed that daptomycin has a potential role in treating these types of infections, with 63% of treatments proving successful overall. Similarly a review by Li highlights in great detail the effective role of polymyxin E (colistin) via inhalation and intravenous administration to treat multi-resistant pseudomonal infections in cystic fibrosis patients [113]. There is a clinical need to improve toxicity, bioavailability, and selectivity profiles. Activity is influenced by the amino acid chain and hydrophobicity, with the length of the conjugated fatty acid chain an influential factor [91].

Research is increasingly focused on the action of antimicrobial peptides against resistant biofilm phenotypes [114]. Evidence shows that peptides interact with polysaccharide components of the biofilm causing break down within the polymeric matrix [115]. Peptides also act synergistically with standardly employed antimicrobials, eradicating the biofilm and membrane barriers, allowing clinically employed antibiotics access to intracellular targets. The antimicrobial peptides magainin-II (amphibian-derived) and cecropin-A (insect-derived) were proven by Cirioni *et al.* to act synergistically with rifampicin against multi-drug resistant *Pseudomonas aeruginosa* in both *in vivo* and *in vitro* models [116]. The lipopeptide polymyxin E demonstrated synergistic efficacy with ticarcillin/clavulanate against *Stenotrophomonas maltophilia* isolated from cystic fibrosis patients [117]. Infectious diseases and their causative pathogens continue to display a profile of increased resistance to standardly employed antimicrobials. A recent investigation in a Spanish hospital urology department showed that approximately 52% of isolated *Escherichia coli* and 36% *Pseudomonas aeruginosa* displayed resistance to fluoroquinolones [118]. There is a pressing need not only to develop new antimicrobials but also to refine the properties of these potentially novel chemotherapeutics so that stability, size, immunogenicity, and cost-effectiveness can be improved [119]. The area of antimicrobial peptides hold much promise in the development of antimicrobial therapeutics and their potential is covered in more detail in reviews by Bahar [47] and our own research group [44].

Ultrashort refers to peptides up to 7 amino acids in length. They have become increasingly attractive in the development of peptide therapeutics due to reduction in associated cost and ease of synthesis. Amino acids are rationally selected in line with a minimum pharmacophore required to permit antimicrobial activity [120]. Residues are selected to achieve an optimal lipophilic-charge balance. Typically, more active short peptides are the result of greater lipophilic bulk provided by non-proteinogenic groups. Strøm and co-workers investigated the effect of ultrashort antimicrobial peptides on a variety of nosocomial bacteria including methicillin resistant and sensitive Staphylococcus aureus, methicillin resistant Staphylococcus epidermidis and Escherichia coli and defined the minimum motif required for activity [106]. They hypothesized that activity in staphylococci required a combination of no more than two units of hydrophobic bulk and two units of charge. The Gram-negative rod required three units of bulk and at least two charged species for antibacterial activity to be observed. Such specificity allows ultrashort antimicrobial peptide therapy to be potentially tailored to causative microorganisms in infectious diseases. Harnessing this theory allowed the development of ultrashort lipopeptide variants. Peptides composed of four amino acids and a general sequence of KXXK (K = lysine, X = one of leucine, alanine, glycine, lysine or glutamic acid) were characterized for activity by the Shai group [108]. Aliphatic chains of various lengths were conjugated to these molecules. The resulting ultrashort lipopeptides were tested against a variety of bacteria, fungi, and yeast: Escherichia coli, Pseudomonas aeruginosa, Staphylococcus aureus, gentamicin-resistant Acinetobacter baumannii, Aspergillus fumigatus, Aspergillus flavus, and Candida albicans. This study resulted in three key findings. (1) The aliphatic side chain compensated for a reduced peptide chain length and contributed to hydrophobicity of the structure and resulting antimicrobial properties; (2) Substrate specificity is linked to the amino acid sequence or aliphatic chain length; (3) Many conventional antimicrobial peptides display activity against specific microbes. Some of the lipopeptides tested displayed activity against fungi as well as bacteria. Our own group used these finding together with the work of Bisht *et al.* to produce a series of ultrashort cationic lipopeptides [107]. Based on an ornithine-ornithine-tryptophan-tryptophan tetrapeptide amide motif, our group sequentially increased the lipophilic tail via conjugation of fatty acids to the ornithine terminus. C_{12}-ornithine-ornithine-tryptophan-tryptophan displayed the most potent activity particularly against Gram-positive bacteria with complete eradication obtained within 24 h exposure against mature biofilms of Staphylococcus epidermidis (ATCC 35984) at concentrations as low as 15 µg/mL [45]. The group demonstrated it was possible to incorporate the peptide and the amphibian peptide maximin-4 into a poly(2-hydroxyethyl methacrylate) hydrogel in order to prevent short-term (24 h) Staphylococcus epidermidis biofilm adherence [46].

An alternative approach is to tag the end of the peptide residues with hydrophobic, bulky aromatics such as phenylalanine and tryptophan. Work on this area has involved ultrashort peptides composed of 4–7 amino acid residues. As with lipopeptides, these compounds are amphiphilic in nature and readily interact with target cell membranes. Of the tagged peptides investigated by Pasupuleti and colleagues [121], the most potent molecule, KNK10-WWWWW, displayed similar antimicrobial activity to human cathelicidin LL-37. Findings were similar for the phenylalanine-tagged peptides. Tagging also gave increased protection against proteolysis, providing an advantage for such compounds over the enzymatically degradable LL-37. This protection may be attributed to steric hindrance resulting from the bulky nature of the tags employed, preventing incorporation of the peptide into the protease active site.

Oligo-acyl-lysines (OAKs) are peptidomimetic molecules that mimic the primary structure and function of naturally occurring peptides. They are composed of acyl-lysines, with the acyl chain length determining hydrophobicity of the molecule and lysine conferring cationic charge for targeting of bacterial membranes or inhibition of cellular processes linked to intracellular DNA [122]. They can be linked to an inert resin to enhance the ability of OAKs to bind and capture bacteria for pathogen detection. A study conducted by Rotem and colleagues demonstrated that resin-bound OAKs have the potential to capture both Gram-positive and Gram-negative bacteria under continuous flow and stationary settings [123]. These molecules may be useful in terms of filtration of contaminated samples including drinking water in a hospital or community setting. Antimicrobial activity of OAKs has also been investigated *in vivo* highlighting their clinical potential. Livne demonstrated OAKs incorporating synergistic erythromycin had improved survival rates in neutropenic mice infected with multi-drug resistant *Escherichia coli* compared to erythromycin or OAK monotherapy [124]. Sarig determined the optimal lipid mixtures in the preparation of OAK-erythromycin cochleates, utilized for drug delivery [125]. Housing OAK molecules in a cochleate drug-delivery vehicle produced molecules with enhanced *in vivo* erythromycin efficacy. Cochleates are a drug delivery vehicle consisting of liposome-like molecules formed by a lipid-based supramolecular assembly of natural products (phosphatidylserine), negatively charged phospholipid and a divalent cation (calcium). The work of Sarig underlines the importance of the drug delivery vehicle in ensuring promising *in vitro* results for antimicrobial peptide-like molecules are translated efficiently to clinical practice. This is the greatest challenge in drug development and is particularly difficult with regard to peptides and proteins which suffer from poor solubility, pharmacokinetic properties, stability and antigenicity issues [126]. Hence antimicrobial peptides are often limited to topical use. The short peptides structures outlined possess many pharmaceutical advantages compared with larger peptide/protein molecules as their macromolecular structure allows for decreased recognition by proteases and antigens, with potential extension of their pharmacokinetic profile [127].

5. Self-Assembled Antimicrobial Peptides

The development of peptides that self-assemble upon exposure to environmental stimuli is of increasing interest in biomedicine. The ability to modify a peptide to assemble on cue provides the peptide with a range of desirable properties and potential applications including targeted drug delivery in the area of antimicrobials. For biomaterials, preventing the formation of a highly resistant biofilm phenotype is pivotal in preventing infection throughout the life of the material [128]. Harnessing environmental changes is a significant strategy to deliver activity when most required. Potential triggers for the formation of an inherently antimicrobial self-assembling hydrogel include: pH and ionic strength [50], temperature [129], light [130] and microbial enzymes [131].

5.1. Self-Assembly via Changes in pH and Ionic Strength

pH and ionic strength are the most commonly utilized methods to achieve assembly and disassembly of peptides on cue. Charge interactions are crucial to the assembly process and are influenced by the pKa of the peptide, the amino acid backbone and substituent functional groups. The effect of salt on pH-triggered assembly is also an important factor in determining the degree of ionic interactions [78]. The Schneider group is responsible for a large body of research in this area. They developed a synthetic peptide MAX-1, which adopted a beta(β)-hairpin structure due to the presence of a central V^{D}PPT peptide motif (V = D-enantiomer of valine, ^{D}P = D-enantiomer of proline, T = threonine) [132]. Lysine and valine amino acid residues flank the type-II β-turn structure in alternating sequences. Basic pH, above the pKa of lysine's primary amine R-group (pH > 9) resulted in self-assembly as intramolecular folding resulted in a hydrophobic valine core surrounded by a hydrophilic lysine surface. Lowering the pH, below the pKa of lysine favored charge repulsion and disassembly. Addition of buffered saline (150 millimolar sodium chloride) or Dulbecco's Modified Eagle's Medium (165 millimolar sodium chloride) to 2% w/v of MAX-1 in water at pH 7.4 directed the formation of a biocompatible hydrogel. Formation of a hydrogel was due to screening of positive charged lysine moieties by chloride ions and alteration of the hydrophobic: charge balance allowing a decrease in solubility, therefore promoting assembly [133].

Replacing lysine with aspartic acid at amino acid position 15 (MAX-8) lowered the overall charge of the molecule by +2 and was sufficient to decrease gelation time from 30 min (for MAX-1) to 1 min [134]. Encapsulation of antimicrobial drugs and/or cells into this matrix could conceivably allow the targeted delivery of a hydrogel dressing for wound application via a syringe. This is especially true as MAX-1 was proven to display inherent antimicrobial properties against a broad spectrum of Gram-positive (*Staphylococcus epidermidis*, *Staphylococcus aureus* and *Streptococcus pyogenes*) and Gram-negative (*Klebsiella pneumoniae* and *Escherichia coli*) bacteria [132]. The results obtained highlight the role of the polycationic lysine surface in compromising negatively charged bacterial membranes resulting in bacterial cell death (Figure 3). The Schneider group altered the MAX1 template further to produce second generation cationic self-assembled antimicrobial hydrogels containing both cationic arginine and lysine residues [132]. MARG1, consisting of two arginine residues, was highly potent against methicillin resistant *Staphylococcus aureus*. A second peptide molecule, PEP6R, consisting of six arginines within its peptide primary structure, demonstrated broad spectrum activity against *Staphylococcus aureus*, *Escherichia coli* and multi-drug resistant *Pseudomonas aeruginosa*. Both were able to form hydrogels at physiological pH.

Figure 3. The antibacterial mechanism of action of self-assembling β-sheet cationic peptides using the example of MAX1 peptide developed by the Schneider group [132]. Basic pH, above the pKa of lysine's primary amine R-group (pH > 9), results in self-assembly of the primary peptide motif into a β-sheet secondary structure. The central V^{D}PPT peptide forms a type II β-turn resulting in the formation of a hydrophobic valine core (blue) and a hydrophilic cationic lysine face (red). The primary amine (−NH$_2$) R-groups of lysine protrude from the β-sheet structure forming a surface of polycationic character that is selective for negatively charged bacterial membranes. Adhesion and biofilm formation is prevented as bacterial membranes are compromised resulting in leakage of cell contents and bacterial cell death. In the hydrogel form the cationic groups may also displace divalent metal ions from the bacterial cell wall causing membrane disruption in biofilm cells, leading to cell death in both Gram-positive and –negative pathogens.

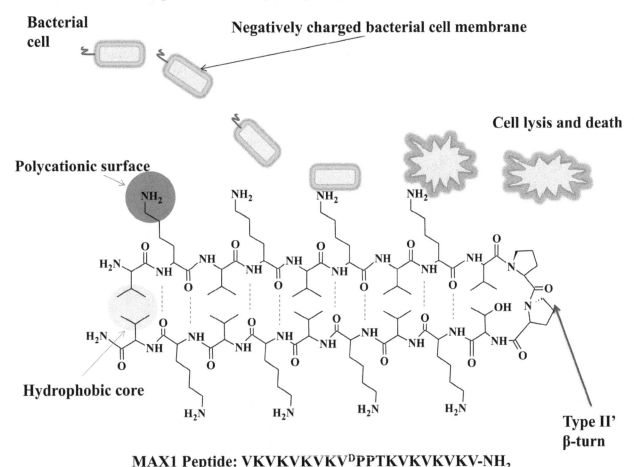

MAX1 Peptide: VKVKVKVKV^{D}PPTKVKVKVKV-NH$_2$

A related arginine rich peptide PEP8R (containing 8 arginine residues) was also created [135]. Variations of PEP8R were prepared, with arginine residues replaced by lysines to determine the optimal number of arginines required to achieve an antimicrobial effect. Decreasing the number of arginine residues formed PEP6R, a peptide that formed more rigid gels. The variants at all percentages tested were active against *Escherichia coli* and *Staphylococcus aureus*. Gels containing only two arginine residues demonstrated limited activity against Gram-negative *Escherichia coli*. Peptide derivatives were more active against Gram-positive bacteria. The presence of divalent ions such as calcium (Ca^{2+}) reduced the peptides antimicrobial activity. The group concluded that in order to achieve optimal antimicrobial activity a minimum of four arginine residues were required.

Recent research by Liu and colleagues demonstrated the rational design of a pH dependent self-assembled antimicrobial peptide (ASCP1) consisting of two peripheral $(KIGAKI)_3$-NH_2 species conjugated to a central tetrapeptide linker (T^DPPG) [50]. Similarly to the MAX peptides, the central motif allowed for the formation of a predominantly β-sheet structure with a central β-hairpin at pH greater than 10. The presence of twelve lysine primary amine side chains created sufficient electrostatic repulsion to prevent self-assembly. Elimination of these net charges via an increase in pH or addition of greater than 40 millimolar sodium chloride permits self-assembly. ASCP1 displayed inherent antibacterial properties against cultures of *Escherichia coli* after 36 h incubation. High bacterial loads (greater than 10^7 colony forming units per mL) resulted in loss of inhibitory capacity. Again membrane disruption due to the presence of polycationic lysine residues was the most plausible mechanism for antibacterial activity.

RADA16 is one of the most comprehensively studied self-assembled peptides due to its ability to self-assemble at physiological pH [136]. Marketed commercially as PuraMatrix™ it has the ability to support cell growth and attachment leading to research into its use as a nanofiber scaffold to support wound healing. It has been hypothesized that functionalisation with antimicrobials and wound healing stimulants, such as epidermal growth factor, provide wound protection while encouraging wound closure [137]. Debnath and co-workers developed antimicrobial peptide amphiphiles which self-assemble at physiological pH [138]. These Fmoc pyridinium functionalised peptides were tested against a variety of Gram-positive (*Bacillus subtilis* and *Staphylococcus aureus*) and Gram-negative (*Escherichia coli* and *Pseudomonas aeruginosa*) bacteria, with minimum inhibitory concentrations determined. Compounds with the most broad-spectrum antimicrobial effect had hydrophobic phenylalanine closely attached to the Fmoc moiety. The close proximity of fluorenyl and phenyl moieties allowed an optimum hydrophobicity, described by the authors as the "threshold hydrophobicity", to be obtained thus allowing significant activity against bacteria via membrane attack.

pH triggered self-assembly has potential to be utilized in antimicrobial therapies. Urinary catheter associated infections are synonymous with an increase in alkaline conditions due to the presence of the enzyme urease synthesized by Gram-negative *Proteus mirabilis*. Urease catalyses the breakdown of urea to ammonia via hydrolysis leading to increased pH at the urine-catheter interface and the precipitation of mineral salts such as calcium phosphate (hydroxyapatite) and magnesium ammonium phosphate (struvite). A combination of encrustation and biofilm formation leads to blockage of the catheter, with removal of the device necessary to resolve infection [139]. We hypothesize a role whereby an antimicrobial peptide may self-assemble at the device surface in response to an increase in pH (or the presence of urease) forming a protective barrier, reducing biofilm formation and encrustation thus preventing the need for catheter removal. This strategy would require the peptide molecule to be attached to the catheter surface, physicochemically stable at pH 7.4 and active against a broad spectrum of urinary pathogens, especially biofilm forms of *Proteus mirabilis.*

5.2. Photo-Activated Self-Assembly

Light may be used as an environmental trigger for the formation of hydrogels. These are typically formed when a water-soluble polymer and photo-initiator are exposed to a specific wavelength of light and crosslinking occurs. The resulting hydrogels display temporal and spatial resolution. Macromolecules are the preferred starting material and these are chosen to achieve the desired crosslinking and mechanical properties for the final hydrogel. The photo-initiator must be sufficiently reactive yet cytocompatible. Exposure to ultraviolet light triggers arrangement of a peptide into β-hairpins and subsequent self-assembly to a hydrogel occurs provided that the side chains permit this. Cysteine is hydrophobic in nature and easily functionalized. Therefore it is a useful side chain component for facilitating assembly. An example of this type of assembly is the 20-residue MAX7CNB peptide [130]. This caged (α- carboxy-2 nitrobenzyl) peptide is unfolded in ambient conditions but exposure to UV light triggers decaging and peptide folding to form a supramolecular hydrogel. There is no specific investigation in the literature for a peptide that induces self-assembly and antimicrobial activity in response to light. The use of light to stimulate antimicrobial delivery has been evaluated previously and therefore may serve as a valid mechanism for future research. McCoy and colleagues, developed an antimicrobial biomaterial containing tetracationic porphyrin, (tetrakis(4-N-methylpyridyl)porphyrin), which binds electrostatically with methacrylate groups of a methacrylic acid or a methyl methacrylate copolymer [140]. Visible light allowed the porphyrin to catalytically generate short-lived singlet oxygen at the device surface, with antimicrobial activity displayed against *Staphylococcus aureus* and *Pseudomonas aeruginosa*.

5.3. Thermo-Responsive Self-Assembly

Temperature can be used as a trigger to form higher assemblies (hydrogel structures) either through cooling or heating of molecules. The degree of hydrophobicity governs the temperature at which folding occurs. Typically, assembly of more hydrophobic molecules takes place at a lower temperature [141]. Schneider and colleagues modified their MAX-1 peptide, which forms a hydrogel at 25 °C and pH 9, by the replacement of two valine residues (at amino acid positions 7 and 16) with threonine [141]. This resulted in a peptide that formed hydrogel structures at higher temperatures (~60 °C). A replacement at position 16 only resulted in a gelation temperature of 40 °C, only slightly above that of normal body temperature, suggesting possible use as a thermo-responsive hydrogel in drug delivery. Liu's ASCP1 peptide displayed similar self-supporting hydrogel structures at higher temperatures (~60 °C) [50]. Temperature change alters the solubility of the hydrophobic amino acid residues in these peptides, thus altering the hydrophobic: hydrophilic balance to favor decreased solubility. The process is thermally-reversible. Temperature-responsive gelation is not only limited to large peptide structures. Tang discovered replacing the terminal phenylalanine residue in Fmoc–FF with glycine (forming FmocFG) created a peptide that also gelled at increased temperatures [142]. Rheological analysis below its *pKa* demonstrated self-assembly had occurred at 25 °C but only sufficient to produce a viscous solution. Gelation occurred between 55 and 80 °C which the authors attributed to dissolution of precipitate, formed due to a low pH, allowing homogenous hydrogels to be formed in solution. Further work by Tang studied glycine and leucine substituted Fmoc dipeptides [143]. In addition, employing pH and temperature to facilitate the formation of Fmoc hydrogels, FmocFG and FmocLG gelation proved also to be temperature-dependent. Both FmocFG and FmocLG hydrogels formed upon heating to 80 °C. Mechanical properties were retained upon subsequent cooling of heated peptides to 25 °C and 4 °C. FmocLG appeared to gel at 25 °C, with further heating and cooling of this gel to 4 °C forming stiffer hydrogel structures. This confirmed that a heating step was shown to improve the homogeneity of the samples without altering the topography of the self-assembled structures. Therefore, hydrophobicity of the peptide molecule, pH and homogeneity in aqueous solutions have to be taken into account in the design of a temperature triggered antimicrobial self-assembly peptide structure.

5.4. Bacterial Enzymatic Self-Assembly

Enzyme mediated self-assembly occurs as a result of catalysis or removal of a blocking group within the peptide primary sequence. It occurs under standard physiological conditions (pH and temperature) [144]. Enzymes such as proteases [145], phosphatases [49] and esterases [146], serve as viable molecules to drive peptide self-assembly. Catalysis occurs due to a thermodynamic shift resulting from condensation or hydrolysis of the peptide bond. In some cases both of these processes may occur in order to form peptide structures that are more stable. Research by Toledano demonstrated environmentally dependent protease triggered reverse hydrolysis of Fmoc amino acids [147]. Enzymes are selected, and the concentrations modified, in order to achieve optimum assembly under a defined set of conditions [148]. Enzymatic approaches to self-assembly are becoming more popular in research due to the abundance of bacterial enzymes, allowing tailored specificity for selected pathogens.

As outlined previously (Section 3), selection of specific amino acid residues and their corresponding properties is crucial in developing ultrashort peptides. Investigations into self-assembling ultrashort antimicrobial peptides are relatively novel but are increasing in the literature, especially in the area of enzyme triggered self-assembly. Removal or addition of one or two amino acid units has a larger influence on the overall properties of short peptide structures, including its solubility and therefore ability to self-assemble. One of the first examples of such research was conducted by the Xu group [49]. They were able to demonstrate that a strain of *Escherichia coli*, that overexpressed a phosphatase enzyme, was able to be selectively inhibited by a short naphthalene containing peptide. Dephosphorylation of soluble phosphorylated NapFFY(p), Nap^{D}F^{D}FY(p) and Nap-β^3-HPhg-β^3-HPhgY(p) (β^3-HPhg: a β-amino acid named β^3-homophenylglycine, p: phosphorylated) occurred in the cell cytoplasm causing inhibition of multiple intracellular processes resulting in a reduction in bacterial viability. Further work by the Xu group demonstrated how peptide self-assembly can be governed by a tyrosine-linked kinase/phosphatase switch [80]. Phosphorylation (via kinase) and dephosphorylation (via phosphatase) of the hydrogelator at the tyrosine terminus regulated the formation of supramolecular hydrogels. Gelation occurred *in vivo* in the presence of phosphatase enzyme, as removal of hydrophilic phosphate groupings increased the hydrophobicity of the molecule, driving self-assembly. The presence of phosphatases have been attributed to medical device related pathogens such as *Escherichia coli*, where alkaline phosphatase is present in the periplasmic space and therefore serves as a valid microbial target [149,150]. The Xu group [151] also produced a NapFF precursor conjugated to a β-lactam ring, capable of hydrogelation in response to the addition of β-lactamase enzymes from cell lysates of *Escherichia coli*. This mechanism has potential to be exploited for the detection of extended spectrum β-lactamases in a clinical setting and allowing screening of potential inhibitors.

Enzymatic assembly of ultrashort peptides, utilizing alkaline phosphatase, has been conducted more recently by the Ulijn group [131]. The Fmoc dipeptides (FY, YT, YS, YN and YQ in a FmocYpX-OH motif, where X = any amino acid) were central to the study, with tyrosine providing the hydroxyl grouping for phosphorylation. Phosphorous nuclear magnetic resonance (^{31}P NMR) allowed determination of the rate of dephosphorylation and inhibition within defined areas of the bacterial cell and enabled the location of formed fibers to be identified. Treatment with alkaline phosphatase facilitates protonation of phosphate groups and the formation of higher assemblies. Peptide hydrogels formed over 24 h. Assembly was evident at a molecular level and there was evidence of β sheets, hydrogen bonding and π-stacking. Ability to assemble *in vivo* was investigated using media with and without the nucleoside inosine, which increases alkaline phosphatase synthesis two-fold. Bacterial cells were treated with a FmocFYp-OH precursor and HPLC analysis showed that the peptide moved into the hydrophobic environment of the bacterial cells. This demonstrated that assembly could occur *in vivo*. Treatment of *Escherichia coli* cells with other precursors showed similar results (self-assembly) however the effect of hydrophobicity on assembly and the resulting location of the formed peptides varied. More hydrophilic peptides were more likely to partition into the surrounding media rather than remaining within the hydrophobic environment of the bacterial cell. The findings indicated that formation of the peptides followed by movement out of the bacterial cells was sufficient to significantly reduce the number of viable bacterial cells. Therefore retention of the formed nanostructure within the cells was not essential to exert an antimicrobial effect. The intracellular and extracellular modes of action of these peptides reduce the ability of bacteria to develop resistance and bode well for their future development as therapeutics. The Ulijn group also employed the esterase subtilisin, obtained from the soil derived bacterium *Bacillus licheniformis*, as a mediator for assembly of Fmoc dipeptide methyl esters proving the versatility of the enzymatic approach to allow self-assembly [146].

6. Future Perspectives and Translation of Peptide Self-Assembly to Antimicrobial Therapeutics

Challenges exist to the use of peptides as antimicrobial therapeutics. There is currently only one licensed self-assembled peptide therapeutic; the injectable β-sheet forming octapeptide lanreotide administered for the relief of neuroendocrine symptoms [152]. The licensing of lanreotide by the Food and Drug administration in 2007 provides great hope that similar molecules can be translated into therapeutics. In antimicrobial drug delivery there is increasing research into the utilization of self-assembled peptides as practical therapeutics. It is becoming increasingly relevant in the innovative production of antimicrobials and their delivery platforms. Peptide self-assembly has been utilized in combination with standardly employed antibiotics. Marchesan *et al.*, produced a macroscopic tripeptide hydrogel (^{D}LFF) at physiological pH which incorporated the sparingly soluble antibiotic ciprofloxacin [153]. The hydrophobic tripeptide acted as a suitable drug delivery vehicle for the release of ciprofloxacin *in vitro*. Mild antibiofilm activity was demonstrated for the tripeptide alone against *Staphylococcus aureus*, *Escherichia coli*, and *Klebsiella pneumoniae*, with significant reduction in viability obtained via inclusion of 30% w/w ciprofloxacin.

Paladini and co-workers investigated the antimicrobial effects of silver incorporated into ultrashort Fmoc diphenylalanine (FmocFF) hydrogels on *Staphylococcus aureus*. [154]. Hydrogels (as detailed in Section 2) are commonly used in wound management and can be impregnated with antimicrobial agents, including silver. The nature of the hydrogels themselves creates a hydrated environment and protects the wound, creating an ideal environment for wound healing. Self-assembling peptide hydrogels such as those formed from assembly of FmocFF create a similar environment, making them ideal candidates for wound dressings. Paladini's 'silver-doped' FmocFF hydrogels are composed of varying concentrations of silver nitrate (0.01%, 0.1%, 2% weight). The hydrogels produced were used to coat flax textiles and exposed to *Staphylococcus aureus* overnight. The work demonstrated the ability of FmocFF to disassemble and reassemble when added to the flax substrates. Scanning electron microscopy suggested that the higher the concentration of silver present, the more uniform the nature of the flax coverage. Precipitates formed with the 2% w/v gels thus homogeneity was not achieved. Antimicrobial studies demonstrated a reduction in bacterial numbers with an increased silver concentration. Bacterial adhesion and biofilm formation was also investigated. Incorporation of silver was necessary to prevent biofilm formation and the minimum concentration of silver needed to achieve this effect was 0.1% weight.

The amphipathic peptide, FmocFFECG, contains both hydrophobic and hydrophilic moieties. The presence of carboxylic acid functionalities allowed adsorption of silver nanoparticles into the peptide motif [155]. Activity was proven against Gram-positive *Bacillus subtilis* and Gram-negative *Escherichia coli* for up to 30 days. Stability was also increased compared with silver nanoparticles alone suggesting the peptide hydrogel protects silver nanoparticles from oxidation. The hydrophobic character of ultrashort self-assembling peptides may also allow the incorporation of other highly lipophilic antimicrobial drugs.

Peptides also provide access to infections in the brain. Research by Liu demonstrated how the peptide CG_3R_6TAT (C = hydrophobic cholesterol, G = glycine spacers, R = cationic arginine residues, TAT = minimal amino acid sequence required for membrane translocation) assembles to form micelles with a hydrophobic cholesterol core and hydrophilic peptide exterior [156]. This peptide displays antimicrobial activity against a range of Gram-positive and Gram–negative bacteria. Ability to cross the blood brain barrier and exert an antimicrobial effect was also demonstrated *in vivo* in an infected *Staphylococcus aureus* induced meningitis rabbit model. This work highlights the ability of assembled peptides as tailored molecules to achieve targeted antimicrobial effects in challenging areas of drug delivery.

Key problems associated with peptide design namely, high manufacturing costs and susceptibility to enzymatic degradation, mean there is still a need to develop compounds that have similar properties to conventional antimicrobial peptides in physiological conditions namely: cationic charge, hydrophobicity and amphiphilic nature to enable antimicrobial action and self-assembly. Peptidomimetics and other synthetic oligomers are thus coming to the forefront of current and future research plans. The design of ultrashort peptides has the potential to create functional peptide molecules with a relatively reasonable manufacturing cost. Our own group has moved research forward in this area with the synthesis of a variety of ultrashort and more cost-effective cationic naphthalene containing peptide hydrogels, which are highly active against biofilm forms of biomaterial related pathogens [157]. The very nature of peptides and their proven activity against pathogenic biofilms renders them useful compounds for prevention and management of nosocomial infections and wound healing. Further development of peptidomimetics will provide novel biomaterial platforms and the development of new molecules with tunable chemical and mechanical properties.

Acknowledgments

The authors acknowledge funding provided by the Queen's University Research Support Package for New Academic Staff for GL and a DEL studentship grant for APM.

References

1. Bryers, J.D. Medical biofilms. *Biotechnol. Bioeng.* **2008**, *100*, 1–18.
2. Ratner, B.D.; Hoffman, A.S.; Schoen, F.J.; Lemons, J.E. Introduction-Biomaterials Science: An Evolving, Multidisciplinary Endeavor. In *Biomaterials Science*; Ratner, B.D., Hoffman, A.S., Schoen, F.J., Lemons, J.E., Eds.; Academic Press Elsevier Inc.: Waltham, MA, USA, 2013; pp. 1–20.
3. Kojic, E.M.; Darouiche, R.O. *Candida* infections of medical devices. *Clin. Microbiol. Rev.* **2004**, *17*, 255–267.
4. Grainger, D.W.; van der Mei, H.C.; Jutte, P.C.; van den Dungen, J.J.; Schultz, M.J.; van der Laan, B.F.; Zaat, S.A.; Busscher, H.J. Critical factors in the translation of improved antimicrobial strategies for medical implants and devices. *Biomaterials* **2013**, *34*, 9237–9243.
5. Zaveri, T.D.; Lewis, J.S.; Dolgova, N.V.; Clare-Salzler, M.J.; Keselowsky, B.G. Integrin-directed modulation of macrophage responses to biomaterials. *Biomaterials* **2014**, *35*, 3504–3515.
6. Anderson, J.M. Biological Responses to Materials. *Annu. Rev. Mater. Res.* **2001**, *31*, 81–110.
7. Darouiche, R.O. Treatment of infections associated with surgical implants. *N. Engl. J. Med.* **2004**, *350*, 1422–1429.
8. Kaplan, J.B. Antibiotic-induced biofilm formation. *Int. J. Artif. Organs* **2011**, *34*, 737–751.
9. Busscher, H.J.; van der Mei, H.C.; Subbiahdoss, G.; Jutte, P.C.; van den Dungen, J.J.; Zaat, S.A.; Schultz, M.J.; Grainger, D.W. Biomaterial-associated infection: Locating the finish line in the race for the surface. *Sci. Transl. Med.* **2012**, *4*, 153rv10.
10. O'Toole, G.; Kaplan, H.B.; Kolter, R. Biofilm formation as microbial development. *Annu. Rev. Microbiol.* **2000**, *54*, 49–79.
11. Gilbert, P.; Maira-Litran, T.; McBain, A.J.; Rickard, A.H.; Whyte, F.W. The physiology and collective recalcitrance of microbial biofilm communities. *Adv. Microb. Physiol.* **2002**, *46*, 202–256.
12. Francolini, I.; Donelli, G. Prevention and control of biofilm-based medical-device-related infections. *FEMS Immunol. Med. Microbiol.* **2010**, *59*, 227–238.
13. Koenig, A.L.; Gambillara, V.; Grainger, D.W. Correlating fibronectin adsorption with endothelial cell adhesion and signaling on polymer substrates. *J. Biomed. Mater. Res. A* **2003**, *64*, 20–37.

14. MacKintosh, E.E.; Patel, J.D.; Marchant, R.E.; Anderson, J.M. Effects of biomaterial surface chemistry on the adhesion and biofilm formation of *Staphylococcus epidermidis in vitro*. *J. Biomed. Mater. Res. A* **2006**, *78*, 836–842.

15. Gottenbos, B.; van der Mei, H.C.; Busscher, H.J. Initial adhesion and surface growth of *Staphylococcus epidermidis* and *Pseudomonas aeruginosa* on biomedical polymers. *J. Biomed. Mater. Res.* **2000**, *50*, 208–214.

16. Hu, J.; Xu, T.; Zhu, T.; Lou, Q.; Wang, X.; Wu, Y.; Huang, R.; Liu, J.; Liu, H.; Yu, F.; *et al.* Monoclonal antibodies against accumulation-associated protein affect EPS biosynthesis and enhance bacterial accumulation of *Staphylococcus epidermidis*. *PLoS One* **2011**, *6*, e20918.

17. Costerton, J.W.; Montanaro, L.; Arciola, C.R. Bacterial communications in implant infections: A target for an intelligence war. *Int. J. Artif. Organs* **2007**, *30*, 757–763.

18. Fux, C.A.; Costerton, J.W.; Stewart, P.S.; Stoodley, P. Survival strategies of infectious biofilms. *Trends Microbiol.* **2005**, *13*, 34–40.

19. Donlan, R.M. Biofilm formation: A clinically relevant microbiological process. *Clin. Infect. Dis.* **2001**, *33*, 1387–1392.

20. Nordmann, P.; Poirel, L.; Toleman, M.A.; Walsh, T.R. Does broad-spectrum beta-lactam resistance due to NDM-1 herald the end of the antibiotic era for treatment of infections caused by Gram-negative bacteria? *J. Antimicrob. Chemother.* **2011**, *66*, 689–692.

21. Brooks, B.D.; Brooks, A.E.; Grainger, D.W. Immunological Aspects and Antimicrobial Strategies, Antimicrobial Medical Devices in Preclinical Development and Clinical Use. In *Biomaterials associated infection*; Moriaty, F.T., Zaat, S.A., Busscher, H.J., Eds.; Springer: New York, NY, USA, 2013; pp. 307–354.

22. World Health Organization. *Antimicrobial Resistance: Global Report on Surveillance*; WHO Press: Geneva, Switzerland, 2014.

23. Crnich, C.J.; Drinka, P. Medical device-associated infections in the long-term care setting. *Infect. Dis. Clin. N. Am.* **2012**, *26*, 143–164.

24. Donlan, R.M. Biofilms and device-associated infections. *Emerg. Infect. Dis.* **2001**, *7*, 277–281.

25. Plowman, R. The socioeconomic burden of hospital acquired infection. *Eur. Surveill.* **2000**, *5*, 4.

26. Pittet, D.; Allegranzi, B.; Boyce, J.; World Health Organization World Alliance for Patient Safety First Global Patient Safety Challenge Core Group of Experts The World Health Organization Guidelines on Hand Hygiene in Health Care and their consensus recommendations. *Infect. Control Hosp. Epidemiol.* **2009**, *30*, 611–622.

27. Langer, R.; Tirrell, D.A. Designing materials for biology and medicine. *Nature* **2004**, *428*, 487–492.

28. Saldarriaga Fernandez, I.C.; van der Mei, H.C.; Lochhead, M.J.; Grainger, D.W.; Busscher, H.J. The inhibition of the adhesion of clinically isolated bacterial strains on multi-component cross-linked poly(ethylene glycol)-based polymer coatings. *Biomaterials* **2007**, *28*, 4105–4112.

29. Zhang, Z.; Nix, C.A.; Ercan, U.K.; Gerstenhaber, J.A.; Joshi, S.G.; Zhong, Y. Calcium binding-mediated sustained release of minocycline from hydrophilic multilayer coatings targeting infection and inflammation. *PLoS One* **2014**, *9*, e84360.

30. Adams, D.J. Dipeptide and tripeptide conjugates as low-molecular-weight hydrogelators. *Macromol. Biosci.* **2011**, *11*, 160–173.

31. Kopecek, J.; Yang, J. Peptide-directed self-assembly of hydrogels. *Acta Biomater.* **2009**, *5*, 805–816.

32. Peppas, N.A.; Bures, P.; Leobandung, W.; Ichikawa, H. Hydrogels in pharmaceutical formulations. *Eur. J. Pharm. Biopharm.* **2000**, *50*, 27–46.

33. Ahearn, D.G.; Grace, D.T.; Jennings, M.J.; Borazjani, R.N.; Boles, K.J.; Rose, L.J.; Simmons, R.B.; Ahanotu, E.N. Effects of hydrogel/silver coatings on *in vitro* adhesion to catheters of bacteria associated with urinary tract infections. *Curr. Microbiol.* **2000**, *41*, 120–125.

34. Wang, Y.; Burgress, D.J.; Aagaard, J. Drug Device Combination Products. In *Drug Device Combination Products: Delivery Technologies and Applications*; Lewis, A., Ed.; Woodhead Publishing Ltd.: Cambridge, UK, 2010; pp. 11–12.

35. Gaonkar, T.A.; Modak, S.M. Comparison of microbial adherence to antiseptic and antibiotic central venous catheters using a novel agar subcutaneous infection model. *J. Antimicrob. Chemother.* **2003**, *52*, 389–396.

36. Yorganci, K.; Krepel, C.; Weigelt, J.A.; Edmiston, C.E. *In vitro* evaluation of the antibacterial activity of three different central venous catheters against Gram-positive bacteria. *Eur. J. Clin. Microbiol. Infect. Dis.* **2002**, *21*, 379–384.

37. Gransden, W.R. Antibiotic resistance. Nosocomial Gram-negative infection. *J. Med. Microbiol.* **1997**, *46*, 436–439.

38. Thomas, W.E.; Trintchina, E.; Forero, M.; Vogel, V.; Sokurenko, E.V. Bacterial adhesion to target cells enhanced by shear force. *Cell* **2002**, *109*, 913–923.

39. Rachid, S.; Ohlsen, K.; Witte, W.; Hacker, J.; Ziebuhr, W. Effect of subinhibitory antibiotic concentrations on polysaccharide intercellular adhesin expression in biofilm-forming *Staphylococcus epidermidis*. *Antimicrob. Agents Chemother.* **2000**, *44*, 3357–3363.

40. Laverty, G.; Gorman, S.P.; Gilmore, B.F. Biomolecular mechanisms of staphylococcal biofilm formation. *Future Microbiol.* **2013**, *8*, 509–524.

41. Danese, P.N. Antibiofilm approaches: Prevention of catheter colonization. *Chem. Biol.* **2002**, *9*, 873–880.

42. Rochford, E.T.J.; Jaekel, D.J.; Hickok, N.J.; Richards, R.G.; Moriarity, T.F.; Poulsson, A.H.C. *PEEK Biomaterials Handbook*; Kurtz, S.M., Ed.; Elsevier: Oxford, UK, 2012; pp. 104–105.

43. Veiga, A.S.; Schneider, J.P. Antimicrobial hydrogels for the treatment of infection. *Biopolymers* **2013**, *100*, 637–644.

44. Laverty, G.; Gorman, S.P.; Gilmore, B.F. The potential of antimicrobial peptides as biocides. *Int. J. Mol. Sci.* **2011**, *12*, 6566–6596.

45. Laverty, G.; McLaughlin, M.; Shaw, C.; Gorman, S.P.; Gilmore, B.F. Antimicrobial activity of short, synthetic cationic lipopeptides. *Chem. Biol. Drug Des.* **2010**, *75*, 563–569.

46. Laverty, G.; Gorman, S.P.; Gilmore, B.F. Antimicrobial peptide incorporated poly(2-hydroxyethyl methacrylate) hydrogels for the prevention of *Staphylococcus epidermidis*-associated biomaterial infections. *J. Biomed. Mater. Res. A* **2012**, *100*, 1803–1814.

47. Bahar, A.A.; Ren, D. Antimicrobial peptides. *Pharmaceuticals [Basel]* **2013**, *6*, 1543–1575.

48. Dasgupta, A.; Mondal, J.H.; Das, D. Peptide hydrogels. *RSC Adv.* **2013**, *3*, 9117–9149.

49. Yang, Z.; Liang, G.; Guo, Z.; Guo, Z.; Xu, B. Intracellular hydrogelation of small molecules inhibits bacterial growth. *Angew. Chem. Int. Ed. Engl.* **2007**, *46*, 8216–8219.

50. Liu, Y.; Yang, Y.; Wang, C.; Zhao, X. Stimuli-responsive self-assembling peptides made from antibacterial peptides. *Nanoscale* **2013**, *5*, 6413–6421.

51. Kushner, D.J. Self-assembly of biological structures. *Bacteriol. Rev.* **1969**, *33*, 302–345.

52. Zhang, S. Fabrication of novel biomaterials through molecular self-assembly. *Nat. Biotechnol.* **2003**, *21*, 1171–1178.

53. Stephanopoulos, N.; Ortony, J.H.; Stupp, S.I. Self-Assembly for the Synthesis of Functional Biomaterials. *Acta Mater.* **2013**, *61*, 912–930.

54. Whitesides, G.M.; Grzybowski, B. Self-assembly at all scales. *Science* **2002**, *295*, 2418–2421.

55. Javid, N.; Roy, S.; Zelzer, M.; Yang, Z.; Sefcik, J.; Ulijn, R.V. Cooperative self-assembly of peptide gelators and proteins. *Biomacromolecules* **2013**, *14*, 4368–4376.

56. Sargent, J.F., Jr. Nanotechnology: A policy primer. Available online: http://digitalcommons.ilr.cornell.edu/cgi/viewcontent.cgi?article=1911&context=key_workplace (accessed on 28 September 2014).

57. Bohorquez, M.; Koch, C.; Trygstad, T.; Pandit, N. A Study of the Temperature-Dependent Micellization of Pluronic F127. *J. Colloid Interface Sci.* **1999**, *216*, 34–40.

58. Nie, S.; Hsiao, W.L.; Pan, W.; Yang, Z. Thermoreversible Pluronic F127-based hydrogel containing liposomes for the controlled delivery of paclitaxel: *In vitro* drug release, cell cytotoxicity, and uptake studies. *Int. J. Nanomed.* **2011**, *6*, 151–166.

59. Liaw, J.; Lin, Y. Evaluation of poly(ethylene oxide)-poly(propylene oxide)-poly(ethylene oxide) (PEO-PPO-PEO) gels as a release vehicle for percutaneous fentanyl. *J. Control. Release* **2000**, *68*, 273–282.

60. Barichello, J.M.; Morishita, M.; Takayama, K.; Nagai, T. Absorption of insulin from pluronic F-127 gels following subcutaneous administration in rats. *Int. J. Pharm.* **1999**, *184*, 189–198.

61. Escobar-Chavez, J.J.; Lopez-Cervantes, M.; Naik, A.; Kalia, Y.N.; Quintanar-Guerrero, D.; Ganem-Quintanar, A. Applications of thermo-reversible Pluronic F-127 gels in pharmaceutical formulations. *J. Pharm. Pharm. Sci.* **2006**, *9*, 339–358.

62. Wesenberg-Ward, K.E.; Tyler, B.J.; Sears, J.T. Adhesion and biofilm formation of *Candida albicans* on native and Pluronic-treated polystyrene. *Biofilms* **2005**, *2*, 63–71.

63. Veyries, M.L.; Faurisson, F.; Joly-Guillou, M.L.; Rouveix, B. Control of staphylococcal adhesion to polymethylmethacrylate and enhancement of susceptibility to antibiotics by poloxamer 407. *Antimicrob. Agents Chemother.* **2000**, *44*, 1093–1096.

64. Leszczynska, K.; Namiot, A.; Cruz, K.; Byfield, F.J.; Won, E.; Mendez, G.; Sokolowski, W.; Savage, P.B.; Bucki, R.; Janmey, P.A. Potential of ceragenin CSA-13 and its mixture with Pluronic F-127 as treatment of topical bacterial infections. *J. Appl. Microbiol.* **2011**, *110*, 229–238.

65. Kant, V.; Gopal, A.; Kumar, D.; Gopalkrishnan, A.; Pathak, N.N.; Kurade, N.P.; Tandan, S.K.; Kumar, D. Topical Pluronic F-127 gel application enhances cutaneous wound healing in rats. *Acta Histochem.* **2014**, *116*, 5–13.

66. Norris, P.; Noble, M.; Francolini, I.; Vinogradov, A.M.; Stewart, P.S.; Ratner, B.D.; Costerton, J.W.; Stoodley, P. Ultrasonically controlled release of ciprofloxacin from self-assembled coatings on poly(2-hydroxyethyl methacrylate) hydrogels for *Pseudomonas aeruginosa* biofilm prevention. *Antimicrob. Agents Chemother.* **2005**, *49*, 4272–4279.

67. Kruszewski, K.M.; Nistico, L.; Longwell, M.J.; Hynes, M.J.; Maurer, J.A.; Hall-Stoodley, L.; Gawalt, E.S. Reducing *Staphylococcus aureus* biofilm formation on stainless steel 316L using functionalized self-assembled monolayers. *Mater. Sci. Eng. C Mater. Biol. Appl.* **2013**, *33*, 2059–2069.

68. Hou, S.; Burton, E.A.; Simon, K.A.; Blodgett, D.; Luk, Y.Y.; Ren, D. Inhibition of *Escherichia coli* biofilm formation by self-assembled monolayers of functional alkanethiols on gold. *Appl. Environ. Microbiol.* **2007**, *73*, 4300–4307.

69. Wang, Q.; Uzunoglu, E.; Wu, Y.; Libera, M. Self-assembled poly(ethylene glycol)-co-acrylic acid microgels to inhibit bacterial colonization of synthetic surfaces. *ACS Appl. Mater. Interfaces* **2012**, *4*, 2498–2506.

70. Zhang, S.; Marini, D.M.; Hwang, W.; Santoso, S. Design of nanostructured biological materials through self-assembly of peptides and proteins. *Curr. Opin. Chem. Biol.* **2002**, *6*, 865–871.

71. Zhang, S.; Holmes, T.; Lockshin, C.; Rich, A. Spontaneous assembly of a self-complementary oligopeptide to form a stable macroscopic membrane. *Proc. Natl. Acad. Sci. USA* **1993**, *90*, 3334–3338.

72. Aggeli, A.; Nyrkova, I.A.; Bell, M.; Harding, R.; Carrick, L.; McLeish, T.C.; Semenov, A.N.; Boden, N. Hierarchical self-assembly of chiral rod-like molecules as a model for peptide beta -sheet tapes, ribbons, fibrils, and fibers. *Proc. Natl. Acad. Sci. USA* **2001**, *98*, 11857–11862.

73. Fields, G.B.; Tirrell, M.V. Self-Assembling Amphiphiles for Construction of Peptide Secondary Structures. Patent, US 08/702,254 and WO 1998007752 A1, 2000.

74. Ghadiri, M.R.; Granja, J.R.; Milligan, R.A.; McRee, D.E.; Khazanovich, N. Self-assembling organic nanotubes based on a cyclic peptide architecture. *Nature* **1993**, *366*, 324–327.

75. Rajagopal, K.; Schneider, J.P. Self-assembling peptides and proteins for nanotechnological applications. *Curr. Opin. Struct. Biol.* **2004**, *14*, 480–486.

76. Ulijn, R.V.; Smith, A.M. Designing peptide based nanomaterials. *Chem. Soc. Rev.* **2008**, *37*, 664–675.

77. Caplan, M.R.; Schwartzfarb, E.M.; Zhang, S.; Kamm, R.D.; Lauffenburger, D.A. Control of self-assembling oligopeptide matrix formation through systematic variation of amino acid sequence. *Biomaterials* **2002**, *23*, 219–227.

78. Hong, Y.; Pritzker, M.D.; Legge, R.L.; Chen, P. Effect of NaCl and peptide concentration on the self-assembly of an ionic-complementary peptide EAK16-II. *Colloids Surf. B Biointerfaces* **2005**, *46*, 152–161.

79. Joshi, N.S.; Whitaker, L.R.; Francis, M.B. A three-component Mannich-type reaction for selective tyrosine bioconjugation. *J. Am. Chem. Soc.* **2004**, *126*, 15942–15943.

80. Yang, Z.; Liang, G.; Wang, L.; Xu, B. Using a kinase/phosphatase switch to regulate a supramolecular hydrogel and forming the supramolecular hydrogel *in vivo*. *J. Am. Chem. Soc.* **2006**, *128*, 3038–3043.

81. Mahalka, A.K.; Kinnunen, P.K. Binding of amphipathic alpha-helical antimicrobial peptides to lipid membranes: Lessons from temporins B and L. *Biochim. Biophys. Acta* **2009**, *1788*, 1600–1609.

82. Paramonov, S.E.; Jun, H.W.; Hartgerink, J.D. Self-assembly of peptide-amphiphile nanofibers: The roles of hydrogen bonding and amphiphilic packing. *J. Am. Chem. Soc.* **2006**, *128*, 7291–7298.

83. Silva, G.A.; Czeisler, C.; Niece, K.L.; Beniash, E.; Harrington, D.A.; Kessler, J.A.; Stupp, S.I. Selective differentiation of neural progenitor cells by high-epitope density nanofibers. *Science* **2004**, *303*, 1352–1355.

84. Gazit, E. Self-assembled peptide nanostructures: The design of molecular building blocks and their technological utilization. *Chem. Soc. Rev.* **2007**, *36*, 1263–1269.

85. Martinez, C.R.; Iverson, B.I. Rethinking the term "pi-stacking". *Chem. Sci.* **2012**, *3*, 2191–2201.

86. Burley, S.K.; Petsko, G.A. Aromatic-aromatic interaction: A mechanism of protein structure stabilization. *Science* **1985**, *229*, 23–28.

87. Reches, M.; Gazit, E. Casting metal nanowires within discrete self-assembled peptide nanotubes. *Science* **2003**, *300*, 625–627.

88. Yang, Z.; Gu, H.; Zhang, Y.; Wang, L.; Xu, B. Small molecule hydrogels based on a class of antiinflammatory agents. *Chem. Commun.* **2004**, *2*, 208–209.

89. Yang, Z.; Liang, G.; Ma, M.; Gao, Y.; Xu, B. Conjugates of naphthalene and dipeptides confer molecular hydrogelators with high efficiency of hydrogelation and superhelical nanofibers. *J. Mater. Chem.* **2007**, *17*, 850–854.

90. Kyle, S.; Aggeli, A.; Ingham, E.; McPherson, M.J. Production of self-assembling biomaterials for tissue engineering. *Trends Biotechnol.* **2009**, *27*, 423–433.

91. Avrahami, D.; Shai, Y. A new group of antifungal and antibacterial lipopeptides derived from non-membrane active peptides conjugated to palmitic acid. *J. Biol. Chem.* **2004**, *279*, 12277–12285.

92. Peschel, A.; Sahl, H.G. The co-evolution of host cationic antimicrobial peptides and microbial resistance. *Nat. Rev. Microbiol.* **2006**, *4*, 529–536.

93. Yeaman, M.R.; Yount, N.Y. Mechanisms of antimicrobial peptide action and resistance. *Pharmacol. Rev.* **2003**, *55*, 27–55.

94. Jenssen, H.; Hamill, P.; Hancock, R.E. Peptide antimicrobial agents. *Clin. Microbiol. Rev.* **2006**, *19*, 491–511.

95. Zasloff, M. Antimicrobial peptides of multicellular organisms. *Nature* **2002**, *415*, 389–395.

96. Matsuzaki, K. Why and how are peptide-lipid interactions utilized for self-defense? Magainins and tachyplesins as archetypes. *Biochim. Biophys. Acta* **1999**, *1462*, 1–10.

97. Park, C.B.; Kim, H.S.; Kim, S.C. Mechanism of action of the antimicrobial peptide buforin II: Buforin II kills microorganisms by penetrating the cell membrane and inhibiting cellular functions. *Biochem. Biophys. Res. Commun.* **1998**, *244*, 253–257.

98. Patrzykat, A.; Friedrich, C.L.; Zhang, L.; Mendoza, V.; Hancock, R.E. Sublethal concentrations of pleurocidin-derived antimicrobial peptides inhibit macromolecular synthesis in *Escherichia coli*. *Antimicrob. Agents Chemother.* **2002**, *46*, 605–614.

99. Hilpert, K.; McLeod, B.; Yu, J.; Elliott, M.R.; Rautenbach, M.; Ruden, S.; Burck, J.; Muhle-Goll, C.; Ulrich, A.S.; Keller, S.; *et al.* Short cationic antimicrobial peptides interact with ATP. *Antimicrob. Agents Chemother.* **2010**, *54*, 4480–4483.

100. Hancock, R.E.; Scott, M.G. The role of antimicrobial peptides in animal defenses. *Proc. Natl. Acad. Sci. USA* **2000**, *97*, 8856–8861.

101. Finlay, B.B.; Hancock, R.E. Can innate immunity be enhanced to treat microbial infections? *Nat. Rev. Microbiol.* **2004**, *2*, 497–504.

102. Harris, F.; Dennison, S.R.; Phoenix, D.A. Anionic antimicrobial peptides from eukaryotic organisms. *Curr. Protein Pept. Sci.* **2009**, *10*, 585–606.

103. Grubor, B.; Meyerholz, D.K.; Ackermann, M.R. Collectins and cationic antimicrobial peptides of the respiratory epithelia. *Vet. Pathol.* **2006**, *43*, 595–612.

104. Brogden, K.A.; Ackermann, M.; McCray, P.B., Jr; Tack, B.F. Antimicrobial peptides in animals and their role in host defences. *Int. J. Antimicrob. Agents* **2003**, *22*, 465–478.

105. Schmidtchen, A.; Frick, I.M.; Andersson, E.; Tapper, H.; Bjorck, L. Proteinases of common pathogenic bacteria degrade and inactivate the antibacterial peptide LL-37. *Mol. Microbiol.* **2002**, *46*, 157–168.

106. Strom, M.B.; Haug, B.E.; Skar, M.L.; Stensen, W.; Stiberg, T.; Svendsen, J.S. The pharmacophore of short cationic antibacterial peptides. *J. Med. Chem.* **2003**, *46*, 1567–1570.

107. Bisht, G.S.; Rawat, D.S.; Kumar, A.; Kumar, R.; Pasha, S. Antimicrobial activity of rationally designed amino terminal modified peptides. *Bioorg. Med. Chem. Lett.* **2007**, *17*, 4343–4346.

108. Makovitzki, A.; Avrahami, D.; Shai, Y. Ultrashort antibacterial and antifungal lipopeptides. *Proc. Natl. Acad. Sci. USA* **2006**, *103*, 15997–16002.

109. Chen, Y.; Vasil, A.I.; Rehaume, L.; Mant, C.T.; Burns, J.L.; Vasil, M.L.; Hancock, R.E.; Hodges, R.S. Comparison of biophysical and biologic properties of alpha-helical enantiomeric antimicrobial peptides. *Chem. Biol. Drug Des.* **2006**, *67*, 162–173.

110. Straus, S.K.; Hancock, R.E. Mode of action of the new antibiotic for Gram-positive pathogens daptomycin: Comparison with cationic antimicrobial peptides and lipopeptides. *Biochim. Biophys. Acta* **2006**, *1758*, 1215–1223.

111. Zavascki, A.P.; Goldani, L.Z.; Li, J.; Nation, R.L. Polymyxin B for the treatment of multidrug-resistant pathogens: A critical review. *J. Antimicrob. Chemother.* **2007**, *60*, 1206–1215.

112. Levine, D.P.; Lamp, K.C. Daptomycin in the treatment of patients with infective endocarditis: Experience from a registry. *Am. J. Med.* **2007**, *120*, S28–S33.

113. Li, J.; Nation, R.L.; Turnidge, J.D.; Milne, R.W.; Coulthard, K.; Rayner, C.R.; Paterson, D.L. Colistin: The re-emerging antibiotic for multidrug-resistant Gram-negative bacterial infections. *Lancet Infect. Dis.* **2006**, *6*, 589–601.

114. Di Luca, M.; Maccari, G.; Nifosi, R. Treatment of microbial biofilms in the post-antibiotic era: Prophylactic and therapeutic use of antimicrobial peptides and their design by bioinformatics tools. *Pathog. Dis.* **2014**, *70*, 257–270.

115. Park, S.C.; Park, Y.; Hahm, K.S. The role of antimicrobial peptides in preventing multidrug-resistant bacterial infections and biofilm formation. *Int. J. Mol. Sci.* **2011**, *12*, 5971–5992.

116. Cirioni, O.; Silvestri, C.; Ghiselli, R.; Orlando, F.; Riva, A.; Mocchegiani, F.; Chiodi, L.; Castelletti, S.; Gabrielli, E.; Saba, V.; *et al.* Protective effects of the combination of alpha-helical antimicrobial peptides and rifampicin in three rat models of *Pseudomonas aeruginosa* infection. *J. Antimicrob. Chemother.* **2008**, *62*, 1332–1338.

117. Milne, K.E.; Gould, I.M. Combination antimicrobial susceptibility testing of multidrug-resistant *Stenotrophomonas maltophilia* from cystic fibrosis patients. *Antimicrob. Agents Chemother.* **2012**, *56*, 4071–4077.

118. Medina-Polo, J.; Jimenez-Alcaide, E.; Garcia-Gonzalez, L.; Guerrero-Ramos, F.; Perez-Cadavid, S.; Arrebola-Pajares, A.; Sopena-Sutil, R.; Benitez-Salas, R.; Diaz-Gonzalez, R.; Tejido-Sanchez, A. Healthcare-associated infections in a department of urology: Incidence and patterns of antibiotic resistance. *Scand. J. Urol.* **2014**, *48*, 203–209.

119. Hancock, R.E.; Sahl, H.G. Antimicrobial and host-defense peptides as new anti-infective therapeutic strategies. *Nat. Biotechnol.* **2006**, *24*, 1551–1557.

120. Haug, B.E.; Stensen, W.; Stiberg, T.; Svendsen, J.S. Bulky nonproteinogenic amino acids permit the design of very small and effective cationic antibacterial peptides. *J. Med. Chem.* **2004**, *47*, 4159–4162.

121. Pasupuleti, M.; Schmidtchen, A.; Chalupka, A.; Ringstad, L.; Malmsten, M. End-tagging of ultra-short antimicrobial peptides by W/F stretches to facilitate bacterial killing. *PLoS One* **2009**, *4*, e5285.

122. Rotem, S.; Radzishevsky, I.S.; Bourdetsky, D.; Navon-Venezia, S.; Carmeli, Y.; Mor, A. Analogous oligo-acyl-lysines with distinct antibacterial mechanisms. *FASEB J.* **2008**, *22*, 2652–2661.

123. Rotem, S.; Raz, N.; Kashi, Y.; Mor, A. Bacterial capture by peptide-mimetic oligoacyllysine surfaces. *Appl. Environ. Microbiol.* **2010**, *76*, 3301–3307.

124. Livne, L.; Epand, R.F.; Papahadjopoulos-Sternberg, B.; Epand, R.M.; Mor, A. OAK-based cochleates as a novel approach to overcome multidrug resistance in bacteria. *FASEB J.* **2010**, *24*, 5092–5101.

125. Sarig, H.; Ohana, D.; Epand, R.F.; Mor, A.; Epand, R.M. Functional studies of cochleate assemblies of an oligo-acyl-lysyl with lipid mixtures for combating bacterial multidrug resistance. *FASEB J.* **2011**, *25*, 3336–3343.

126. Jain, A.; Jain, A.; Gulbake, A.; Shilpi, S.; Hurkat, P.; Jain, S.K. Peptide and protein delivery using new drug delivery systems. *Crit. Rev. Ther. Drug Carrier Syst.* **2013**, *30*, 293–329.

127. Karin, N.; Binah, O.; Grabie, N.; Mitchell, D.J.; Felzen, B.; Solomon, M.D.; Conlon, P.; Gaur, A.; Ling, N.; Steinman, L. Short peptide-based tolerogens without self-antigenic or pathogenic activity reverse autoimmune disease. *J. Immunol.* **1998**, *160*, 5188–5194.

128. Mack, D.; Rohde, H.; Harris, L.G.; Davies, A.P.; Horstkotte, M.A.; Knobloch, J.K. Biofilm formation in medical device-related infection. *Int. J. Artif. Organs* **2006**, *29*, 343–359.

129. Rughani, R.V.; Salick, D.A.; Lamm, M.S.; Yucel, T.; Pochan, D.J.; Schneider, J.P. Folding, self-assembly, and bulk material properties of a *de novo* designed three-stranded beta-sheet hydrogel. *Biomacromolecules* **2009**, *10*, 1295–1304.

130. Haines, L.A.; Rajagopal, K.; Ozbas, B.; Salick, D.A.; Pochan, D.J.; Schneider, J.P. Light-activated hydrogel formation via the triggered folding and self-assembly of a designed peptide. *J. Am. Chem. Soc.* **2005**, *127*, 17025–17029.

131. Hughes, M.; Debnath, S.; Knapp, C.W.; Ulijn, R.V. Antimicrobial properties of enzymatically triggered self-assembling aromatic peptide amphiphiles. *Biomater. Sci.* **2013**, *1*, 1138–1142.

132. Schneider, J.P.; Pochan, D.J.; Ozbas, B.; Rajagopal, K.; Pakstis, L.; Kretsinger, J. Responsive hydrogels from the intramolecular folding and self-assembly of a designed peptide. *J. Am. Chem. Soc.* **2002**, *124*, 15030–15037.

133. Kretsinger, J.K.; Haines, L.A.; Ozbas, B.; Pochan, D.J.; Schneider, J.P. Cytocompatibility of self-assembled beta-hairpin peptide hydrogel surfaces. *Biomaterials* **2005**, *26*, 5177–5186.

134. Haines-Butterick, L.; Rajagopal, K.; Branco, M.; Salick, D.; Rughani, R.; Pilarz, M.; Lamm, M.S.; Pochan, D.J.; Schneider, J.P. Controlling hydrogelation kinetics by peptide design for three-dimensional encapsulation and injectable delivery of cells. *Proc. Natl. Acad. Sci. USA* **2007**, *104*, 7791–7796.

135. Veiga, A.S.; Sinthuvanich, C.; Gaspar, D.; Franquelim, H.G.; Castanho, M.A.; Schneider, J.P. Arginine-rich self-assembling peptides as potent antibacterial gels. *Biomaterials* **2012**, *33*, 8907–8916.

136. Yokoi, H.; Kinoshita, T.; Zhang, S. Dynamic reassembly of peptide RADA16 nanofiber scaffold. *Proc. Natl. Acad. Sci. USA* **2005**, *102*, 8414–8419.

137. Schneider, A.; Garlick, J.A.; Egles, C. Self-assembling peptide nanofiber scaffolds accelerate wound healing. *PLoS One* **2008**, *3*, e1410.

138. Debnath, S.; Shome, A.; Das, D.; Das, P.K. Hydrogelation through self-assembly of fmoc-peptide functionalized cationic amphiphiles: Potent antibacterial agent. *J. Phys. Chem. B* **2010**, *114*, 4407–4415.

139. Williams, G.J.; Stickler, D.J. Some observations on the migration of *Proteus mirabilis* and other urinary tract pathogens over foley catheters. *Infect. Control Hosp. Epidemiol.* **2008**, *29*, 443–445.

140. McCoy, C.P.; Craig, R.A.; McGlinchey, S.M.; Carson, L.; Jones, D.S.; Gorman, S.P. Surface localisation of photosensitisers on intraocular lens biomaterials for prevention of infectious endophthalmitis and retinal protection. *Biomaterials* **2012**, *33*, 7952–7958.

141. Pochan, D.J.; Schneider, J.P.; Kretsinger, J.; Ozbas, B.; Rajagopal, K.; Haines, L. Thermally reversible hydrogels via intramolecular folding and consequent self-assembly of a *de novo* designed peptide. *J. Am. Chem. Soc.* **2003**, *125*, 11802–11803.

142. Tang, C.; Ulijn, R.V.; Saiani, A. Effect of glycine substitution on Fmoc-diphenylalanine self-assembly and gelation properties. *Langmuir* **2011**, *27*, 14438–14449.

143. Tang, C.; Ulijn, R.V.; Saiani, A. Self-assembly and gelation properties of glycine/leucine Fmoc-dipeptides. *Eur. Phys. J. E.* **2013**, *36*, 111.

144. Wu, L.Q.; Payne, G.F. Biofabrication: Using biological materials and biocatalysts to construct nanostructured assemblies. *Trends Biotechnol.* **2004**, *22*, 593–599.

145. Hughes, M.; Frederix, P.W.J.M.; Raeburn, J.; Birchall, L.S.; Sadownik, J.; Coomer, F.C.; Lin, I.H.; Cussen, E.J.; Hunt, N.T.; Tuttle, T.; *et al.* Sequence/structure relationships in aromatic dipeptide hydrogels formed under thermodynamic control by enzyme-assisted self-assembly. *Soft Matter* **2012**, *8*, 5595–5602.

146. Hughes, M.; Birchall, L.S.; Zuberi, K.; Aitken, L.A.; Debnath, S.; Javida, N.; Ulijn, R.V. Differential supramolecular organization of Fmoc-dipeptides with hydrophilic terminal amino acid residues by biocatalytic self-assembly. *Soft Matter* **2012**, *8*, 11565–11574.

147. Toledano, S.; Williams, R.J.; Jayawarna, V.; Ulijn, R.V. Enzyme-triggered self-assembly of peptide hydrogels via reversed hydrolysis. *J. Am. Chem. Soc.* **2006**, *128*, 1070–1071.

148. Wang, H.; Yang, C.; Tan, M.; Wang, L.; Konga, D.; Yang, Z. A structure–gelation ability study in a short peptide-based 'Super Hydrogelator' system. *Soft Matter* **2011**, *7*, 1070–1071.

149. Derman, A.I.; Beckwith, J. *Escherichia coli* alkaline phosphatase localized to the cytoplasm slowly acquires enzymatic activity in cells whose growth has been suspended: A caution for gene fusion studies. *J. Bacteriol.* **1995**, *177*, 3764–3770.

150. Yang, K.; Metcalf, W.W. A new activity for an old enzyme: *Escherichia coli* bacterial alkaline phosphatase is a phosphite-dependent hydrogenase. *Proc. Natl. Acad. Sci. USA* **2004**, *101*, 7919–7924.

151. Yang, Z.; Ho, P.K.; Liang, G.; Chow, K.H.; Wang, Q.; Cao Y.; Guo, Z.; Xu, B. Using β-lactamase to trigger supramolecular hydrogelation. *J. Am. Chem. Soc.* **2007**, *129*, 266–267.

152. Valery, C.; Paternostre, M.; Robert, B.; Gulik-Krzywicki, T.; Narayanan, T.; Dedieu, J.C.; Keller, G.; Torres, M.L.; Cherif-Cheikh, R.; Calvo, P.; *et al.* Biomimetic organization: Octapeptide self-assembly into nanotubes of viral capsid-like dimension. *Proc. Natl. Acad. Sci. USA* **2003**, *100*, 10258–10262.

153. Marchesan, S.; Qu, Y.; Waddington, L.J.; Easton, C.D.; Glattauer, V.; Lithgow, T.J.; McLean, K.M.; Forsythe, J.S.; Hartley, P.G. Self-assembly of ciprofloxacin and a tripeptide into an antimicrobial nanostructured hydrogel. *Biomaterials* **2013**, *34*, 3678–3687.

154. Paladini, F.; Meikle, S.T.; Cooper, I.R.; Lacey, J.; Perugini, V.; Santin, M. Silver-doped self-assembling di-phenylalanine hydrogels as wound dressing biomaterials. *J. Mater. Sci. Mater. Med.* **2013**, *24*, 2461–2472.

155. Wang, Y.; Cao, L.; Guan, S.; Shi, G.; Luo, Q.; Miao, L.; Thistlethwaite, I.; Huang, Z.; Xu, J.; Liu, J. Silver mineralization on self-assembled peptide nanofibers for long term antimicrobial effect. *J. Mater. Chem.* **2012**, *22*, 2575–2581.

156. Liu, L.; Xu, K.; Wang, H.; Tan, P.K.; Fan, W.; Venkatraman, S.S.; Li, L.; Yang, Y.Y. Self-assembled cationic peptide nanoparticles as an efficient antimicrobial agent. *Nat. Nanotechnol.* **2009**, *4*, 457–463.

157. Laverty, G.; McCloskey, A.; Gilmore, B.F.; Jones, D.S.; Zhou, J.; Xu, B. Ultrashort cationic naphthalene-derived self-Assembled peptides as antimicrobial nanomaterials. *Biomacromolecules* **2014**, *15*, 3429–3439.

6

Biomolecular Mechanisms of *Pseudomonas aeruginosa* and *Escherichia coli* Biofilm Formation

Garry Laverty *, Sean P. Gorman and Brendan F. Gilmore

Biomaterials, Biofilm and Infection Control Research Group, School of Pharmacy, Queen's University Belfast, Medical Biology Centre, 97 Lisburn Road, Belfast BT9 7BL, UK; E-Mails: s.gorman@qub.ac.uk (S.P.G.); b.gilmore@qub.ac.uk (B.F.G.)

* Author to whom correspondence should be addressed; E-Mail: garry.laverty@qub.ac.uk;

Abstract: *Pseudomonas aeruginosa* and *Escherichia coli* are the most prevalent Gram-negative biofilm forming medical device associated pathogens, particularly with respect to catheter associated urinary tract infections. In a similar manner to Gram-positive bacteria, Gram-negative biofilm formation is fundamentally determined by a series of steps outlined more fully in this review, namely adhesion, cellular aggregation, and the production of an extracellular polymeric matrix. More specifically this review will explore the biosynthesis and role of pili and flagella in Gram-negative adhesion and accumulation on surfaces in *Pseudomonas aeruginosa* and *Escherichia coli*. The process of biofilm maturation is compared and contrasted in both species, namely the production of the exopolysaccharides via the polysaccharide synthesis locus (*Psl*), pellicle Formation (*Pel*) and alginic acid synthesis in *Pseudomonas aeruginosa,* and UDP-4-amino-4-deoxy-L-arabinose and colonic acid synthesis in *Escherichia coli*. An emphasis is placed on the importance of the LuxR homologue *sdiA*; the *luxS*/autoinducer-II; an autoinducer-III/epinephrine/norepinephrine and indole mediated Quorum sensing systems in enabling Gram-negative bacteria to adapt to their environments. The majority of Gram-negative biofilms consist of polysaccharides of a simple sugar structure (either homo- or heteropolysaccharides) that provide an optimum environment for the survival and maturation of bacteria, allowing them to display increased resistance to antibiotics and predation.

Keywords: bacteria; biofilm; biomaterial; Gram-negative; infection; quorum sensing

1. Introduction

Pseudomonas aeruginosa and *Escherichia coli* are the most prevalent Gram-negative biofilm forming medical device associated pathogens [1,2]. Nosocomial infections are estimated to occur annually in 1.75 million hospitalized patients throughout Europe, resulting in 175,000 deaths [3]. *Pseudomonas aeruginosa* accounts for 10%–20% of all hospital-acquired infections [4]. *Pseudomonas aeruginosa* is notoriously difficult to eradicate when colonizing the lungs of cystic fibrosis patients, forming thick antibiotic resistant biofilms that also guard from host immune defenses, lowering of the long-term prognosis of the infected patient [5]. *Escherichia coli* is the most frequently implicated bacteria in urinary catheter related infections, accounting for 50% of such all infections [6,7]. Urinary catheter related infections are the most common form of nosocomial infection with over one million cases a year in the United States alone [7]. In a similar manner to Gram-positive bacteria [8], Gram-negative biofilm formation is determined by the processes of adhesion, cellular aggregation, and the production of an extracellular polymeric matrix with the majority of Gram-negative polysaccharides having a simple structure consisting of either homo- or heteropolysaccharides [9]. The following review will highlight the importance of these stages, and their control at a molecular level, in the production of highly antimicrobial resistant biofilm architectures.

2. Adhesion in the Gram-Negative Bacteria *Pseudomonas aeruginosa* and *Escherichia coli*

The successful adhesion of Gram-negative bacteria to surfaces is largely dependent on the presence of cell appendages such as flagella, pili, and fimbriae [10]. The presence of functional flagella enables the bacterium to swim and overcome repulsive electrostatic forces that may exist between the cell surface and the surface of material or the host's conditioning film [11]. In both *Pseudomonas aeruginosa* and *Escherichia coli* the flagellum-associated hook protein 1 is encoded by the *flgK* gene with a 40% correlation between the nucleotide sequences of the two species [12]. The processes of adhesion and accumulation in both species are outlined below.

2.1. Pseudomonas aeruginosa Adhesion and Accumulation

In *Pseudomonas aeruginosa*, type IV pili aid in surface adhesion. Type IV pili are constructed from a single protein subunit, PilA, that is exported out of the cell by the secretin, PilQ, to form a polymer fimbrial strand. PilA and PilQ are derived from preplins (molecules of short peptide sequences) whose synthesis is positively controlled by the *algR* regulator [13]. The *fimU-pilVWXY1Y2E* operon codes for type IV pili prepilins that gather in the periplasmic space to be cleaved and methylated by type IV prepilin peptidase [14]. Encoded in this sequence are PilY1, PilY2, and the six minor prepilins FimT, FimU, PilV, PilW, PilX, and PilE [15]. Required for pilus biosynthesis, the minor preplins are located in the cell membrane, they are not incorporated into the pili structure and are normally associated with assembly, transport, localization, maturation, and secretion of bacterial proteins [16].

PilY1 and PilY2 are also required for the formation of pili [17]. PilY1 is a large protein located both in the membrane and as part of the pili, with involvement in fimbrial assembly. PilY2 is a small protein involved in fimbrial biosynthesis. The formation of genetic mutants that lack the necessary genes to form flagella and pili/fimbriae have been shown to be surface attachment deficient with little or no biofilm formation when compared to wild-type form, thus highlighting the importance of these bacterial appendages in the adhesion process [11,18].

In *Pseudomonas aeruginosa* type-IV pili are present to aid initial adhesion in combination with two forms of the *O*-polysaccharide chain of lipopolysaccharide, labeled A and B [19]. Makin *et al.*, utilizing *Pseudomonas aeruginosa* PAO1 discovered based on environmental factors that *Pseudomonas aeruginosa* could alter its phenotypic lipopolysaccharide composition to enhance adherence, thus favoring survival and biofilm formation on a variety of biomaterial surfaces. The production of lipopolysaccharide-A increased the hydrophobicity of the cell surface and increased adhesion to hydrophobic surfaces such as polystyrene [19]. The opposite was true of lipopolysaccharide-B with increased hydrophilicity and adhesion to hydrophilic glass observed. After initial adhesion, a monolayer of *Pseudomonas aeruginosa* forms at the material surface. Movement of bacteria across the surface continues via twitching motility carried out by extension and contraction type IV pili [20]. The importance of type IV pili in biofilm architecture is demonstrated by the formation of a capped portion in the mushroom-shaped structures synonymous with *Pseudomonas aeruginosa* biofilms. These occur due to type IV pili-linked bacterial migration [21].

Intercellular adhesion of *Pseudomonas aeruginosa* cells is increased by the production of lectins, such as PA-IL and PA-IIL (also known as LecA and LecB) synthesized in the cytoplasm of planktonic cells [22]. These two internal lectins are synthesized when the cell population cannot support itself, as in the decline phase of bacterial growth or upon subjection to environmental stress. A proportion of the total bacterial population lyses, releasing these internal lectins. These newly available lectins weakly bind to healthy, uncompromised, bacterial cells with adherence to the glycoconjugate substrata. To aid in adherence PA-IL and PA-IIL are positioned in the outer membrane of biofilm bacteria [23]. PA-IL binds preferentially to galactose whereas PA-IIL has a high affinity for monosaccharides especially fucose, thus contributing to biofilm formation [24]. In *Pseudomonas aeruginosa* these lectins are soluble, with evidence to suggest they are involved in both strengthening of established biofilms and adhesion to the airways of cystic fibrosis patients [25]. Competitive inhibition of the lectin binding site, using alternative glycans such as fucose and galactose, has been studied as a potential strategy to reduce *Pseudomonas aeruginosa* exacerbations in cystic fibrosis patients [26]. Delivered as an inhalation therapy, fucose and galactose provided promising results when utilized as monotherapy or in conjunction with intravenous antibiotics. Improved lectin binding affinity was demonstrated when glycans were attached to multivalent dendrimers, suggesting a promising role as future therapeutics [27]. *Rhl* quorum sensing pathways and the stationary phase sigma factor RpoS both directly regulate the transcription of lectin-related genes (*lecA* and *lecB*) in *Pseudomonas aeruginosa* and also serve as potential therapeutic targets in the prevention of *Pseudomonas aeruginosa* biofilm formation [28].

2.2. Escherichia Coli Adhesion and Accumulation

Escherichia coli encode for pili via transcription of the *fim* gene operon with adhesion due partly to the production of type I, type IV and P pili [29]. *Escherichia coli* possess a mannose-specific FimH receptor on the tip of their type I pili that is responsible for invasion and persistence of bacteria in target cells [30]. Mannose-specific receptors aid adhesion to host tissue surfaces such as the bladder epithelium, resulting in cystitis [31]. Evidence provided by Mobley and colleagues showed that *Escherichia coli* isolates from established long-term bacteriuria, greater than 12 weeks, expressed more type I fimbriae (92% of isolates) than those in short term infections of a duration of less than 1 week (59% of isolates) [32]. A study of P fimbriae did not demonstrate persistence in the urinary tract, however proof was provided for an increase in adherence to ureteral stents when isolates possessing P fimbriae were present [33]. These results demonstrate the importance of the bacterial isolate/strain of *Escherichia coli* in the establishment of different infections. Strains of *Escherichia coli* with type I predominate in bladder infections, with P fimbriae strains usually present in kidney infections.

The assembly of type I pili is controlled by the periplasmic FimC protein. FimC accelerates the folding of pilus subunits in the periplasm for delivery to the outer membrane protein FimD, where these subunits then dissociate to form the mature pilus [34] (Figure 1). FimC is termed the periplasmic chaperone and FimD the outer membrane assembly platform or usher, based on how they control type I pili synthesis [35]. FimF and FimG are linear connective proteins present in the fibrillum tip allowing the projection of the adhesin FimH that occurs only on the outer surface of the pilus [36].

As discussed, other forms of pili exist in *Escherichia coli* namely: P pili and type IV pili. P pili are chaperone-usher assembly mediated pili, encoded by the *pap* locus and contain galabiose specific receptors (Gal(α1–4)Gal-) on a distal PapG unit (Figure 2) [37]. This allows *Escherichia coli* to colonize the upper urinary tract, causing pyelonephritis, by binding of galabiose specific receptors (Gal(α1–4)Gal-) to the glycolipid galabiose on urinary tract tissue [38]. The fibrillum tip of P pili is composed of repeating subunits of PapE protein, with the rod consisting of PapA. PapF, PapK, and PapH proteins are also present in low quantities. PapF and PapK act as protein initiators and coordinators for assembly. PapF also acts as a linker in the fibrillum tip to PapG and PapK, thus attaching the fibrillum tip to the rod protein PapA [39]. PapH acts as the rod terminus linking it to the outer membrane surface [40]. The protein PapD acts as the periplasmic chaperone in a similar manner to FimC in type I pili [41] with PapC, like FimD, acting as the outer membrane usher [42]. Type IV pili in *Escherichia coli* are formed independently of a chaperone-usher system and are coded for by the *bfp* operon [43]. Also termed bundle-forming pili, their properties are associated with swarming and twitching motility, unlike type I and P pili, as well as adhesion [44]. Relative to type I and P pili, the formation of type IV pili is less characterized. Ramer and colleagues discovered that a *bfp* encoded assembly complex spans the entire periplasmic space and associated proteins, such as BfpU and BfpL, are present at both the inner and outer membranes [45]. They observed that a type IV related assembly complex consisted of an inner membrane component composed of three pilin-like proteins, BfpI, BfpJ and BfpK. These proteins were localized with BfpE, BfpL, and BfpA forming the major pilin subunit. BfpI, BfpJ, and BfpK were also associated with an outer membrane, secretin-like component, BfpB and BfpG, and a periplasmic component composed of BfpU. Together they create the bundle-forming pilus.

Figure 1. The assembly of the type I pilus. The periplasmic protein FimC binds secreted pilus subunits, from the SecYEG translocon based in the internal membrane, to the periplasm. A process of accelerated subunit folding by FimC (periplasmic chaperone) occurs, followed by delivery to the usher outer assembly platform FimD, also performed by FimC. These FimC-subunit complexes are recognized and bind to the *N*-terminal domain of the usher: $FimD_N$. Uncomplexed FimC is then released to the periplasm when subunits are assembled into the pilus. The tip of the pilus (fibrillum) consists of the protein adhesins FimF, FimG, and FimH, with FimA forming the bulk of the pilus rod. Adapted from Capitani, 2006 [37].

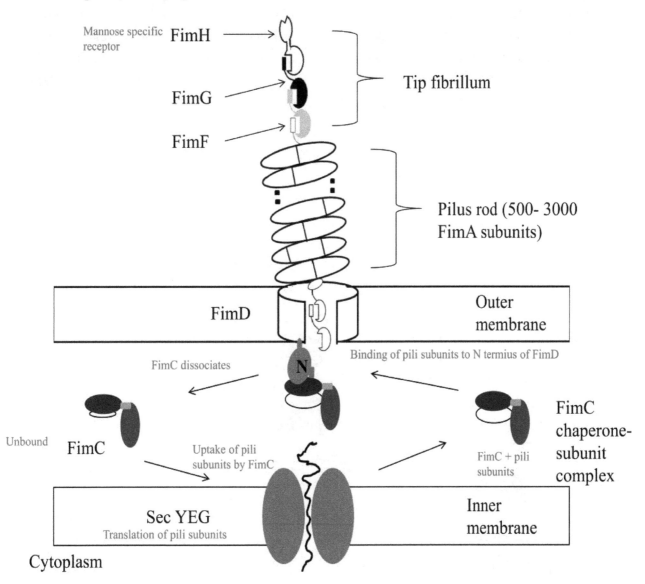

Figure 2. Structure of *Escherichia coli* Type P pili encompassing the PapG unit containing galabiose specific receptors (Gal(α1–4)Gal-) for attachment to urinary tract tissue. The pilus is anchored to the membrane by PapH, whose location is yet to be characterized fully but has been hypothesized by Verger and colleagues to terminate the pilus structure at the base as shown, allowing anchoring to the membrane [46]. Type P pili subunits enter the periplasm by the Sec transport system. In the presence of PapD, stable chaperone-subunit complexes are formed via attachment to the hydrophobic C-terminus of pili subunits [47]. PapD acts as the chaperone to assemble and deliver pili subunits to the outer membrane usher PapC. PapC is a pore forming protein that facilitates pilus assembly by creating a narrow channel across the outer membrane. Assembly of subunits from the outer membrane PapC occurs through a donor strand exchange mechanism. PapA forms a tightly wound helix fiber on the external cell and provides a driving force for the translocation of pili subunits across the outer membrane, facilitating outward pilus growth [48]. Adapted from Mu and Bullitt, 2006 [48] and Mu, 2005 [49].

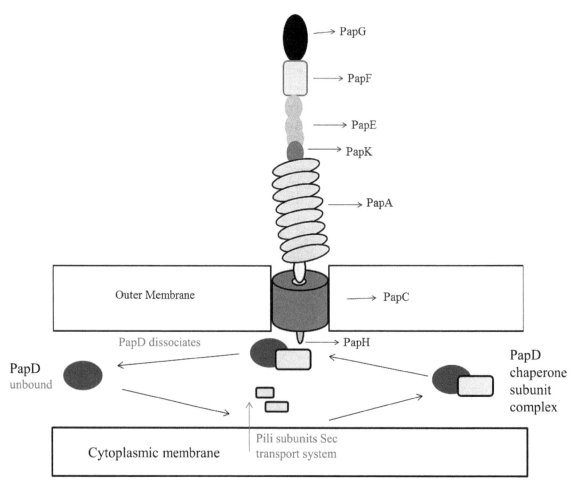

Curli fibers are organelles associated with the early stages of *Escherichia coli* adhesion and virulence. They consist of proteinaceous adhesive filaments that form a coil-like structure on the surface of *Salmonella* and *Escherichia coli*. They have an affinity for proteins such as fibronectin and are responsible for cell to cell adhesion [50]. The production of curli fibers is regulated by transcription of the *csgD* gene. CsgD protein is derived from the LuxR family of transcriptional regulators and is the activator and transcription regulator of the *csgBAC* gene operon. It is at the *csgBAC* gene loci that the protein subunits that form curli fibers are encoded [51]. CsgD also controls cellulose production, through *adrA* gene transcription, which itself is linked to the formation of an extracellular matrix [52]. Control of curli production is a very complex process with two separate gene loci required for effective curli synthesis and multiple regulatory pathways controlling their expression [53,54]. The *csgDEFG* operon encodes both the transcription of CsgD and also a curli-specific transport system mediated by CsgEFG proteins. The curli structural subunits, encoded by upregulation of the *csgBAC* gene locus, are produced in the presence of cellular and environmental stress such as low temperature (<32 °C), lack of nutrients, low osmolarity, and iron shock [55–57]. Limited expression of curli related genes, such as the *csgA* gene, correlates to reduced biofilm formation due to a lowering in production of the main curlin protein subunit CsgA [58]. Their importance as therapeutic targets is demonstrated by the work of Cegelski and colleagues [59]. They produced a series of ring-fused 2-pyridone containing peptidomimetic molecules (FN075 and BibC6), which prevented macromolecular assembly of the major curli subunit protein CsgA and inhibited *Escherichia coli* curli biogenesis. This resulted in reduced *Escherichia coli* colonization in the bladder of *in vivo* mouse models. These so-called curlicides also prevented type I pilus biogenesis via blockage of the FimC chaperone. Delivery of such molecules at therapeutically relevant concentrations remains a challenge that prohibits their clinical development. Changes in environmental stresses affect biofilm formation in *Escherichia coli* via the two-component regulatory system CpxA/CpxR. The CpxA/CpxR system negatively controls the transcription of the *csg*, *pap*, *bfp,* and *flgM* (*flg* are involved in flagella protein transcription and motility together with *fli*) operons [60]. CpxA is a histidine kinase involved in the transfer of a phosphate group to the regulatory protein CpxR, allowing it to bind specifically to sequences of bacterial DNA that regulate gene transcription [61]. The CpxA/CpxR system senses changes in the environmental surroundings of the periplasm, outer membrane, and bacterial envelope. Activation occurs at low nutrient concentrations, high osmolarity and high temperatures due to their effects on lipopolysaccharide and exopolysaccharide biosynthesis and the outer membrane structure [62,63]. Transcription of *CpxA/CpxR* system genes is controlled by the general stress response factor RpoS (stationary phase sigma factor) [64]. RpoS, also known as the alternative subunit of RNA polymerase (σ^S), is a protein encoded by the *rpoS* gene that controls the overall response of *Escherichia coli* to environmental stress, with a sharp increase in concentrations shown at the onset of the stationary phase of growth [65]. Negative regulation of curli occurs by binding of phosphorylated CpxR to the *csgD* promoter therefore switching *csgD* expression off. In mature biofilm cells a majority of CpxA/CpxR are activated [66]. The events of initial adhesion have already occurred; therefore many of the adhesion-related appendages are not required. CpxA/CpxR expression correlates to an upregulation of genes corresponding to resistance pathways, such as the *mdtA* gene, responsible for the efflux and resistance against many β-lactam antibiotics [67]. Therefore the positive role of CpxA/CpxR is more likely to be associated with dormant or persister *Escherichia coli* cells. CpxA/CpxR is unlikely to be associated with the dispersal of biofilm cells, to facilitate recolonization of new surfaces, as genes related to motility such as flagella-related genes (*flgM*) have also been shown to be downregulated by the CpxA/CpxR system [68].

Positive regulation of curli fiber production is controlled by the EnvZ/OmpR two-component regulatory system. The OmpR protein binds to the same promoter region of *csgD* as CpxR but it is still not fully established whether they actively compete for this binding site [69]. EnvZ is a histidine kinase that controls the phosphorylation and binding-affinity of OmpR to CsgD, with phosphorylation in the presence of environmental stimuli such as high osmolarity [70]. CpxA plays a similar activating role with CpxR via a process of phosphorylation [71]. Most recently Ogasawara and colleagues analyzed mRNA of mutant *Escherichia coli* and *csgD* to indicate that CpxR and H-NS acted as repressor molecules with OmpR, an acid-stress response regulator termed RstA and IHF acting as activators within a five component system. They concluded these five factors bonded to the same narrow gene operon region of approximately 200 base pairs, upstream from the *csgD* promoter [72]. Despite the promising results obtained, the biomolecular and transcription mechanism of the *csgD* operon has not been fully elucidated. Their work showed the presence of competitive positive and negative factors but also cooperation between the positive and negative factor groups. Regulation of the *csg* loci is also controlled by the global regulatory gene *hns* [73]. The gene regulator *hns* has an established negative effect on adhesion due to upregulation of genes responsible for flagella synthesis, in comparison to *ompR,* the conclusive positive regulator of curli production [69,74].

3. Biofilm Maturation in *Pseudomonas Aeruginosa* and *Escherichia Coli*

Accumulation and ultimately maturation of the biofilm corresponds to the increased production of the major extracellular polymeric substance alginate in *Pseudomonas aeruginosa* [75] and colanic acid in *Escherichia coli* [76]. These compounds are important in forming the respective biofilm architecture of these microorganisms but they are not essential for biofilm formation to occur. Both species exhibit similar three-dimensional structures possessing water channels; micro and macrocolonies of significant heterogeneity and a thick biofilm matrix. Both microorganisms display downregulation of genes required for motility apparatus, specifically flagella-related genes, and upregulation in genes for extracellular polymeric substance production in the maturation stage of growth [77]. Bacterial maturation in both these Gram-negative bacteria is tightly controlled by quorum sensing systems involving *N*-acyl-l-homoserine lactone as signaling molecules, together with long-chain hydrocarbon structures derived from fatty acids, fatty acid methyl esters, peptides, γ-butyrolactones, 2-alkyl-4-quinolones, furanones, and the 4,5-dihydroxy-2,3-pentandione derivatives, collectively referred to as autoinducer-II and autoinducer-III [78–82].

3.1. Pseudomonas aeruginosa Biofilm Maturation: Production of Exopolysaccharides via the Polysaccharide Synthesis Locus (Psl), Pellicle Formation (Pel), and Alginic Acid Synthesis

The extracellular polymeric substance of *Pseudomonas aeruginosa* biofilm, in line with the majority of bacterial biofilms, consists mainly of polysaccharide, proteins, and nucleic acids [83–85]. In mucoid strains of *Pseudomonas aeruginosa*, isolated from cystic fibrosis patients, the most prevalent exopolysaccharide produced is alginic acid, an *O*-acetylated linear polymer of β-1,4-linked D-mannuronic acid with a C-5 epimer, L-guluronic acid [86]. Interestingly non-mucoid strains have been shown to contain low levels of alginate, with biofilm formation retained [87]. Only 1% of strains isolated from sites other than the lungs of cystic fibrosis patients are mucoid [88], therefore in relation to medical device related infection, alginic acid is not necessarily the most common exopolysaccharide present.

3.1.1. Production of the Psl and Pel Exopolysaccharides by Non-Mucoid *Pseudomonas aeruginosa*

Adherence, aggregation, maturation, and formation of the biofilm architecture are also due to production the exopolysaccharides Psl and Pel. The proteins, enzymes, and transporter molecules required for Psl and Pel synthesis and pellicle formation (thin biofilm surrounding cells that assembles at the air-liquid interface) are encoded by the genes *pslA-O* and *pelA-G,* respectively, in *Pseudomonas aeruginosa* PAO1 [89]. Upon analysis of PelA-G proteins it was observed that PelA is a cytosolic protein and an oligogalacturonide lyase; Pel B functions as an outer membrane protein; PelC is a glycosyltransferase present in the periplasm; both PelD and PelE are large cytosolic proteins located on the inner membrane, with PelD an inner membrane located transmembrane protein; PelF is a glycosyltransferases and PelG is a 12-transmembrane inner membrane protein [90].

Psl proteins are not as well defined in the literature as Pel in terms of individual functions [91]. PslA was identified as a putative UDP-glucose carrier protein essential to biofilm formation in strains of *Pseudomonas aeruginosa* such as PAO1 [92]. Observations of the extracellular polymeric substances present in *Pseudomonas aeruginosa* PAO1 show that the main carbohydrate constituents are glucose, mannose, and rhamnose and not the alginic acid components mannuronate or guluronate [93]. Psl is rich in sugars, particularly mannose, with glucose, galactose, rhamnose, and a limited quantity of xylose also present [91]. The gene locus *pslA-G* is present in some strains, for example *Pseudomonas aeruginosa* PAO1, but not PA14 strains [94,95]. Pel is a glucose-rich polymer and although the genes encoding its production (*pel*) have been shown to be present in all identified strains of *Pseudomonas aeruginosa*, their expression is limited in laboratory conditions [94]. Psl is located mainly in the peripheral regions of the biofilm matrix and may have a role in attracting free-flowing planktonic bacteria to form part of the biofilm structure [84,96]. The reason for this peripheral localization is, as yet, unproven but an increase in nutrients; metabolism; DNA and protein synthesis at the outer extremities of the biofilm and/or a breakdown of Psl in the center of the matrix by the production of enzymes may contribute to this observation [97]. An interesting study by DiGiandomenico and co-workers highlighted the potential of monoclonal antibodies in combating exopolysaccharides such as Psl [98]. By performing phenotypic screening they discovered that Psl was an antibody-accessible antigen that allowed targeted monoclonal antibody mediated opsonophagocytic killing of *Pseudomonas aeruginosa*. Reduced bacterial attachment was shown with cultured lung epithelial cells and prophylactic protection provided in infected animal models. Use of such techniques may have potential for future prophylaxis against *Pseudomonas aeruginosa* infections in high-risk patients.

The production of the secondary messenger molecule bis-(3',5')-cyclic-dimeric-guanosine monophosphate (c-di-GMP) is linked to the maturation of biofilms and production of exopolysaccharides in many species of bacteria including *Pseudomonas aeruginosa*. Its production is regulated by the action of diguanylate cyclase enzymes. Cleavage of, or a decrease in, c-di-GMP production is linked to the expression of motility factors and virulence, with phosphodiesterases also linked to c-di-GMP degradation [99,100]. High levels of c-di-GMP are associated with an increase in biofilm-related traits (attachment and accumulation) [101]. A c-di-GMP binding site has also been identified on the cytosolic inner membrane protein PelD, therefore linking this molecule to Pel synthesis in *Pseudomonas aeruginosa* [90]. There has been an increasing interest in targeting c-di-GMP, or more specifically the proteins that are involved in the biosynthesis of c-di-GMP, in order to prevent biofilm formation [102]. C-di-GMP is produced from two guanosine triphosphate molecules and its synthesis is controlled by the enzyme diguanylate cyclase [103]. Irie and colleagues recently discovered that although Psl formation is controlled by c-di-GMP, it also acts as a positive feedback signal and stimulates the production of two diguanylate cyclases, SiaD and SadC, resulting in increased formation of c-di-GMP [104]. Eukaryotes do not express diguanylate cyclase, therefore it serves as an excellent target for antibacterial drug development [105]. Analogues of c-di-GMP, for example the monophosphorothioic acid of c-di-GMP (c-GpGps), display antibiofilm activity against *Pseudomonas aeruginosa* and *Staphylococcus aureus in vitro* [106]. Biofilm dispersal and an increased sensitivity to antimicrobials have also been attributed to low concentrations of nitric oxide in *Pseudomonas aeruginosa*. Barraud *et al.* uncovered a possible molecular link between nitrous oxide, reduced levels of c-di-GMP and biofilm dispersion due to an increase in phosphodiesterase activity [107]. C-di-GMP also has potential as a vaccine molecule due to its immunostimulatory and adjuvant properties [108]. The translation of such therapies to clinical practice is limited at present, as the role of c-di-GMP in biofilm formation has not been fully established. Concerns may also exist with regard to the affect such therapies may have on commensal microorganisms.

Extracellular DNA also plays an important role in biofilm maturation and stabilization of non mucoid *Pseudomonas aeruginosa* strains such as PAO1, compensating for a lack of alginate [109]. Matsukawa *et al.* showed that in the matrix of mature *Pseudomonas aeruginosa*, PAO1 extracellular DNA was the most prevalent polymer and that exopolysaccharides were of great importance with regard to structural integrity [85]. Whitchurch and colleagues demonstrated that DNase could dissolve young *Pseudomonas aeruginosa* PAO1 biofilms, but matured biofilms showed only small dissolution. This suggests that early biofilms are held together by extracellular DNA, but mature PAO1 biofilms are held together by other compounds, namely exopolysaccharides [110]. Research by Ma demonstrated extracellular DNA to be present mostly in the stalk region of mature biofilm colonies, and spatially separate from Psl proteins [111]. Differences in the prevalence of extracellular DNA in *in vitro* and *in vivo* biofilms may be attributed to the stage of biofilm growth. Extracellular DNA may also play a role in increasing resistance of biofilm forms of *Pseudomonas aeruginosa* toward cationic antimicrobials, such as antimicrobial peptides. Extracellular DNA is a cation chelator and acts to sequester cations from the surrounding environment. It also plays a role in the modification of the cationic antimicrobial peptide binding site lipid A by the sugar dehydrogenases enzyme UDP-glucose dehydrogenase (Ugd) and covalent binding to 4-amino-4-deoxy-L-arabinose [112].

3.1.2. Production of the Exopolysaccharide Alginic Acid by Mucoid *Pseudomonas aeruginosa*

Slime production by mucoid forming strains of *Pseudomonas aeruginosa* is important for the colonization of both medical devices and cell surfaces, such as the lungs in cystic fibrosis patients [113]. The formation of this slime, composed of mainly alginic acid, is important in protecting *Pseudomonas aeruginosa* from antimicrobials and host defense mechanisms by restricted penetration of these molecules through the biofilm matrix [114]. Synthesis of alginic acid, commonly known as alginate, is controlled by the *algACD* operon present in *Pseudomonas aeruginosa*. Upregulation of alginate-related genes is dependent on multiple environmental factors including: high oxygen concentration, high osmolarity, lack of nitrogen, and the presence of ethanol [115,116]. In general the production of alginic acid by the *algACD* gene locus is similar to the regulation of the *icaADBC* operon, responsible for polysaccharide intercellular adhesin production in staphylococci.

Of high importance to alginic acid production are the *algA*, *algC,* and *algD* genes that transcribe the enzymes required for the production of the alginate precursor guanosine diphosphate (GDP)-mannuronic acid [117]. A combination of the transmembrane transporter proteins Alg44 and Alg8, which are normally not active in non-mucoid *Pseudomonas aeruginosa*, allows the movement of this alginate precursor across the inner membrane for polymerization [118]. AlgA-X are alginate enzymes involved in the polymerization and biosynthesis processes that result in the formation of alginate (Figure 3). The role of alginate lyase, at the maturation stage, is unclear although it may allow the production of short oligomers that prime polymerization and may also allow the breakdown of alginate at the cell detachment phase of biofilm growth [119]. AlgG interacts with AlgK and AlgX. They have an important role in protecting the production of the alginate polymer by forming a scaffold in the periplasm surrounding newly formed polymer molecules [120]. Epimerization of polymerized mannuronate residues is controlled by AlgG, a C-5-epimerase enzyme [121]. Acetylation of these mannuronate residues also occurs via the enzymes AlgF, AlgJ, and AlgI at O2 and/or O3 positions [122]. AlgF is located in the periplasm. AlgJ is a type II membrane protein with an uncleaved signal peptide portion linked to the inner membrane with a remaining portion in the periplasm, whereas AlgI is an integral transmembrane helix that accepts an acetyl group form an unknown donor [123]. When the process of *O*-acetylation is concluded, transportation of alginate out of the cell is mediated by AlgE present on the outer membrane forming the majority of the extracellular polymeric matrix substance of mucoid producing *Pseudomonas aeruginosa* [124].

Figure 3. The synthesis and polymerization mechanism involved in the production of *Pseudomonas aeruginosa* alginate. The letters A–X and numbers 8 and 44 correlate to alginate biosynthetic enzymes that are preceded by Alg (for example A = AlgA). AlgA, AlgC, and AlgD control the production of the alginate precursor GDP-mannuronic acid. Both Alg8 and Alg44 transport this molecule for polymerization in the periplasm. Alginate lysase (AlgL) produces short oligomers that prime polymerization. AlgG interacts with AlgK and AlgX protecting the production of the alginate polymer by forming a scaffold in the periplasm. Epimerization of polymerized mannuronate residues is also controlled by AlgG, a C-5-epimerase. Acetylation of some mannuronate residues occurs via the enzymes AlgF, AlgJ, and AlgI at O2 and/or O3 positions, with AlgE transporting the formed alginate out of the cell. Adapted from Franklin and Ohman 2002 [122], Ramsey 2005 [125], and Gimmestad, 2003 [126].

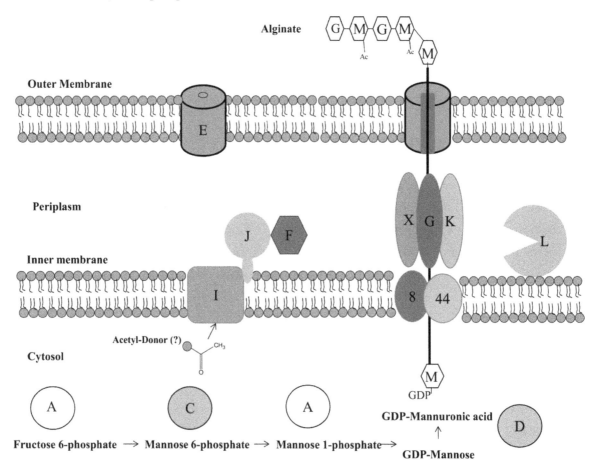

AlgA, AlgC, and AlgD are important enzymes in the production of GDP-mannuronic acid. AlgA is involved in alginate biosynthesis catalyzing both the production of mannose-6-phosphate from fructose-6-phosphate and GDP-mannose from mannose-1-phosphate, as a phosphomannose isomerase and GDP-mannose pyrophosphorylase, respectively [127]. AlgC is a phosphomannomutase and phosphoglucomutae enzyme that catalyses the reversible production of mannose-6-phosphate to mannose-1-phosphate (Figure 3). AlgC has also been shown to be important in lipopolysaccharide synthesis, with its preference for both mannose and glucose containing substrates allowing it to possess a diverse mechanism of action [128].

AlgD is a rate-limiting GDP-mannose dehydrogenase that catalyses the production of GDP-mannuronic acid from GDP-mannose [129]. Control of alginate biosynthesis and the transcription of the Alg proteins are therefore mediated by the *algD* operon, which is responsible for the final production of GDP-mannuronic acid, the foundation molecule for polymerization and alginate synthesis. A regulatory cascade consisting of an alternative sigma factor AlgT, also known as AlgU or σ^{22} and encoded by *algT* controls the transcription of *algD* [130]. Autoregulation of *algT* and upregulation of the alginate-linked gene loci *algR*, *algB*, *algZ* are also performed by σ^{22} [131]. AlgR regulates both *algC* and *algD* transcription by binding to sites upstream of their genes [132]. AlgB also activates *algD* transcription but by an undefined method that has previously been thought to be related to indirect action of the promoter region of *algD* [133]. However, Leech and colleagues observed, through DNA binding and transcriptome analysis, that AlgB bound directly to the promoter region of the *algD* operon [134]. Transcription of *algZ*, also known as *amrZ*, leads to the activation of *algD* by binding to sequences upstream of the *algD* promoter [135]. It also inhibits transcription of the gene loci *fleQ* related to the control of flagella-related genes [136]. This demonstrates the complex systems involved in the transcription of alginate-related genes, such as *algD*, with multiple pathways involved in its transcription.

The action of σ^{22} is itself controlled by the regulatory protein products of *mucABCD* transcription [137]. The inner membrane protein MucA is an anti-sigma factor that complexes to the periplasmic protein MucB. The MucA portion then directly binds to σ^{22} after *algT* transcription to negatively regulate its activity [138]. Rowen *et al.* suggested that σ^{22} associates with the periphery of the inner membrane by interacting with RNA polymerase or MucA, or by an unknown independent mechanism blocking the action of σ^{22} [139]. MucC's role is relatively uncharacterized, however, it is hypothesized to be an inner membrane protein that may act synergistically with both MucA and MucB in the negative regulation of σ^{22} [140]. MucD is an endoprotease that negatively regulates σ^{22} by the removal of activating factors present in σ^{22} [141]. Inactivation of *mucA* or *mucB* via mutations in non-mucoid *Pseudomonas aeruginosa* strains has been shown to induce alginate synthesis leading to an overexpression in alginate-related genes. Clinical isolates from cystic fibrosis patients have also been shown to possess mutations in *mucA*, causing an exponential increase in alginate synthesis [142,143].

3.2. Escherichia coli Biofilm Maturation

The process of biofilm maturation in *Escherichia coli* is very similar to *Pseudomonas aeruginosa* in that genes that encode for flagella mediated motility (*fli* and *flg*) are downregulated with corresponding upregulation of genes corresponding to the exopolysaccharide colanic acid (*wca*), porin (*ompC*) production, tripeptidase T, and synthesis of a nickel and glycine betaine high-affinity transport system [144]. As previously discussed (Section 2.2.), the Cpx/CpxR two component regulatory system, controlled by the general stress response factor RpoS (stationary phase sigma factor) [64], is responsible for the upregulation of many of the genes implicated in biofilm maturation [66].

The production of the exopolysaccharide colanic acid is essential for the maturation and complex three-dimensional structure of *Escherichia coli* biofilms but not the process of initial adhesion [145]. Colanic acid consists of hexasaccharide subunits with a high prevalence of fucose and glucuronic acid [146]. The physical barrier presented by colanic acid production and the negative charge that it possesses allows *Escherichia coli* biofilms to resist large changes in osmotic stress, oxidative stress (by hydrogen peroxide), and temperature [76]. Generally colanic acid is only produced at temperatures above 30 °C and is thought to be important in capsule formation and ultimately survival of *Escherichia coli* outside of the host [147]. The gene operon *wca*, also known as *cps*, encodes for polymerase enzymes that regulate colanic acid synthesis from sugars by a pathways that has not been elucidated fully. The transcription of the *wca* genes is controlled by the *rcsABCF* gene loci, and this pathway is more fully understood. After phosphorylation of the response regulator RcsB by the sensor kinase RscC, the accessory positive regulator RcsA binds to RcsB to form the heterodimer RcsA-RscB, which activates *wca* transcription [148]. RscF is hypothesized to promote the phosphorylation of RscB by RscC [149]. The processes and signals that cause the activation of RscC are relatively unknown [147]. It has been suggested that environmental stimuli, such as osmotic shock, play a role in the upregulation of *rscC* via changes in membrane-bound protein MdoH, which is involved in the production of membrane-derived oligosaccharides [150]. RscC senses changes in these membrane-derived oligosaccharides to initiate a response [151]. RcsA is present normally in low amounts at 37 °C due to low levels of synthesis and the presence of the protease Lon, a negative regulator of *wca* transcription [152]. The minimal level of RcsA production is due transcriptional silencing by the histone-like protein H-NS, that is negated by overproduction of a small RNA molecule known as DsrA [153].

The *wca* operon consists of 19 genes with the third gene in order of transcription being the *wzc* gene. *Wzc* has been shown to encode a membrane bound autophosphorylated protein-tyrosine kinase [154]. Upstream of this *wcz* locus, the *wca* operon codes for a phosphotyrosine phosphatase (PTP), Wcz, that has the ability to specifically dephosphorylate a corresponding protein-tyrosine kinase and is otherwise defined as a BY-kinase, a newly defined group of enzymes involved in protein-tyrosine phosphorylation [155]. Although the mechanism is unclear, dephosphorylation of Wzc tends to lead to increased colonic acid production and provides a means by which exopolysaccharides are transported out of the cell [156]. Wzc has also been shown to phosphorylate the sugar dehydrogenase enzyme Uridine diphosphate (UDP)-glucose dehydrogenase, allowing it to mediate the construction of extracellular polysaccharide precursors, such as UDP-glucuronic acid.

Etk, like Wzc, is a BY-kinase of *Escherichia coli* and is involved in the production of the group IV capsule surrounding the *Escherichia coli* bacterial cell membrane [157]. Etk is coded for by the *etk* gene present on the *ymc* operon of some pathogenic strains of *Escherichia coli* [158]. The mechanism and use of the *ymc* operon itself is unknown, although it could possibly be a promoter of *etk* expression [159]. Etk is also involved in the phosphorylation of UDP-glucose dehydrogenase allowing for the production of UDP-4-amino-4-deoxy-L-arabinose, a compound that allows *Escherichia coli* to become resistant to cationic antimicrobial peptides and polymixin-B [159].

The two-component systems PhoP/PhoQ and PmrA/PmrB are induced by limitation of magnesium and calcium ions or the RcsA/RcsB/RcsC system leading to upregulation of the genes involved in UDP-4-amino-4-deoxy-L-arabinose biosynthesis. The gene loci *arn* is controlled by both the PhoP/PhoQ and PmrA/PmrB pathways. Transcription of *arn* leads to the synthesis of UDP-4-amino-4-deoxy-L-arabinose via *arn*-linked enzymes, however synthesis of UDP-4-amino-4-deoxy-L-arabinose is also due to RcsA/RcsB/RcsC or PhoP/PhoQ and PmrA/PmrB mediated transcription of *ugd*. The protein Ugd, when phosphorylated via Etk, forms UDP-Glucuronic acid from the precursor UDP-Glucose. Formation of UDP-4-amino-4-deoxy-L-arabinose is mediated by a series of *arn* encoded enzymes [160]. Meredith *et al.* hypothesized that Ugd synthesis of colonic acid (in this case defined as M-antigen) also affects the production of lipopolysaccharides in the cell membrane via the formation of a complex lipopolysaccharide glycoform termed M_{LPS} [161]. Resistance develops against cationic antimicrobial peptides and polymyxin due to covalent modifications of lipid A, the hydrophobic anchor of the lipopolysaccharide membrane and the cationic antimicrobial binding site, by UDP-4-amino-4-deoxy-L-arabinose [160].

4. Quorum Sensing in Gram-Negative Bacteria: *Pseudomonas aeruginosa* and *Escherichia coli*

Quorum sensing is a system whereby bacterial cells communicate in order to act as a community of cells. This maximizes the potential of their mutualistic survival strategies, allowing selective benefits to be conferred to the bacterial population that would otherwise not be present as individual cells. Quorum sensing is of great importance in the production of bacterial biofilms and the up and down regulation of related genes [7].

4.1. Quorum Sensing in Pseudomonas aeruginosa

In *Pseudomonas aeruginosa* there are currently three identified quorum sensing systems. These are; the *las*-based system controlled via *N*-(3-oxododecanoyl)-L-homoserine lactone production by *lasRI* gene loci [162]; the *rhl* system regulated by *N*-butyryl-homoserine lactone produced by the *rhlRI* operon [163] and the *pqs* system that controls the *las* and *rhl* quorum sensing through 2-heptyl-3-hydroxy-4-quinolone production [164]. The *rhl* system is controlled by the *las* system as LasR-*N*-(3-oxododecanoyl)-L-homoserine lactone activates the transcription of *rhlR* and *rhlI* meaning these two systems are interlinked [165].

As for all microorganisms that demonstrate quorum sensing pathways, these signals allow for the control of phenotypic expressions such as virulence, biofilm formation, and resistance to antimicrobials [166]. In *Pseudomonas aeruginosa* quorum sensing controls the production of exoenzymes and secreted toxins, such as elastase and exotoxin A [162,167,168], and also directs biofilm formation [169]. Cells lacking in the *las* system have been shown to be flat rather than the atypical mushroom-like shape of mature *Pseudomonas aeruginosa* biofilms, with increased sensitivity to antibiotics also demonstrated [168]. It is hypothesized that the transcription of the exopolysaccharide-related *pelA-G* gene loci is controlled indirectly by *las* and *rhl* quorum sensing systems through transcriptional factors; however this process is as yet largely undefined [170]. Quorum sensing has also been shown to regulate the production of extracellular DNA in *Pseudomonas aeruginosa* biofilms [83]. The most defined quorum sensing pathways in *Pseudomonas aeruginosa* are the *las* and *rhl* systems.

The *las* system comprises of the transcriptional activator protein LasR and the autoinducer synthase enzyme LasI, coded for by *lasR* and *lasI,* respectively. The transcription of *lasI* results in the formation of the enzyme LasI that directs the synthesis of *N*-(3-oxododecanoyl)-L-homoserine lactone, an important acyl-homoserine lactone of *Pseudomonas aeruginosa*, otherwise known as autoinducer-III [171]. Increased cell density of *Pseudomonas aeruginosa* correlates to an increase in autoinducer-III concentration and when a threshold value is reached the binding of autoinducer-III to its specific target protein LasR will result in the transcription of multiple virulent and biofilm-related genes mediated by *las*. These genes include those responsible for the production of multiple enzymes such as exotoxin A (*toxA*), elastase (*lasB*), the LasA protease (*lasA*), and alkaline protease (*aprA*) [172]. The binding of autoinducer-III to LasR also results in further transcription of *lasI*, thus proving *N*-(3-oxododecanoyl)-L-homoserine lactone to be an autoinducing peptide [173]. The activation of the *las* system also results in activation of the *rhl* quorum sensing system, resulting in the production of a second autoinducer *N*-butyryl-homoserine lactone. It is therefore believed, through this mechanism, that the *las* system controls regulatory protein (RhlR) production both before and after transcription [163,173].

The *rhl* system consists of the transcriptional activator protein RhlR and the synthase RhlI that regulate *N*-butyryl-homoserine lactone production [165]. The *rhl* pathway is responsible for the production of amphiphilic biosurfactants, known as rhamnolipids (heat stable haemolysin), in the latter stages of biofilm development that aid in the maintenance of macrocolonies and fluid-filled channels [174]. The *rhl* system is also responsible for the production of multiple extracellular enzymes along with secondary metabolites such as pyocyanin, hydrogen cyanide and pyoverdin [175]. In *Pseudomonas aeruginosa* there is a high correlation between biofilm architecture and quorum sensing, with little or no influence on biofilm adhesion and motility [176].

Figure 4. The *las*, *pqs,* and *rhl* interlinked quorum sensing systems in *Pseudomonas aeruginosa*. The *las* system consists of the proteins LasR (transcriptional activator) and LasI (synthase enzyme) coded for by *lasR* and *lasI* respectively. The *rhl* system consists of RhlR (transcriptional activator) and RhlI (synthase enzyme) coded for by *rhlR* and *rhlI*. Adapted from Raina, 2009 [177].

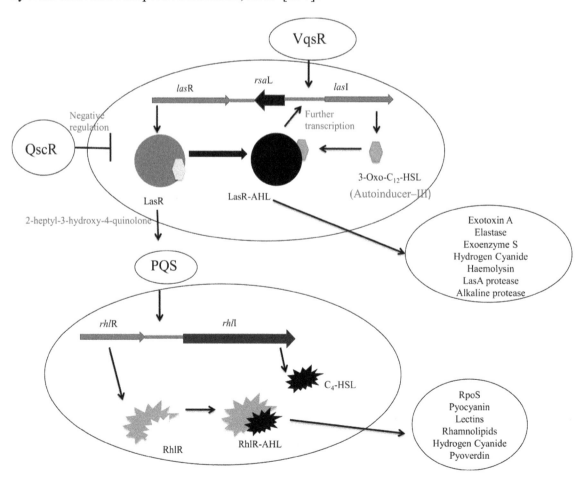

The third quorum sensing system identified in *Pseudomonas aeruginosa* is the *pqs* system that utilizes 2-heptyl-3-hydroxy-4-quinolone, also known as *Pseudomonas* quinolone signal. The *pqs* system has particular importance for the production of *rhl*-dependent exoproducts at the beginning of the stationary phase of growth [177]. The production of 2-heptyl-3-hydroxy-4-quinolone is related to the activation of *lasR* and is therefore thought to operate between the *las* and *rhl* systems (Figure 4) [178]. The 2-heptyl-3-hydroxy-4-quinolone molecule differs from that of acyl-homoserine lactone in that it is capable of overcoming cell density dependent production of exoproducts but not growth-phase dependent production [179]. *Pseudomonas aeruginosa* mutants defective at producing 2-heptyl-3-hydroxy-4-quinolone have lower levels of exoproducts but similar levels of the lectin adhesin PA-IL as the wild type [180]. By supplying exogenous 2-heptyl-3-hydroxy-4-quinolone exoproduct levels are restored to wild type [181]. The similar levels of lectin adhesin (PA-IL) present in mutant defective *Pseudomonas aeruginosa* suggest its control via *lecA* transcription may be due in part to an alternative system, namely the stationary phase sigma factor RpoS [28].

The *las* system is regulated directly by a variety of complex factors. Two LuxR homologues, known as quorum sensing control repressor (QscR) and virulence quorum sensing regulator (VqsR), are responsible for the negative and positive regulation of the *las* system, respectively, by unquantified mechanisms [182]. It is hypothesized that QscR negatively regulates *las* by repressing *lasI* transcription in the lag phase of growth when the concentration of autoinducing signal molecules has not reached its threshold for quorum sensing activation. QscR is thought to achieve repression by forming heterodimers of both LasR and RglR that are inactive but compete with acyl-homoserine lactones for binding to their relative cognate response regulator up to the threshold concentration. Above the threshold concentration these heterodimers dissociate allowing the formation of active LasR and RhlR homodimers [183].

VqsR allows positive regulation of quorum sensing pathways. Mutant strains of *Pseudomonas aeruginosa*, with no *vqsR* gene, show a lack of acyl-homoserine lactone production corresponding to a reduction in virulence and pathogenicity by an as yet unestablished mechanism [182]. The complexity of quorum sensing control is shown by the multitude of factors controlling its regulation. RsaI is a transcriptional regulator that acts to block *lasI* transcription by competitively binding to LasI and thus preventing LasR-*N*-(3-oxododecanoyl)-L-homoserine lactone complexes from autoinducing LasI production [172]. This is likely to occur below threshold concentrations of *N*-(3-oxododecanoyl)-L-homoserine lactone in response to an uncharacterized environmental or metabolic stimulus [184,185]. There are a variety of accounts in the literature were synthetic derivatives of *N*-L-homoserine lactones result in inhibition of quorum sensing pathways and reduced biofilm development. Of particular relevance is the study by Hentzer and colleagues [186]. They demonstrated that synthesized compounds based on natural furanones were shown to be potent antagonists of *las* and *rhl* quorum sensing in *Pseudomonas aeruginosa*. Similarly Geske *et al.* synthesized small molecular weight, non-native *N*-L-homoserine lactone derivatives that blocked natural signals via binding to LasR in *Pseudomonas aeruginosa* [187].

4.2. RpoS and Quorum Sensing

RpoS, also known as the alternative subunit of RNA polymerase or the stationary phase sigma factor, is a protein encoded by the *rpoS* gene and controls the overall response of both *Pseudomonas aeruginosa* and *Escherichia coli* to environmental stress. A sharp increase in RpoS concentration has been demonstrated at the onset of the stationary phase of growth [75]. In *Pseudomonas aeruginosa*, mutation of *rpoS* leads to enhanced susceptibility of stationary-phase cells to heat, high osmolarity, acidic (low) pH, hydrogen peroxide, and ethanol [188]. The stationary phase sigma factor RpoS is also controlled directly by the *rhl* system and therefore indirectly by *las*, enabling the quorum sensing control of genes at the stationary phase [165,188–190]. Their interaction is complex, a relationship has been observed but no obvious mechanism apparent. Whiteley *et al.* suggest RpoS is responsible for negatively regulating *rhlI* transcription, especially in hydrogen cyanide (*hcnABC*) and phenazine (*phzABC*) genes [190]. The production of the lectin adhesin PA-IL and possibly PA-IL, encoded by *lecA* and *lecB*, respectively, are mediated both directly by the *rhl*-dependent regulation of the *lecA* and indirectly by *rhl* though RpoS [28]. Other studies, such as those by Medina *et al.*, suggest RpoS partially activate the *rhlAB* genes that transcribe rhamnolipid production with a possibility that RpoS activates quorum sensing linked genes required in the stationary phase only [191]. Schuster *et al.* proposed that RpoS acts by repressing *rhlI* at the log phase of growth thus decreasing *N*-butyryl-homoserine lactone production, with loss of this repression at the late logarithmic to stationary phase of growth [192].

4.3. Quorum Sensing in Escherichia coli

Quorum sensing in *Escherichia coli* occurs via four different systems; the LuxR homologue *sdiA* system [193,194]; the *luxS*/autoinducer-II system [195]; an autoinducer-III/epinephrine/norepinephrine system [78], and an indole mediated system [196].

4.3.1. sdiA Quorum Sensing System

The *sdiA* quorum sensing system provides a means by which *Escherichia coli* can sense the autoinducer *N*-acyl-l-homoserine lactone from other species of microorganisms. SdiA is a LuxR homologue that binds to *N*-acyl-l-homoserine lactone and has links to the upregulation of the cell division gene operon *ftsQAZ* [197]. In other microorganisms, such as *Vibrio fischeri*, the LuxI protein [198] (encoded by *luxI*) allows the formation of *N*-acyl-l-homoserine lactone. The *luxI* gene is not present in *Escherichia coli* and thus *N*-acyl-l-homoserine lactone must be synthesized by other microorganisms [199]. This quorum sensing system of importance to *Escherichia coli* is present in the gut microflora, where other species of *N*-acyl-l-homoserine lactone producing bacteria are prevalent. Nature is proving to be a ubiquitous source of quorum sensing inhibitors. Research performed recently by Ravichandiran demonstrated that extracts from seeds of the Melia dubia plant contained compounds that competitively inhibited SdiA, resulting in reduced biofilm formation in *Escherichia coli* [200]. Other natural sources of quorum sensing inhibitors include garlic, marine algae, and soil bacteria [201–203]. Difficulties remain with regard to identification, structural elucidation, isolation, and purification of natural sourced components.

4.3.2. *luxS* Quorum Sensing System

The *luxS* system in *Escherichia coli* has autoinducer-II as its mediating quorum-sensing molecule, and synthesis of autoinducer-II is as described for the staphylococcal *luxS* system [7]. The *luxS* system may also have a role in cell metabolism through the intracellular activated methyl cycle, together with up and downregulation of quorum sensing-related genes [80,204]. Concentration of extracellular autoinducer-II reaches a peak at the mid- to late-exponential phase with a large decrease as bacteria enter the stationary phase, but there is no relative decrease in LuxS protein levels at the stationary phase of growth [205,206]. Decrease in the concentration of extracellular autoinducer-II, at the onset of the stationary phase, corresponds to an increase in autoinducer-II uptake into cells via an ATP-binding cassette deemed the Lsr transporter that is itself *luxS*-regulated [206]. Uptake of autoinducer-II, via an alternative active transport mechanism or diffusion, may be due to the bacteria requiring autoinducer-II to regulate gene expression and therefore switch off external metabolic and cellular responses. The Lsr transporter is encoded by the *lsrABCD* operon, with LsrB required for autoinducer-II transport into the cell, and whose transcription itself is regulated via the proteins LsrK and LsrR (transcribed from *lsrRK* operon) [207]. LsrK, present in the cytoplasm, is a kinase that donates a phosphate group to autoinducer-II, allowing the phosphorylated autoinducer-II to bind to the *lsr* repressor LsrR (Figure 5). Phosphorylation may act to sequester autoinducer-II activity within the cell, although its purpose is generally undefined [193]. Mutants of *lsrK*, deficient in LsrK production, have shown the Lsr transporter to be repressed, thus autoinducer-II remains in the extracellular fluid [207]. Mutants of *lsrR* express Lsr transporter and therefore autoinducer-II is imported into the cell cytoplasm continuously [208].

LsrK and LsrR are both quorum sensing regulators. A study of how the separate deletion of each corresponded to the resulting phenotypic profile was conducted by Li *et al.* [209]. They observed that genes associated with adhesion, such as the curli-related genes CsgA, CsgE, CsgF, and CsgG, together with the pili gene *htrE*, a homolog of *papD*, were all downregulated with increased intracellular autoinducer-II in *lsrR* mutants [210,211]. In *lsrK* mutants, fimbrial genes were downregulated with two putative fimbrial proteins, *yadK* and *yadN*, repressed. The large complexity of colonic acid synthesis and *luxS* quorum sensing in general is shown by upregulation of the *wza* gene in both mutants with *wcaA* upregulation in *lsrR* mutants corresponding to an increase in intracellular autoinducer-II. The complexity involved in having extracellular and intracellular, as well as both quorum sensing and metabolic roles for autoinducer-II, is further demonstrated by the work of DeLisa *et al.* [212]. They observed that autoinducer-II upregulated a series of genes involved in fimbriae (*yadK* and *yadN*, putative fimbrial proteins), curli fiber (*crl*, the transcriptional regulator of cryptic *csgA* gene), and colonic acid production (*wzb*, a probable protein-tyrosine-phosphatase and *rscB*), with associated down regulation of genes linked to flagella synthesis (*flgN*). No link to either the intracellular or extracellular action of autoinducer-II was provided.

Figure 5. Summary of the *LuxS* Quorum sensing system of *Escherichia coli*. Autoinducer-II, represented by pentagons, is formed from a LuxS catalyzed cleavage reaction of *S*-ribosylhomocysteine to 4,5-dihydroxy 2,3-pentanedione and homocysteine [213]. Key: AIP-II: Autoinducer-II: ● DPD: 4,5-dihydroxy-2,3-pentanedione. Adapted from Li, 2007 [184].

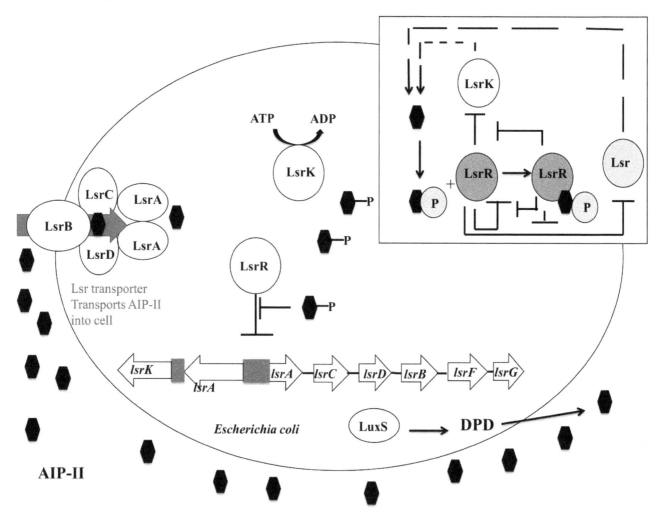

Further reactions form autoinducer-II. LsrR acts as the autoinducer-II uptake repressor repressing the *lsrACDBFG* and *lsrRK* operons [207]. At early and mid-exponential phases, the intracellular and extracellular autoinducer-II levels are low, thus LsrR can bind to and repress these genes [206]. As the levels of autoinducer-II increase extracellularly, active transport and diffusion of this molecule into the cell occurs by an uncharacterized non-Lsr related pathway [195]. Non-phosphorylated autoinducer-II binds to LsrR to depress many quorum sensing and biofilm forming genes including; *lsrR* itself; *flu* which is responsible for the phase-variable protein antigen 43 linked to autoaggregation; *wza* the gene linked to colonic acid synthesis; *dsrA* which encodes a small RNA molecule known as DsrA resulting in increased RcsA and upregulation of the colonic acid producing *wca* operon [153]. Lsr autoinducer-II uptake remains repressed until the late exponential phase whereby a threshold concentration of autoinducer-II is reached, corresponding to nutrient depletion, and leading to rapid autoinducer-II uptake by the Lsr transporter. Autoinducer-II is phosphorylated by LsrK (boxed section) with binding of this molecule to LsrR causing a cessation of *lsr* repression [214]. Transcription of the *lsr* operon acts as a positive feedback loop, importing more autoinducer-II in response to detection of phosphorylated autoinducer-II [215]. This leads to a relative decrease in LsrR/autoinducer-II quorum sensing and an increase in the LsrR/Phosphorylated autoinducer-II quorum sensing system, triggering the expression of biofilm linked genes.

4.3.3. Autoinducer-III/Epinephrine/Norepinephrine and Indole Quorum Sensing Systems

The LuxS enzyme is also responsible for the formation of another 4,5-dihydroxy-2,3-pentandione derivative, autoinducer-III [216]. This system is present within enterohemorrhagic *Escherichia coli,* which causes bloody diarrhoea linked to haemorrhagic colitis and haemolytic-uremic syndrome [217]. The formation of autoinducer-III is not fully reliant on LuxS. A *luxS* mutation leaves the cell with only one pathway to produce homocysteine, a molecule required for autoinducer-III synthesis, and produced by other microorganisms present as part of the normal microbial gut flora [218]. Autoinducer-III is not linked directly to biofilm formation in *Escherichia coli.* Its use is mainly focused on genes related to virulence factors, adhesion in the large intestine (*LEE* operon and attaching and effacing lesions) and motility (flagella) [219]. The catecholamine class of hormones also act as agonists to this system, in particular epinephrine and norepinephrine, which are produced by the colonized host [78,220]. The autoinducer-III/epinephrine/norepinephrine quorum sensing system involves a set of regulon. The QsecC regulon autophosphorylates in the presence of both autoinducer-III and epinephrine, phosphorylating the QseB response regulator to activate the genes responsible for flagella synthesis [221]. The attaching and effacing lesions required for intestinal attachment are controlled by a similar QseE and QseF system [222]. Two LysR transcriptional factors, QseA and QseD control *LEE* transcription [223]. The indole mediated quorum sensing signal is thought to allow *Escherichia coli* to adapt to environments where nutrients are poor and the breakdown of amino acids serves as an energy source. Indole itself is formed from the breakdown of tryptophan by the tryptophanase enzyme encoded by the *tna* gene. The production of indole activates this *tna* gene and also the *astD* and *gabT* genes, which code for enzymes that control the degradation of amino acids to pyruvate or succinate [196,224].

5. Conclusions

The biomolecular processes that govern biofilm formation in Gram-negative *Escherichia coli* and *Pseudomonas aeruginosa* display intricate differences and are excellent examples as to the complexities that govern the survival of microbial communities. Antimicrobial resistance is increasing worldwide. This together with a relative lack of innovative antimicrobials being released to the pharmaceutical market has led to real concerns from the World Health Organization. Their 2014 global report on surveillance of antimicrobial resistance outlined the real possibility of a future whereby common infections and minor injuries can kill, including those by Gram-negative bacteria such as *Escherichia coli* [225]. Biofilm formation is one of the most important phenotypic traits in determining the resistance characteristics of microbial communities to current therapeutic strategies [226]. Therefore a comprehensive understanding of the biomolecular mechanisms allows targeted therapies to be developed in order to prevent the development of, or to eradicate, established biofilms. Thereby limiting pathogenicity in areas such as medical device related infections. O'Loughlin and colleagues recently demonstrated that small synthetically produced molecules, such as meta-bromo-thiolactone, were able to inhibit both *Pseudomonas aeruginosa* LasR and RhlR *in vitro* and *in vivo* resulting in inhibition of biofilm formation [227]. Major challenges still exist with regard to translating these molecules to produce effective therapeutic applications. One significant obstacle is that blocking a biofilm linked pathway may lead to upregulation of genes involved in the production of virulent factors [228]. Processes such as quorum sensing are often strain or isolate specific. Further research is required into control and feedback mechanisms of each biomolecular system and how they are inherently interlinked to produce phenotypic traits. Sophisticated control and modulation, rather than a policy of complete negation, of multiple pathways will be required tailored individual etiology of the infectious disease.

Author Contributions

G.L. conceived the study and wrote the review. S.P.G. and B.F.G. contributed to literature search, technical support and constructive discussions to form the review article.

References

1.   Christensen, L.D.; Moser, C.; Jensen, P.O.; Rasmussen, T.B.; Christophersen, L.; Kjelleberg, S.; Kumar, N.; Hoiby, N.; Givskov, M.; Bjarnsholt, T. Impact of *Pseudomonas aeruginosa* Quorum Sensing on Biofilm Persistence in an *in Vivo* Intraperitoneal Foreign-Body Infection Model. *Microbiology* **2007**, *153*, 2312–2320.

2.   Cole, S.J.; Records, A.R.; Orr, M.W.; Linden, S.B.; Lee, V.T. Catheter-Associated Urinary Tract Infection by *Pseudomonas aeruginosa* is Mediated by Exopolysaccharide-Independent Biofilms. *Infect. Immun.* **2014**, *82*, 2048–2058.

3.   Guggenbichler, J.P.; Assadian, O.; Boeswald, M.; Kramer, A. Incidence and Clinical Implication of Nosocomial Infections Associated with Implantable Biomaterials—Catheters, Ventilator-Associated Pneumonia, Urinary Tract Infections. *GMS Krankenhhyg. Interdiszip.* **2011**, *6*, 1-19.

4.   Ramos, G.P.; Rocha, J.L.; Tuon, F.F. Seasonal Humidity may Influence *Pseudomonas aeruginosa* Hospital-Acquired Infection Rates. *Int. J. Infect. Dis.* **2013**, *17*, e757–e761.

5.   Hoiby, N.; Ciofu, O.; Bjarnsholt, T. *Pseudomonas aeruginosa* Biofilms in Cystic Fibrosis. *Future Microbiol.* **2010**, *5*, 1663–1674.

6.   Jacobsen, S.M.; Stickler, D.J.; Mobley, H.L.; Shirtliff, M.E. Complicated Catheter-Associated Urinary Tract Infections due to *Escherichia coli* and *Proteus mirabilis*. *Clin. Microbiol. Rev.* **2008**, *21*, 26–59.

7.   Foxman, B.; Brown, P. Epidemiology of Urinary Tract Infections: Transmission and Risk Factors, Incidence, and Costs. *Infect. Dis. Clin. N. Am.* **2003**, *17*, 227–241.

8.   Laverty, G.; Gorman, S.P.; Gilmore, B.F. Biomolecular Mechanisms of Staphylococcal Biofilm Formation. *Future Microbiol.* **2013**, *8*, 509–524.

9.   Sutherland, I.W. Microbial Polysaccharides from Gram-negative Bacteria. *Int. Dairy J.* **2001**, *11*, 663–674.

10.   Lejeune, P. Contamination of Abiotic Surfaces: What a Colonizing Bacterium Sees and how to Blur it. *Trends Microbiol.* **2003**, *11*, 179–184.

11.   O'Toole, G.A.; Kolter, R. Flagellar and Twitching Motility are Necessary for *Pseudomonas aeruginosa* Biofilm Development. *Mol. Microbiol.* **1998**, *30*, 295–304.

12.   Dunne, W.M., Jr. Bacterial Adhesion: Seen any Good Biofilms Lately? *Clin. Microbiol. Rev.* **2002**, *15*, 155–166.

13.   Bohn, Y.S.; Brandes, G.; Rakhimova, E.; Horatzek, S.; Salunkhe, P.; Munder, A.; van Barneveld, A.; Jordan, D.; Bredenbruch, F.; Haussler, S.; *et al.* Multiple Roles of *Pseudomonas aeruginosa* TBCF10839 PilY1 in Motility, Transport and Infection. *Mol. Microbiol.* **2009**, *71*, 730–747.

14.   Strom, M.S.; Nunn, D.N.; Lory, S. Posttranslational Processing of Type IV Prepilin and Homologs by PilD of *Pseudomonas aeruginosa*. *Methods Enzymol.* **1994**, *235*, 527–540.

15.   Mattick, J.S. Type IV Pili and Twitching Motility. *Ann. Rev. Microbiol.* **2002**, *56*, 289–314.

16.   Nunn, D.; Bergman, S.; Lory, S. Products of Three Accessory Genes, *pilB*, *pilC*, and *pilD*, are Required for Biogenesis of *Pseudomonas aeruginosa* Pili. *J. Bacteriol.* **1990**, *172*, 2911–2919.

17.   Alm, R.A.; Hallinan, J.P.; Watson, A.A.; Mattick, J.S. Fimbrial Biogenesis Genes of *Pseudomonas aeruginosa*: *pilW* and *pilX* Increase the Similarity of Type 4 Fimbriae to the GSP Protein-Secretion Systems and *pilY1* Encodes a Gonococcal PilC Homologue. *Mol. Microbiol.* **1996**, *22*, 161–173.

18.   Murray, T.S.; Kazmierczak, B.I. *Pseudomonas aeruginosa* Exhibits Sliding Motility in the Absence of Type IV Pili and Flagella. *J. Bacteriol.* **2008**, *190*, 2700–2708.

19.   Makin, S.A.; Beveridge, T.J. The Influence of A-Band and B-Band Lipopolysaccharide on the Surface Characteristics and Adhesion of *Pseudomonas aeruginosa* to Surfaces. *Microbiology* **1996**, *142*, 299–307.

20.   Darzins, A.; Russell, M.A. Molecular Genetic Analysis of Type-4 Pilus Biogenesis and Twitching Motility using *Pseudomonas aeruginosa* as a Model System-a Review. *Gene* **1997**, *192*, 109–115.

21.   Barken, K.B.; Pamp, S.J.; Yang, L.; Gjermansen, M.; Bertrand, J.J.; Klausen, M.; Givskov, M.; Whitchurch, C.B.; Engel, J.N.; Tolker-Nielsen, T. Roles of Type IV Pili, Flagellum-Mediated Motility and Extracellular DNA in the Formation of Mature Multicellular Structures in *Pseudomonas aeruginosa* Biofilms. *Environ. Microbiol.* **2008**, *10*, 2331–2343.

22.   Wentworth, J.S.; Austin, F.E.; Garber, N.; Gilboa-Garber, N.; Paterson, C.A.; Doyle, R.J. Cytoplasmic Lectins Contribute to the Adhesion of *Pseudomonas aeruginosa*. *Biofouling* **1991**, *4*, 99–104.

23.   Tielker, D.; Hacker, S.; Loris, R.; Strathmann, M.; Wingender, J.; Wilhelm, S.; Rosenau, F.; Jaeger, K.E. *Pseudomonas aeruginosa* Lectin LecB is Located in the Outer Membrane and is Involved in Biofilm Formation. *Microbiology* **2005**, *151*, 1313–1323.

24.   Adam, J.; Pokorna, M.; Sabin, C.; Mitchell, E.P.; Imberty, A.; Wimmerova, M. Engineering of PA-IIL Lectin from *Pseudomonas aeruginosa*—Unravelling the Role of the Specificity Loop for Sugar Preference. *BMC Struct. Biol.* **2007**, *7*, 36.

25.   Mewe, M.; Tielker, D.; Schonberg, R.; Schachner, M.; Jaeger, K.E.; Schumacher, U. *Pseudomonas aeruginosa* Lectins I and II and their Interaction with Human Airway Cilia. *J. Laryngol. Otol.* **2005**, *119*, 595–599.

26.   Hauber, H.P.; Schulz, M.; Pforte, A.; Mack, D.; Zabel, P.; Schumacher, U. Inhalation with Fucose and Galactose for Treatment of *Pseudomonas aeruginosa* in Cystic Fibrosis Patients. *Int. J. Med. Sci.* **2008**, *5*, 371–376.

27.   Kolomiets, E.; Swiderska, M.A.; Kadam, R.U.; Johansson, E.M.; Jaeger, K.E.; Darbre, T.; Reymond, J.L. Glycopeptide Dendrimers with High Affinity for the Fucose-Binding Lectin LecB from *Pseudomonas aeruginosa*. *ChemMedChem* **2009**, *4*, 562–569.

28.   Winzer, K.; Falconer, C.; Garber, N.C.; Diggle, S.P.; Camara, M.; Williams, P. The *Pseudomonas aeruginosa* Lectins PA-IL and PA-IIL are Controlled by Quorum Sensing and by RpoS. *J. Bacteriol.* **2000**, *182*, 6401–6411.

29.   Hull, R.A.; Gill, R.E.; Hsu, P.; Minshew, B.H.; Falkow, S. Construction and Expression of Recombinant Plasmids Encoding Type 1 Or D-Mannose-Resistant Pili from a Urinary Tract Infection *Escherichia coli* Isolate. *Infect. Immun.* **1981**, *33*, 933–938.

30.   Baorto, D.M.; Gao, Z.; Malaviya, R.; Dustin, M.L.; van der Merwe, A.; Lublin, D.M.; Abraham, S.N. Survival of FimH-Expressing Enterobacteria in Macrophages Relies on Glycolipid Traffic. *Nature* **1997**, *389*, 636–639.

31.   Connell, I.; Agace, W.; Klemm, P.; Schembri, M.; Marild, S.; Svanborg, C. Type 1 Fimbrial Expression Enhances *Escherichia coli* Virulence for the Urinary Tract. *Proc. Natl. Acad. Sci. USA* **1996**, *93*, 9827–9832.

32.   Mobley, H.L.; Chippendale, G.R.; Tenney, J.H.; Hull, R.A.; Warren, J.W. Expression of Type 1 Fimbriae may be Required for Persistence of *Escherichia coli* in the Catheterized Urinary Tract. *J. Clin. Microbiol.* **1987**, *25*, 2253–2257.

33.   Cormio, L.; Vuopio-Varkila, J.; Siitonen, A.; Talja, M.; Ruutu, M. Bacterial Adhesion and Biofilm Formation on various Double-J Stents *in Vivo* and *in Vitro*. *Scand. J. Urol. Nephrol.* **1996**, *30*, 19–24.

34.   Vetsch, M.; Puorger, C.; Spirig, T.; Grauschopf, U.; Weber-Ban, E.U.; Glockshuber, R. Pilus Chaperones Represent a New Type of Protein-Folding Catalyst. *Nature* **2004**, *431*, 329–333.

35.   Sauer, F.G.; Barnhart, M.; Choudhury, D.; Knight, S.D.; Waksman, G.; Hultgren, S.J. Chaperone-Assisted Pilus Assembly and Bacterial Attachment. *Curr. Opin. Struct. Biol.* **2000**, *10*, 548–556.

36.   Gossert, A.D.; Bettendorff, P.; Puorger, C.; Vetsch, M.; Herrmann, T.; Glockshuber, R.; Wuthrich, K. NMR Structure of the *Escherichia coli* Type 1 Pilus Subunit FimF and its Interactions with Other Pilus Subunits. *J. Mol. Biol.* **2008**, *375*, 752–763.

37.   Capitani, G.; Eidam, O.; Glockshuber, R.; Grutter, M.G. Structural and Functional Insights into the Assembly of Type 1 Pili from *Escherichia coli*. *Microbes Infect.* **2006**, *8*, 2284–2290.

38.   Lugmaier, R.A.; Schedin, S.; Kuhner, F.; Benoit, M. Dynamic Restacking of *Escherichia coli* P-Pili. *Eur. Biophys. J.* **2008**, *37*, 111–120.

39.   Jacob-Dubuisson, F.; Heuser, J.; Dodson, K.; Normark, S.; Hultgren, S. Initiation of Assembly and Association of the Structural Elements of a Bacterial Pilus Depend on Two Specialized Tip Proteins. *EMBO J.* **1993**, *12*, 837–847.

40. Baga, M.; Norgren, M.; Normark, S. Biogenesis of *E. coli* Pap Pili: PapH, a Minor Pilin Subunit Involved in Cell Anchoring and Length Modulation. *Cell* **1987**, *49*, 241–251.

41. Jones, C.H.; Danese, P.N.; Pinkner, J.S.; Silhavy, T.J.; Hultgren, S.J. The Chaperone-Assisted Membrane Release and Folding Pathway is Sensed by Two Signal Transduction Systems. *EMBO J.* **1997**, *16*, 6394–6406.

42. Thanassi, D.G.; Saulino, E.T.; Lombardo, M.J.; Roth, R.; Heuser, J.; Hultgren, S.J. The PapC Usher Forms an Oligomeric Channel: Implications for Pilus Biogenesis Across the Outer Membrane. *Proc. Natl. Acad. Sci. USA* **1998**, *95*, 3146–3151.

43. Anantha, R.P.; Stone, K.D.; Donnenberg, M.S. Effects of *bfp* Mutations on Biogenesis of Functional Enteropathogenic *Escherichia coli* Type IV Pili. *J. Bacteriol.* **2000**, *182*, 2498–2506.

44. Strom, M.S.; Lory, S. Structure-Function and Biogenesis of the Type IV Pili. *Ann. Rev. Microbiol.* **1993**, *47*, 565–596.

45. Ramer, S.W.; Schoolnik, G.K.; Wu, C.Y.; Hwang, J.; Schmidt, S.A.; Bieber, D. The Type IV Pilus Assembly Complex: Biogenic Interactions among the Bundle-Forming Pilus Proteins of Enteropathogenic *Escherichia coli*. *J. Bacteriol.* **2002**, *184*, 3457–3465.

46. Sauer, F.G.; Knight, S.D.; Waksman and, G.J.; Hultgren, S.J. PapD-Like Chaperones and Pilus Biogenesis. *Semin. Cell Dev. Biol.* **2000**, *11*, 27–34.

47. Verger, D.; Miller, E.; Remaut, H.; Waksman, G.; Hultgren, S. Molecular Mechanism of P Pilus Termination in Uropathogenic *Escherichia coli*. *EMBO Rep.* **2006**, *7*, 1228–1232.

48. Mu, X.Q.; Bullitt, E. Structure and Assembly of P-Pili: A Protruding Hinge Region used for Assembly of a Bacterial Adhesion Filament. *Proc. Natl. Acad. Sci. USA* **2006**, *103*, 9861–9866.

49. Mu, X.Q.; Jiang, Z.G.; Bullitt, E. Localization of a Critical Interface for Helical Rod Formation of Bacterial Adhesion P-Pili. *J. Mol. Biol.* **2005**, *346*, 13–20.

50. Olsen, A.; Arnqvist, A.; Hammar, M.; Sukupolvi, S.; Normark, S. The RpoS Sigma Factor Relieves H-NS-Mediated Transcriptional Repression of *csgA*, the Subunit Gene of Fibronectin-Binding Curli in *Escherichia coli*. *Mol. Microbiol.* **1993**, *7*, 523–536.

51. Arnqvist, A.; Olsen, A.; Normark, S. Sigma S-Dependent Growth-Phase Induction of the *csgBA* Promoter in *Escherichia coli* can be Achieved *in Vivo* by Sigma 70 in the Absence of the Nucleoid-Associated Protein H-NS. *Mol. Microbiol.* **1994**, *13*, 1021–1032.

52. Romling, U.; Rohde, M.; Olsen, A.; Normark, S.; Reinkoster, J. AgfD, the Checkpoint of Multicellular and Aggregative Behaviour in *Salmonella typhimurium* Regulates at Least Two Independent Pathways. *Mol. Microbiol.* **2000**, *36*, 10–23.

53. Brown, P.K.; Dozois, C.M.; Nickerson, C.A.; Zuppardo, A.; Terlonge, J.; Curtiss, R., 3rd. MlrA, a Novel Regulator of Curli (AgF) and Extracellular Matrix Synthesis by *Escherichia coli* and *Salmonella enterica* Serovar Typhimurium. *Mol. Microbiol.* **2001**, *41*, 349–363.

54. Gerstel, U.; Park, C.; Romling, U. Complex Regulation of *csgD* Promoter Activity by Global Regulatory Proteins. *Mol. Microbiol.* **2003**, *49*, 639–654.

55. Gerstel, U.; Romling, U. Oxygen Tension and Nutrient Starvation are Major Signals that Regulate *agfD* Promoter Activity and Expression of the Multicellular Morphotype in *Salmonella typhimurium*. *Environ. Microbiol.* **2001**, *3*, 638–648.

56. Olsen, A.; Arnqvist, A.; Hammar, M.; Normark, S. Environmental Regulation of Curli Production in *Escherichia coli*. *Infect. Agents Dis.* **1993**, *2*, 272–274.

57. Romling, U.; Sierralta, W.D.; Eriksson, K.; Normark, S. Multicellular and Aggregative Behaviour of *Salmonella typhimurium* Strains is Controlled by Mutations in the *agfD* Promoter. *Mol. Microbiol.* **1998**, *28*, 249–264.

58. Dorel, C.; Vidal, O.; Prigent-Combaret, C.; Vallet, I.; Lejeune, P. Involvement of the Cpx Signal Transduction Pathway of *E. coli* in Biofilm Formation. *FEMS Microbiol. Lett.* **1999**, *178*, 169–175.

59. Cegelski, L.; Pinkner, J.S.; Hammer, N.D.; Cusumano, C.K.; Hung, C.S.; Chorell, E.; Aberg, V.; Walker, J.N.; Seed, P.C.; Almqvist, F.; *et al.* Small-Molecule Inhibitors Target *Escherichia coli* Amyloid Biogenesis and Biofilm Formation. *Nat. Chem. Biol.* **2009**, *5*, 913–919.

60. Dorel, C.; Lejeune, P.; Rodrigue, A. The Cpx System of *Escherichia coli*, a Strategic Signaling Pathway for Confronting Adverse Conditions and for Settling Biofilm Communities? *Res. Microbiol.* **2006**, *157*, 306–314.

61. Landini, P. Cross-Talk Mechanisms in Biofilm Formation and Responses to Environmental and Physiological Stress in *Escherichia coli*. *Res. Microbiol.* **2009**, *160*, 259–266.

62. Danese, P.N.; Oliver, G.R.; Barr, K.; Bowman, G.D.; Rick, P.D.; Silhavy, T.J. Accumulation of the Enterobacterial Common Antigen Lipid II Biosynthetic Intermediate Stimulates *degP* Transcription in *Escherichia coli*. *J. Bacteriol.* **1998**, *180*, 5875–5884.

63. Prigent-Combaret, C.; Brombacher, E.; Vidal, O.; Ambert, A.; Lejeune, P.; Landini, P.; Dorel, C. Complex Regulatory Network Controls Initial Adhesion and Biofilm Formation in *Escherichia coli* Via Regulation of the *csgD* Gene. *J. Bacteriol.* **2001**, *183*, 7213–7223.

64. De Wulf, P.; Kwon, O.; Lin, E.C. The CpxRA Signal Transduction System of *Escherichia coli*: Growth-Related Autoactivation and Control of Unanticipated Target Operons. *J. Bacteriol.* **1999**, *181*, 6772–6778.

65. Becker, G.; Klauck, E.; Hengge-Aronis, R. Regulation of RpoS Proteolysis in *Escherichia coli*: The Response Regulator RssB is a Recognition Factor that Interacts with the Turnover Element in RpoS. *Proc. Natl. Acad. Sci. USA* **1999**, *96*, 6439–6444.

66. Beloin, C.; Valle, J.; Latour-Lambert, P.; Faure, P.; Kzreminski, M.; Balestrino, D.; Haagensen, J.A.; Molin, S.; Prensier, G.; Arbeille, B.; Ghigo, J.M. Global Impact of Mature Biofilm Lifestyle on *Escherichia coli* K-12 Gene Expression. *Mol. Microbiol.* **2004**, *51*, 659–674.

67. Hirakawa, H.; Inazumi, Y.; Masaki, T.; Hirata, T.; Yamaguchi, A. Indole Induces the Expression of Multidrug Exporter Genes in *Escherichia coli*. *Mol. Microbiol.* **2005**, *55*, 1113–1126.

68. De Wulf, P.; McGuire, A.M.; Liu, X.; Lin, E.C. Genome-Wide Profiling of Promoter Recognition by the Two-Component Response Regulator CpxR-P in *Escherichia coli*. *J. Biol. Chem.* **2002**, *277*, 26652–26661.

69. Jubelin, G.; Vianney, A.; Beloin, C.; Ghigo, J.M.; Lazzaroni, J.C.; Lejeune, P.; Dorel, C. CpxR/OmpR Interplay Regulates Curli Gene Expression in Response to Osmolarity in *Escherichia coli*. *J. Bacteriol.* **2005**, *187*, 2038–2049.

70. Rampersaud, A.; Harlocker, S.L.; Inouye, M. The OmpR Protein of *Escherichia coli* Binds to Sites in the *ompF* Promoter Region in a Hierarchical Manner Determined by its Degree of Phosphorylation. *J. Biol. Chem.* **1994**, *269*, 12559–12566.

71. Yamamoto, K.; Hirao, K.; Oshima, T.; Aiba, H.; Utsumi, R.; Ishihama, A. Functional Characterization *in Vitro* of all Two-Component Signal Transduction Systems from *Escherichia coli*. *J. Biol. Chem.* **2005**, *280*, 1448–1456.

72. Ogasawara, H.; Yamada, K.; Kori, A.; Yamamoto, K.; Ishihama, A. Regulation of the *Escherichia coli csgD* Promoter: Interplay between Five Transcription Factors. *Microbiology* **2010**, *156*, 2470–2483.

73. Vidal, O.; Longin, R.; Prigent-Combaret, C.; Dorel, C.; Hooreman, M.; Lejeune, P. Isolation of an *Escherichia coli* K-12 Mutant Strain Able to Form Biofilms on Inert Surfaces: Involvement of a New *ompR* Allele that Increases Curli Expression. *J. Bacteriol.* **1998**, *180*, 2442–2449.

74. Landini, P.; Zehnder, A.J. The Global Regulatory *hns* Gene Negatively Affects Adhesion to Solid Surfaces by Anaerobically Grown *Escherichia coli* by Modulating Expression of Flagellar Genes and Lipopolysaccharide Production. *J. Bacteriol.* **2002**, *184*, 1522–1529.

75. Evans, L.R.; Linker, A. Production and Characterization of the Slime Polysaccharide of *Pseudomonas aeruginosa*. *J. Bacteriol.* **1973**, *116*, 915–924.

76. Chen, J.; Lee, S.M.; Mao, Y. Protective Effect of Exopolysaccharide Colanic Acid of *Escherichia coli* O157:H7 to Osmotic and Oxidative Stress. *Int. J. Food Microbiol.* **2004**, *93*, 281–286.

77. Zhao, K.; Liu, M.; Burgess, R.R. Adaptation in Bacterial Flagellar and Motility Systems: From Regulon Members to Foraging-Like Behavior in *E. coli*. *Nucl. Acids Res.* **2007**, *35*, 4441–4452.

78. Sperandio, V.; Torres, A.G.; Jarvis, B.; Nataro, J.P.; Kaper, J.B. Bacteria-Host Communication: The Language of Hormones. *Proc. Natl. Acad. Sci. USA* **2003**, *100*, 8951–8956.

79. Winzer, K.; Williams, P. *Escherichia coli* Gets the Message. *Nat. Med.* **2003**, *9*, 1118–1119.

80. Vendeville, A.; Winzer, K.; Heurlier, K.; Tang, C.M.; Hardie, K.R. Making "Sense" of Metabolism: Autoinducer-2, LuxS and Pathogenic Bacteria. *Nat. Rev. Microbiol.* **2005**, *3*, 383–396.

81. Williams, P.; Winzer, K.; Chan, W.C.; Camara, M. Look Who's Talking: Communication and Quorum Sensing in the Bacterial World. *Philos. Trans. R. Soc. Lond. Ser. B Biol. Sci.* **2007**, *362*, 1119–1134.

82. Winzer, K.; Hardie, K.R.; Williams, P. Bacterial Cell-to-Cell Communication: Sorry, can't Talk Now—Gone to Lunch! *Curr. Opin. Microbiol.* **2002**, *5*, 216–222.

83. Allesen-Holm, M.; Barken, K.B.; Yang, L.; Klausen, M.; Webb, J.S.; Kjelleberg, S.; Molin, S.; Givskov, M.; Tolker-Nielsen, T.A. Characterization of DNA Release in *Pseudomonas aeruginosa* Cultures and Biofilms. *Mol. Microbiol.* **2006**, *59*, 1114–1128.

84. Branda, S.S.; Vik, S.; Friedman, L.; Kolter, R. Biofilms: The Matrix Revisited. *Trends Microbiol.* **2005**, *13*, 20–26.

85. Matsukawa, M.; Greenberg, E.P. Putative Exopolysaccharide Synthesis Genes Influence *Pseudomonas aeruginosa* Biofilm Development. *J. Bacteriol.* **2004**, *186*, 4449–4456.

86. Deretic, V.; Govan, J.R.; Konyecsni, W.M.; Martin, D.W. Mucoid *Pseudomonas aeruginosa* in Cystic Fibrosis: Mutations in the *muc* Loci Affect Transcription of the *algR* and *algD* Genes in Response to Environmental Stimuli. *Mol. Microbiol.* **1990**, *4*, 189–196.

87. Stapper, A.P.; Narasimhan, G.; Ohman, D.E.; Barakat, J.; Hentzer, M.; Molin, S.; Kharazmi, A.; Hoiby, N.; Mathee, K. Alginate Production Affects *Pseudomonas aeruginosa* Biofilm

Development and Architecture, but is Not Essential for Biofilm Formation. *J. Med. Microbiol.* **2004**, *53*, 679–690.

88. Doggett, R.G.; Harrison, G.M.; Stillwell, R.N.; Wallis, E.S. An Atypical *Pseudomonas aeruginosa* Associated with Cystic Fibrosis of the Pancreas. *J. Pediatr.* **1966**, *68*, 215–221.

89. Friedman, L.; Kolter, R. Two Genetic Loci Produce Distinct Carbohydrate-Rich Structural Components of the *Pseudomonas aeruginosa* Biofilm Matrix. *J. Bacteriol.* **2004**, *186*, 4457–4465.

90. Lee, V.T.; Matewish, J.M.; Kessler, J.L.; Hyodo, M.; Hayakawa, Y.; Lory, S. A Cyclic-Di-GMP Receptor Required for Bacterial Exopolysaccharide Production. *Mol. Microbiol.* **2007**, *65*, 1474–1484.

91. Byrd, M.S.; Sadovskaya, I.; Vinogradov, E.; Lu, H.; Sprinkle, A.B.; Richardson, S.H.; Ma, L.; Ralston, B.; Parsek, M.R.; Anderson, E.M.; *et al.* Genetic and Biochemical Analyses of the *Pseudomonas aeruginosa* Psl Exopolysaccharide Reveal Overlapping Roles for Polysaccharide Synthesis Enzymes in Psl and LPS Production. *Mol. Microbiol.* **2009**, *73*, 622–638.

92. Overhage, J.; Schemionek, M.; Webb, J.S.; Rehm, B.H. Expression of the *psl* Operon in *Pseudomonas aeruginosa* PAO1 Biofilms: PslA Performs an Essential Function in Biofilm Formation. *Appl. Environ. Microbiol.* **2005**, *71*, 4407–4413.

93. Wozniak, D.J.; Wyckoff, T.J.; Starkey, M.; Keyser, R.; Azadi, P.; O'Toole, G.A.; Parsek, M.R. Alginate is Not a Significant Component of the Extracellular Polysaccharide Matrix of PA14 and PAO1 *Pseudomonas aeruginosa* Biofilms. *Proc. Natl. Acad. Sci. USA* **2003**, *100*, 7907–7912.

94. Friedman, L.; Kolter, R. Genes Involved in Matrix Formation in *Pseudomonas aeruginosa* PA14 Biofilms. *Mol. Microbiol.* **2004**, *51*, 675–690.

95. Stewart, P.S.; Franklin, M.J. Physiological Heterogeneity in Biofilms. *Nat. Rev. Microbiol.* **2008**, *6*, 199–210.

96. Ma, L.; Lu, H.; Sprinkle, A.; Parsek, M.R.; Wozniak, D.J. *Pseudomonas aeruginosa* Psl is a Galactose- and Mannose-Rich Exopolysaccharide. *J. Bacteriol.* **2007**, *189*, 8353–8356.

97. Rani, S.A.; Pitts, B.; Beyenal, H.; Veluchamy, R.A.; Lewandowski, Z.; Davison, W.M.; Buckingham-Meyer, K.; Stewart, P.S. Spatial Patterns of DNA Replication, Protein Synthesis, and Oxygen Concentration within Bacterial Biofilms Reveal Diverse Physiological States. *J. Bacteriol.* **2007**, *189*, 4223–4233.

98. DiGiandomenico, A.; Warrener, P.; Hamilton, M.; Guillard, S.; Ravn, P.; Minter, R.; Camara, M.M.; Venkatraman, V.; Macgill, R.S.; Lin, J.; *et al.* Identification of Broadly Protective Human Antibodies to *Pseudomonas aeruginosa* Exopolysaccharide Psl by Phenotypic Screening. *J. Exp. Med.* **2012**, *209*, 1273–1287.

99. Christen, B.; Christen, M.; Paul, R.; Schmid, F.; Folcher, M.; Jenoe, P.; Meuwly, M.; Jenal, U. Allosteric Control of Cyclic Di-GMP Signaling. *J. Biol. Chem.* **2006**, *281*, 32015–32024.

100. Kulasakara, H.; Lee, V.; Brencic, A.; Liberati, N.; Urbach, J.; Miyata, S.; Lee, D.G.; Neely, A.N.; Hyodo, M.; Hayakawa, Y.; *et al.* Analysis of *Pseudomonas aeruginosa* Diguanylate Cyclases and Phosphodiesterases Reveals a Role for Bis-(3'-5')-Cyclic-GMP in Virulence. *Proc. Natl. Acad. Sci. USA* **2006**, *103*, 2839–2844.

101. Belas, R. Biofilms, flagella, and mechanosensing of surfaces by bacteria. *Trends Microbiol.* **2014**, doi:10.1016/j.tim.2014.05.002.

102. Sintim, H.O.; Smith, J.A.; Wang, J.; Nakayama, S.; Yan, L. Paradigm Shift in Discovering Next-Generation Anti-Infective Agents: Targeting Quorum Sensing, c-Di-GMP Signaling and Biofilm Formation in Bacteria with Small Molecules. *Future Med. Chem.* **2010**, *2*, 1005–1035.

103. Castiglione, N.; Stelitano, V.; Rinaldo, S.; Giardina, G.; Caruso, M.; Cutruzzolà, F. Metabolism of Cyclic-Di-GMP in Bacterial Biofilms: From a General Overview to Biotechnological Applications. *Indian J. Biotechnol.* **2011**, *10*, 423–431.

104. Irie, Y.; Borlee, B.R.; O'Connor, J.R.; Hill, P.J.; Harwood, C.S.; Wozniak, D.J.; Parsek, M.R. Self-Produced Exopolysaccharide is a Signal that Stimulates Biofilm Formation in *Pseudomonas aeruginosa*. *Proc. Natl. Acad. Sci. USA* **2012**, *109*, 20632–20636.

105. Anantharaman, V.; Iyer, L.M.; Aravind, L. Presence of a Classical RRM-Fold Palm Domain in Thg1-Type 3'- 5'Nucleic Acid Polymerases and the Origin of the GGDEF and CRISPR Polymerase Domains. *Biol. Direct* **2010**, *5*, 43.

106. Mano, E.; Hyodo, M.; Sato, Y.; Ishihara, Y.; Ohta, M.; Hayakawa, Y. Synthesis of Cyclic Bis(3'-5')-2'-deoxyguanylic/guanylic Acid (c-dGpGp) and its Biological Activities to Microbes. *ChemMedChem* **2007**, *2*, 1410–1413.

107. Barraud, N.; Schleheck, D.; Klebensberger, J.; Webb, J.S.; Hassett, D.J.; Rice, S.A.; Kjelleberg, S. Nitric Oxide Signaling in *Pseudomonas aeruginosa* Biofilms Mediates Phosphodiesterase Activity, Decreased Cyclic Di-GMP Levels, and Enhanced Dispersal. *J. Bacteriol.* **2009**, *191*, 7333–7342.

108. Yan, H.; Wang, X.; KuoLee, R.; Chen, W. Synthesis and Immunostimulatory Properties of the Phosphorothioate Analogues of cdiGMP. *Bioorg. Med. Chem. Lett.* **2008**, *18*, 5631–5634.

109. Ghafoor, A.; Hay, I.D.; Rehm, B.H. Role of Exopolysaccharides in *Pseudomonas aeruginosa* Biofilm Formation and Architecture. *Appl. Environ. Microbiol.* **2011**, *77*, 5238–5246.

110. Whitchurch, C.B.; Tolker-Nielsen, T.; Ragas, P.C.; Mattick, J.S. Extracellular DNA Required for Bacterial Biofilm Formation. *Science* **2002**, *295*, 1487.

111. Ma, L.; Jackson, K.D.; Landry, R.M.; Parsek, M.R.; Wozniak, D.J. Analysis of *Pseudomonas aeruginosa* Conditional Psl Variants Reveals Roles for the Psl Polysaccharide in Adhesion and Maintaining Biofilm Structure Postattachment. *J. Bacteriol.* **2006**, *188*, 8213–8221.

112. Mulcahy, H.; Charron-Mazenod, L.; Lewenza, S. Extracellular DNA Chelates Cations and Induces Antibiotic Resistance in *Pseudomonas aeruginosa* Biofilms. *PLoS Pathog.* **2008**, *4*, e1000213.

113. May, T.B.; Shinabarger, D.; Maharaj, R.; Kato, J.; Chu, L.; DeVault, J.D.; Roychoudhury, S.; Zielinski, N.A.; Berry, A.; Rothmel, R.K. Alginate Synthesis by *Pseudomonas aeruginosa*: A Key Pathogenic Factor in Chronic Pulmonary Infections of Cystic Fibrosis Patients. *Clin. Microbiol. Rev.* **1991**, *4*, 191–206.

114. Kumon, H.; Tomochika, K.; Matunaga, T.; Ogawa, M.; Ohmori, H. A Sandwich Cup Method for the Penetration Assay of Antimicrobial Agents through *Pseudomonas* Exopolysaccharides. *Microbiol. Immunol.* **1994**, *38*, 615–619.

115. DeVault, J.D.; Kimbara, K.; Chakrabarty, A.M. Pulmonary Dehydration and Infection in Cystic Fibrosis: Evidence that Ethanol Activates Alginate Gene Expression and Induction of Mucoidy in *Pseudomonas aeruginosa*. *Mol. Microbiol.* **1990**, *4*, 737–745.

116. Zielinski, N.A.; Maharaj, R.; Roychoudhury, S.; Danganan, C.E.; Hendrickson, W.; Chakrabarty, A.M. Alginate Synthesis in *Pseudomonas aeruginosa*: Environmental Regulation of the *algC* Promoter. *J. Bacteriol.* **1992**, *174*, 7680–7688.

117. Gacesa, P. Bacterial Alginate Biosynthesis-Recent Progress and Future Prospects. *Microbiology* **1998**, *144*, 1133–1143.

118. Maharaj, R.; May, T.B.; Wang, S.K.; Chakrabarty, A.M. Sequence of the *alg*8 and *alg*44 Genes Involved in the Synthesis of Alginate by *Pseudomonas aeruginosa*. *Gene* **1993**, *136*, 267–269.

119. Boyd, A.; Chakrabarty, A.M. Role of Alginate Lyase in Cell Detachment of *Pseudomonas aeruginosa*. *Appl. Environ. Microbiol.* **1994**, *60*, 2355–2359.

120. Robles-Price, A.; Wong, T.Y.; Sletta, H.; Valla, S.; Schiller, N.L. AlgX is a Periplasmic Protein Required for Alginate Biosynthesis in *Pseudomonas aeruginosa*. *J. Bacteriol.* **2004**, *186*, 7369–7377.

121. Douthit, S.A.; Dlakic, M.; Ohman, D.E.; Franklin, M.J. Epimerase Active Domain of *Pseudomonas aeruginosa* AlgG, a Protein that Contains a Right-Handed Beta-Helix. *J. Bacteriol.* **2005**, *187*, 4573–4583.

122. Franklin, M.J.; Ohman, D.E. Mutant Analysis and Cellular Localization of the AlgI, AlgJ, and AlgF Proteins Required for O Acetylation of Alginate in *Pseudomonas aeruginosa*. *J. Bacteriol.* **2002**, *184*, 3000–3007.

123. Franklin, M.J.; Douthit, S.A.; McClure, M.A. Evidence that the *algI/algJ* Gene Cassette, Required for O Acetylation of *Pseudomonas aeruginosa* Alginate, Evolved by Lateral Gene Transfer. *J. Bacteriol.* **2004**, *186*, 4759–4773.

124. Rehm, B.H.; Valla, S. Bacterial Alginates: Biosynthesis and Applications. *Appl. Microbiol. Biotechnol.* **1997**, *48*, 281–288.

125. Ramsey, D.M.; Wozniak, D.J. Understanding the Control of *Pseudomonas aeruginosa* Alginate Synthesis and the Prospects for Management of Chronic Infections in Cystic Fibrosis. *Mol. Microbiol.* **2005**, *56*, 309–322.

126. Gimmestad, M.; Sletta, H.; Ertesvag, H.; Bakkevig, K.; Jain, S.; Suh, S.J.; Skjak-Braek, G.; Ellingsen, T.E.; Ohman, D.E.; Valla, S. The *Pseudomonas* Fluorescens AlgG Protein, but Not its Mannuronan C-5-Epimerase Activity, is Needed for Alginate Polymer Formation. *J. Bacteriol.* **2003**, *185*, 3515–3523.

127. Shinabarger, D.; Berry, A.; May, T.B.; Rothmel, R.; Fialho, A.; Chakrabarty, A.M. Purification and Characterization of Phosphomannose Isomerase-Guanosine Diphospho-D-Mannose Pyrophosphorylase. A Bifunctional Enzyme in the Alginate Biosynthetic Pathway of *Pseudomonas aeruginosa*. *J. Biol. Chem.* **1991**, *266*, 2080–2088.

128. Regni, C.; Naught, L.; Tipton, P.A.; Beamer, L.J. Structural Basis of Diverse Substrate Recognition by the Enzyme PMM/PGM from *P. aeruginosa*. *Structure* **2004**, *12*, 55–63.

129. Govan, J.R.; Deretic, V. Microbial Pathogenesis in Cystic Fibrosis: Mucoid *Pseudomonas aeruginosa* and *Burkholderia. cepacia*. *Microbiol. Rev.* **1996**, *60*, 539–574.

130. DeVries, C.A.; Ohman, D.E. Mucoid-to-Nonmucoid Conversion in Alginate-Producing *Pseudomonas aeruginosa* often Results from Spontaneous Mutations in *algT*, Encoding a Putative Alternate Sigma Factor, and shows Evidence for Autoregulation. *J. Bacteriol.* **1994**, *176*, 6677–6687.

131. Wozniak, D.J.; Sprinkle, A.B.; Baynham, P.J. Control of *Pseudomonas aeruginosa algZ* Expression by the Alternative Sigma Factor AlgT. *J. Bacteriol.* **2003**, *185*, 7297–7300.

132. Nikolskaya, A.N.; Galperin, M.Y. A Novel Type of Conserved DNA-Binding Domain in the Transcriptional Regulators of the AlgR/AgrA/LytR Family. *Nucl. Acids Res.* **2002**, *30*, 2453–2459.

133. Woolwine, S.C.; Wozniak, D.J. Identification of an *Escherichia coli pepA* Homolog and its Involvement in Suppression of the *algB* Phenotype in Mucoid *Pseudomonas aeruginosa*. *J. Bacteriol.* **1999**, *181*, 107–116.

134. Leech, A.J.; Sprinkle, A.; Wood, L.; Wozniak, D.J.; Ohman, D.E. The NtrC Family Regulator AlgB, which Controls Alginate Biosynthesis in Mucoid *Pseudomonas aeruginosa*, Binds Directly to the *algD* Promoter. *J. Bacteriol.* **2008**, *190*, 581–589.

135. Baynham, P.J.; Wozniak, D.J. Identification and Characterization of AlgZ, an AlgT-Dependent DNA-Binding Protein Required for *Pseudomonas aeruginosa algD* Transcription. *Mol. Microbiol.* **1996**, *22*, 97–108.

136. Tart, A.H.; Blanks, M.J.; Wozniak, D.J. The AlgT-Dependent Transcriptional Regulator AmrZ (AlgZ) Inhibits Flagellum Biosynthesis in Mucoid, Nonmotile *Pseudomonas aeruginosa* Cystic Fibrosis Isolates. *J. Bacteriol.* **2006**, *188*, 6483–6489.

137. Mathee, K.; McPherson, C.J.; Ohman, D.E. Posttranslational Control of the *algT* (*algU*)-Encoded sigma22 for Expression of the Alginate Regulon in *Pseudomonas aeruginosa* and Localization of its Antagonist Proteins MucA and MucB (AlgN). *J. Bacteriol.* **1997**, *179*, 3711–3720.

138. Schurr, M.J.; Yu, H.; Martinez-Salazar, J.M.; Boucher, J.C.; Deretic, V. Control of AlgU, a Member of the Sigma E-Like Family of Stress Sigma Factors, by the Negative Regulators MucA and MucB and *Pseudomonas aeruginosa* Conversion to Mucoidy in Cystic Fibrosis. *J. Bacteriol.* **1996**, *178*, 4997–5004.

139. Rowen, D.W.; Deretic, V. Membrane-to-Cytosol Redistribution of ECF Sigma Factor AlgU and Conversion to Mucoidy in *Pseudomonas aeruginosa* Isolates from Cystic Fibrosis Patients. *Mol. Microbiol.* **2000**, *36*, 314–327.

140. Boucher, J.C.; Schurr, M.J.; Yu, H.; Rowen, D.W.; Deretic, V. *Pseudomonas aeruginosa* in Cystic Fibrosis: Role of *mucC* in the Regulation of Alginate Production and Stress Sensitivity. *Microbiology* **1997**, *143*, 3473–3480.

141. Wood, L.F.; Ohman, D.E. Independent Regulation of MucD, an HtrA-Like Protease in *Pseudomonas aeruginosa*, and the Role of its Proteolytic Motif in Alginate Gene Regulation. *J. Bacteriol.* **2006**, *188*, 3134–3137.

142. Goldberg, J.B.; Gorman, W.L.; Flynn, J.L.; Ohman, D.E. A Mutation in *algN* Permits Trans Activation of Alginate Production by *algT* in *Pseudomonas* Species. *J. Bacteriol.* **1993**, *175*, 1303–1308.

143. Martin, D.W.; Schurr, M.J.; Mudd, M.H.; Deretic, V. Differentiation of *Pseudomonas aeruginosa* into the Alginate-Producing Form: Inactivation of *mucB* Causes Conversion to Mucoidy. *Mol. Microbiol.* **1993**, *9*, 497–506.

144. Prigent-Combaret, C.; Vidal, O.; Dorel, C.; Lejeune, P. Abiotic Surface Sensing and Biofilm-Dependent Regulation of Gene Expression in *Escherichia coli*. *J. Bacteriol.* **1999**, *181*, 5993–6002.

145. Danese, P.N.; Pratt, L.A.; Kolter, R. Exopolysaccharide Production is Required for Development of *Escherichia coli* K12 Biofilm Architecture. *J. Bacteriol.* **2000**, *182*, 3593–3596.

146. Obadia, B.; Lacour, S.; Doublet, P.; Baubichon-Cortay, H.; Cozzone, A.J.; Grangeasse, C. Influence of Tyrosine-Kinase Wzc Activity on Colanic Acid Production in *Escherichia coli* K12 Cells. *J. Mol. Biol.* **2007**, *367*, 42–53.

147. Whitfield, C.; Roberts, I.S. Structure, Assembly and Regulation of Expression of Capsules in *Escherichia coli*. *Mol. Microbiol.* **1999**, *31*, 1307–1319.

148. Ebel, W.; Trempy, J.E. *Escherichia coli* RcsA, a Positive Activator of Colanic Acid Capsular Polysaccharide Synthesis, Functions to Activate its Own Expression. *J. Bacteriol.* **1999**, *181*, 577–584.

149. Gervais, F.G.; Drapeau, G.R. Identification, Cloning, and Characterization of *rcsF*, a New Regulator Gene for Exopolysaccharide Synthesis that Suppresses the Division Mutation ftsZ84 in *Escherichia coli* K-12. *J. Bacteriol.* **1992**, *174*, 8016–8022.

150. Lacroix, J.M.; Loubens, I.; Tempete, M.; Menichi, B.; Bohin, J.P. The *mdoA* Locus of *Escherichia coli* Consists of an Operon Under Osmotic Control. *Mol. Microbiol.* **1991**, *5*, 1745–1753.

151. Ebel, W.; Vaughn, G.J.; Peters, H.K., 3rd; Trempy, J.E. Inactivation of *mdoH* Leads to Increased Expression of Colanic Acid Capsular Polysaccharide in *Escherichia coli*. *J. Bacteriol.* **1997**, *179*, 6858–6861.

152. Sailer, F.C.; Meberg, B.M.; Young, K.D. Beta-Lactam Induction of Colanic Acid Gene Expression in *Escherichia coli*. *FEMS Microbiol. Lett.* **2003**, *226*, 245–249.

153. Sledjeski, D.; Gottesman, S. A Small RNA Acts as an Antisilencer of the H-NS-Silenced *rcsA* Gene of *Escherichia coli*. *Proc. Natl. Acad. Sci. USA* **1995**, *92*, 2003–2007.

154. Vincent, C.; Doublet, P.; Grangeasse, C.; Vaganay, E.; Cozzone, A.J.; Duclos, B. Cells of *Escherichia coli* Contain a Protein-Tyrosine Kinase, Wzc, and a Phosphotyrosine-Protein Phosphatase, Wzb. *J. Bacteriol.* **1999**, *181*, 3472–3477.

155. Grangeasse, C.; Cozzone, A.J.; Deutscher, J.; Mijakovic, I. Tyrosine Phosphorylation: An Emerging Regulatory Device of Bacterial Physiology. *Trends Biochem. Sci.* **2007**, *32*, 86–94.

156. Mijakovic, I.; Poncet, S.; Boel, G.; Maze, A.; Gillet, S.; Jamet, E.; Decottignies, P.; Grangeasse, C.; Doublet, P.; le Marechal, P.; Deutscher, J. Transmembrane Modulator-Dependent Bacterial Tyrosine Kinase Activates UDP-Glucose Dehydrogenases. *EMBO J.* **2003**, *22*, 4709–4718.

157. Lee, D.C.; Zheng, J.; She, Y.M.; Jia, Z. Structure of *Escherichia coli* Tyrosine Kinase Etk Reveals a Novel Activation Mechanism. *EMBO J.* **2008**, *27*, 1758–1766.

158. Peleg, A.; Shifrin, Y.; Ilan, O.; Nadler-Yona, C.; Nov, S.; Koby, S.; Baruch, K.; Altuvia, S.; Elgrably-Weiss, M.; Abe, C.M.; Knutton, S.; Saper, M.A.; Rosenshine, I. Identification of an *Escherichia coli* Operon Required for Formation of the *O*-Antigen Capsule. *J. Bacteriol.* **2005**, *187*, 5259–5266.

159. Lacour, S.; Bechet, E.; Cozzone, A.J.; Mijakovic, I.; Grangeasse, C. Tyrosine Phosphorylation of the UDP-Glucose Dehydrogenase of *Escherichia coli* is at the Crossroads of Colanic Acid Synthesis and Polymyxin Resistance. *PLoS One* **2008**, *3*, e3053.

160. Raetz, C.R.; Reynolds, C.M.; Trent, M.S.; Bishop, R.E. Lipid A Modification Systems in Gram-negative Bacteria. *Ann. Rev. Biochem.* **2007**, *76*, 295–329.

161. Meredith, T.C.; Mamat, U.; Kaczynski, Z.; Lindner, B.; Holst, O.; Woodard, R.W. Modification of Lipopolysaccharide with Colanic Acid (M-Antigen) Repeats in *Escherichia coli*. *J. Biol. Chem.* **2007**, *282*, 7790–7798.

162. Passador, L.; Cook, J.M.; Gambello, M.J.; Rust, L.; Iglewski, B.H. Expression of *Pseudomonas aeruginosa* Virulence Genes Requires Cell-to-Cell Communication. *Science* **1993**, *260*, 1127–1130.

163. Ochsner, U.A.; Reiser, J. Autoinducer-Mediated Regulation of Rhamnolipid Biosurfactant Synthesis in *Pseudomonas aeruginosa*. *Proc. Natl. Acad. Sci. USA* **1995**, *92*, 6424–6428.

164. Diggle, S.P.; Cornelis, P.; Williams, P.; Camara, M. 4-Quinolone Signalling in *Pseudomonas aeruginosa*: Old Molecules, New Perspectives. *Int. J. Med. Microbiol.* **2006**, *296*, 83–91.

165. Latifi, A.; Foglino, M.; Tanaka, K.; Williams, P.; Lazdunski, A. A Hierarchical Quorum-Sensing Cascade in *Pseudomonas aeruginosa* Links the Transcriptional Activators LasR and RhlR (VsmR) to Expression of the Stationary-Phase Sigma Factor RpoS. *Mol. Microbiol.* **1996**, *21*, 1137–1146.

166. Wagner, V.E.; Bushnell, D.; Passador, L.; Brooks, A.I.; Iglewski, B.H. Microarray Analysis of *Pseudomonas aeruginosa* Quorum-Sensing Regulons: Effects of Growth Phase and Environment. *J. Bacteriol.* **2003**, *185*, 2080–2095.

167. Winson, M.K.; Camara, M.; Latifi, A.; Foglino, M.; Chhabra, S.R.; Daykin, M.; Bally, M.; Chapon, V.; Salmond, G.P.; Bycroft, B.W. Multiple *N*-Acyl-L-Homoserine Lactone Signal Molecules Regulate Production of Virulence Determinants and Secondary Metabolites in *Pseudomonas aeruginosa*. *Proc. Natl. Acad. Sci. USA* **1995**, *92*, 9427–9431.

168. Davies, D.G.; Parsek, M.R.; Pearson, J.P.; Iglewski, B.H.; Costerton, J.W.; Greenberg, E.P. The Involvement of Cell-to-Cell Signals in the Development of a Bacterial Biofilm. *Science* **1998**, *280*, 295–298.

169. Hentzer, M.; Eberl, L.; Nielsen, J.; Givskov, M. Quorum Sensing: A Novel Target for the Treatment of Biofilm Infections. *BioDrugs* **2003**, *17*, 241–250.

170. Sakuragi, Y.; Kolter, R. Quorum-Sensing Regulation of the Biofilm Matrix Genes (*pel*) of *Pseudomonas aeruginosa*. *J. Bacteriol.* **2007**, *189*, 5383–5386.

171. Pearson, J.P.; Gray, K.M.; Passador, L.; Tucker, K.D.; Eberhard, A.; Iglewski, B.H.; Greenberg, E.P. Structure of the Autoinducer Required for Expression of *Pseudomonas aeruginosa* Virulence Genes. *Proc. Natl. Acad. Sci. USA* **1994**, *91*, 197–201.

172. De Kievit, T.R.; Iglewski, B.H. Bacterial Quorum Sensing in Pathogenic Relationships. *Infect. Immun.* **2000**, *68*, 4839–4849.

173. Pesci, E.C.; Iglewski, B.H. The Chain of Command in *Pseudomonas* Quorum Sensing. *Trends Microbiol.* **1997**, *5*, 132–135.

174. Davey, M.E.; Caiazza, N.C.; O'Toole, G.A. Rhamnolipid Surfactant Production Affects Biofilm Architecture in *Pseudomonas aeruginosa* PAO1. *J. Bacteriol.* **2003**, *185*, 1027–1036.

175. Williams, P.; Camara, M. Quorum Sensing and Environmental Adaptation in *Pseudomonas aeruginosa*: A Tale of Regulatory Networks and Multifunctional Signal Molecules. *Curr. Opin. Microbiol.* **2009**, *12*, 182–191.

176. Beatson, S.A.; Whitchurch, C.B.; Semmler, A.B.; Mattick, J.S. Quorum Sensing is Not Required for Twitching Motility in *Pseudomonas aeruginosa*. *J. Bacteriol.* **2002**, *184*, 3598–3604.

177. Raina, S.; de Vizio, D.; Odell, M.; Clements, M.; Vanhulle, S.; Keshavarz, T. Microbial Quorum Sensing: A Tool Or a Target for Antimicrobial Therapy? *Biotechnol. Appl. Biochem.* **2009**, *54*, 65–84.

178. McKnight, S.L.; Iglewski, B.H.; Pesci, E.C. The *Pseudomonas* Quinolone Signal Regulates *rhl* Quorum Sensing in *Pseudomonas aeruginosa. J. Bacteriol.* **2000**, *182*, 2702–2708.

179. Diggle, S.P.; Winzer, K.; Chhabra, S.R.; Worrall, K.E.; Camara, M.; Williams, P. The *Pseudomonas aeruginosa* Quinolone Signal Molecule Overcomes the Cell Density-Dependency of the Quorum Sensing Hierarchy, Regulates *rhl*-Dependent Genes at the Onset of Stationary Phase and can be Produced in the Absence of LasR. *Mol. Microbiol.* **2003**, *50*, 29–43.

180. Pesci, E.C.; Milbank, J.B.; Pearson, J.P.; McKnight, S.; Kende, A.S.; Greenberg, E.P.; Iglewski, B.H. Quinolone Signaling in the Cell-to-Cell Communication System of *Pseudomonas aeruginosa. Proc. Natl. Acad. Sci. USA* **1999**, *96*, 11229–11234.

181. Aendekerk, S.; Diggle, S.P.; Song, Z.; Hoiby, N.; Cornelis, P.; Williams, P.; Camara, M. The MexGHI-OpmD Multidrug Efflux Pump Controls Growth, Antibiotic Susceptibility and Virulence in *Pseudomonas aeruginosa* Via 4-Quinolone-Dependent Cell-to-Cell Communication. *Microbiology* **2005**, *151*, 1113–1125.

182. Juhas, M.; Wiehlmann, L.; Huber, B.; Jordan, D.; Lauber, J.; Salunkhe, P.; Limpert, A.S.; von Gotz, F.; Steinmetz, I.; Eberl, L.; Tummler, B. Global Regulation of Quorum Sensing and Virulence by VqsR in *Pseudomonas aeruginosa. Microbiology* **2004**, *150*, 831–841.

183. Ledgham, F.; Ventre, I.; Soscia, C.; Foglino, M.; Sturgis, J.N.; Lazdunski, A. Interactions of the Quorum Sensing Regulator QscR: Interaction with itself and the Other Regulators of *Pseudomonas aeruginosa* LasR and RhlR. *Mol. Microbiol.* **2003**, *48*, 199–210.

184. Rampioni, G.; Bertani, I.; Zennaro, E.; Polticelli, F.; Venturi, V.; Leoni, L. The Quorum-Sensing Negative Regulator RsaL of *Pseudomonas aeruginosa* Binds to the *lasI* Promoter. *J. Bacteriol.* **2006**, *188*, 815–819.

185. Rampioni, G.; Polticelli, F.; Bertani, I.; Righetti, K.; Venturi, V.; Zennaro, E.; Leoni, L. The *Pseudomonas* Quorum-Sensing Regulator RsaL Belongs to the Tetrahelical Superclass of H-T-H Proteins. *J. Bacteriol.* **2007**, *189*, 1922–1930.

186. Hentzer, M.; Wu, H.; Andersen, J.B.; Riedel, K.; Rasmussen, T.B.; Bagge, N.; Kumar, N.; Schembri, M.A.; Song, Z.; Kristoffersen, P.; *et al.* Attenuation of *Pseudomonas aeruginosa* Virulence by Quorum Sensing Inhibitors. *EMBO J.* **2003**, *22*, 3803–3815.

187. Geske, G.D.; Wezeman, R.J.; Siegel, A.P.; Blackwell, H.E. Small Molecule Inhibitors of Bacterial Quorum Sensing and Biofilm Formation. *J. Am. Chem. Soc.* **2005**, *127*, 12762–12763.

188. Jorgensen, F.; Bally, M.; Chapon-Herve, V.; Michel, G.; Lazdunski, A.; Williams, P.; Stewart, G.S. RpoS-Dependent Stress Tolerance in *Pseudomonas aeruginosa. Microbiology* **1999**, *145*, 835–844.

189. Kojic, M.; Venturi, V. Regulation of *rpoS* Gene Expression in *Pseudomonas*: Involvement of a TetR Family Regulator. *J. Bacteriol.* **2001**, *183*, 3712–3720.

190. Whiteley, M.; Parsek, M.R.; Greenberg, E.P. Regulation of Quorum Sensing by RpoS in *Pseudomonas aeruginosa. J. Bacteriol.* **2000**, *182*, 4356–4360.

191. Medina, G.; Juarez, K.; Soberon-Chavez, G. The *Pseudomonas aeruginosa rhlAB* Operon is Not Expressed during the Logarithmic Phase of Growth Even in the Presence of its Activator RhlR and the Autoinducer *N*-Butyryl-Homoserine Lactone. *J. Bacteriol.* **2003**, *185*, 377–380.

192. Schuster, M.; Hawkins, A.C.; Harwood, C.S.; Greenberg, E.P. The *Pseudomonas aeruginosa* RpoS Regulon and its Relationship to Quorum Sensing. *Mol. Microbiol.* **2004**, *51*, 973–985.

193. Ahmer, B.M. Cell-to-Cell Signalling in *Escherichia coli* and *Salmonella enterica*. *Mol. Microbiol.* **2004**, *52*, 933–945.

194. Van Houdt, R.; Aertsen, A.; Moons, P.; Vanoirbeek, K.; Michiels, C.W. *N*-Acyl-L-Homoserine Lactone Signal Interception by *Escherichia coli*. *FEMS Microbiol. Lett.* **2006**, *256*, 83–89.

195. De Keersmaecker, S.C.; Sonck, K.; Vanderleyden, J. Let LuxS Speak Up in AI-2 Signaling. *Trends Microbiol.* **2006**, *14*, 114–119.

196. Walters, M.; Sperandio, V. Quorum Sensing in *Escherichia coli* and *Salmonella*. *Int. J. Med. Microbiol.* **2006**, *296*, 125–131.

197. Kanamaru, K.; Kanamaru, K.; Tatsuno, I.; Tobe, T.; Sasakawa, C. SdiA, an *Escherichia coli* Homologue of Quorum-Sensing Regulators, Controls the Expression of Virulence Factors in Enterohaemorrhagic *Escherichia coli* O157:H7. *Mol. Microbiol.* **2000**, *38*, 805–816.

198. Nealson, K.H.; Platt, T.; Hastings, J.W. Cellular Control of the Synthesis and Activity of the Bacterial Luminescent System. *J. Bacteriol.* **1970**, *104*, 313–322.

199. Michael, B.; Smith, J.N.; Swift, S.; Heffron, F.; Ahmer, B.M. SdiA of *Salmonella enterica* is a LuxR Homolog that Detects Mixed Microbial Communities. *J. Bacteriol.* **2001**, *183*, 5733–5742.

200. Ravichandiran, V.; Shanmugam, K.; Solomon, A.P. Screening of SdiA Inhibitors from Melia Dubia Seeds Extracts Towards the Hold Back of Uropathogenic *E. Coli* Quorum Sensing-Regulated Factors. *J. Med. Chem.* **2013**, *9*, 819–827.

201. Chong, T.M.; Koh, C.L.; Sam, C.K.; Choo, Y.M.; Yin, W.F.; Chan, K.G. Characterization of Quorum Sensing and Quorum Quenching Soil Bacteria Isolated from Malaysian Tropical Montane Forest. *Sensors* **2012**, *12*, 4846–4859.

202. Bjarnsholt, T.; Jensen, P.O.; Rasmussen, T.B.; Christophersen, L.; Calum, H.; Hentzer, M.; Hougen, H.P.; Rygaard, J.; Moser, C.; Eberl, L.; *et al.* Garlic Blocks Quorum Sensing and Promotes Rapid Clearing of Pulmonary *Pseudomonas aeruginosa* Infections. *Microbiology* **2005**, *151*, 3873–3880.

203. Jha, B.; Kavita, K.; Westphal, J.; Hartmann, A.; Schmitt-Kopplin, P. Quorum Sensing Inhibition by *Asparagopsis. taxiformis*, a Marine Macro Alga: Separation of the Compound that Interrupts Bacterial Communication. *Mar. Drugs* **2013**, *11*, 253–265.

204. March, J.C.; Bentley, W.E. Quorum Sensing and Bacterial Cross-Talk in Biotechnology. *Curr. Opin. Biotechnol.* **2004**, *15*, 495–502.

205. Hardie, K.R.; Cooksley, C.; Green, A.D.; Winzer, K. Autoinducer 2 Activity in *Escherichia coli* Culture Supernatants can be Actively Reduced Despite Maintenance of an Active Synthase, LuxS. *Microbiology* **2003**, *149*, 715–728.

206. Xavier, K.B.; Bassler, B.L. Regulation of Uptake and Processing of the Quorum-Sensing Autoinducer AI-2 in *Escherichia coli*. *J. Bacteriol.* **2005**, *187*, 238–248.

207. Wang, L.; Li, J.; March, J.C.; Valdes, J.J.; Bentley, W.E. *luxS*-Dependent Gene Regulation in *Escherichia coli* K-12 Revealed by Genomic Expression Profiling. *J. Bacteriol.* **2005**, *187*, 8350–8360.

208. Taga, M.E.; Miller, S.T.; Bassler, B.L. Lsr-Mediated Transport and Processing of AI-2 in *Salmonella typhimurium*. *Mol. Microbiol.* **2003**, *50*, 1411–1427.

209. Li, J.; Attila, C.; Wang, L.; Wood, T.K.; Valdes, J.J.; Bentley, W.E. Quorum Sensing in *Escherichia coli* is Signaled by AI-2/LsrR: Effects on Small RNA and Biofilm Architecture. *J. Bacteriol.* **2007**, *189*, 6011–6020.

210. Robinson, L.S.; Ashman, E.M.; Hultgren, S.J.; Chapman, M.R. Secretion of Curli Fibre Subunits is Mediated by the Outer Membrane-Localized CsgG Protein. *Mol. Microbiol.* **2006**, *59*, 870–881.

211. Barnhart, M.M.; Chapman, M.R. Curli Biogenesis and Function. *Ann. Rev. Microbiol.* **2006**, *60*, 131–147.

212. DeLisa, M.P.; Wu, C.F.; Wang, L.; Valdes, J.J.; Bentley, W.E. DNA Microarray-Based Identification of Genes Controlled by Autoinducer 2-Stimulated Quorum Sensing in *Escherichia coli*. *J. Bacteriol.* **2001**, *183*, 5239–5247.

213. Schauder, S.; Shokat, K.; Surette, M.G.; Bassler, B.L. The LuxS Family of Bacterial Autoinducers: Biosynthesis of a Novel Quorum-Sensing Signal Molecule. *Mol. Microbiol.* **2001**, *41*, 463–476.

214. Diaz, Z.; Xavier, K.B.; Miller, S.T. The Crystal Structure of the *Escherichia coli* Autoinducer-2 Processing Protein LsrF. *PLoS One* **2009**, *4*, e6820.

215. Xavier, K.B.; Miller, S.T.; Lu, W.; Kim, J.H.; Rabinowitz, J.; Pelczer, I.; Semmelhack, M.F.; Bassler, B.L. Phosphorylation and Processing of the Quorum-Sensing Molecule Autoinducer-2 in Enteric Bacteria. *ACS Chem. Biol.* **2007**, *2*, 128–136.

216. Kendall, M.M.; Rasko, D.A.; Sperandio, V. Global Effects of the Cell-to-Cell Signaling Molecules Autoinducer-2, Autoinducer-3, and Epinephrine in a *luxS* Mutant of Enterohemorrhagic *Escherichia coli*. *Infect. Immun.* **2007**, *75*, 4875–4884.

217. Kaper, J.B.; Nataro, J.P.; Mobley, H.L. Pathogenic *Escherichia coli*. *Nat. Rev. Microbiol.* **2004**, *2*, 123–140.

218. Walters, M.; Sircili, M.P.; Sperandio, V. AI-3 Synthesis is Not Dependent on *luxS* in *Escherichia coli*. *J. Bacteriol.* **2006**, *188*, 5668–5681.

219. Sperandio, V.; Torres, A.G.; Giron, J.A.; Kaper, J.B. Quorum Sensing is a Global Regulatory Mechanism in Enterohemorrhagic *Escherichia coli* O157:H7. *J. Bacteriol.* **2001**, *183*, 5187–5197.

220. Freestone, P.P.; Lyte, M.; Neal, C.P.; Maggs, A.F.; Haigh, R.D.; Williams, P.H. The Mammalian Neuroendocrine Hormone Norepinephrine Supplies Iron for Bacterial Growth in the Presence of Transferrin Or Lactoferrin. *J. Bacteriol.* **2000**, *182*, 6091–6098.

221. Sperandio, V.; Torres, A.G.; Kaper, J.B. Quorum Sensing Escherichia Coli Regulators B and C (QseBC): A Novel Two-Component Regulatory System Involved in the Regulation of Flagella and Motility by Quorum Sensing in *E. Coli*. *Mol. Microbiol.* **2002**, *43*, 809–821.

222. Reading, N.C.; Rasko, D.A.; Torres, A.G.; Sperandio, V. The Two-Component System QseEF and the Membrane Protein QseG Link Adrenergic and Stress Sensing to Bacterial Pathogenesis. *Proc. Natl. Acad. Sci. USA* **2009**, *106*, 5889–5894.

223. Sperandio, V.; Li, C.C.; Kaper, J.B. Quorum-Sensing *Escherichia coli* Regulator A: A Regulator of the LysR Family Involved in the Regulation of the Locus of Enterocyte Effacement Pathogenicity Island in Enterohemorrhagic *E. coli. Infect. Immun.* **2002**, *70*, 3085–3093.

224. Wang, D.; Ding, X.; Rather, P.N. Indole can Act as an Extracellular Signal in *Escherichia coli. J. Bacteriol.* **2001**, *183*, 4210–4216.

225. World Health Organization. *Antimicrobial Resistance: Global Report on Surveillance 2014*; WHO: Geneva, Switzerland, 2014.

226. Ito, A.; Taniuchi, A.; May, T.; Kawata, K.; Okabe, S. Increased Antibiotic Resistance of *Escherichia coli* in Mature Biofilms. *Appl. Environ. Microbiol.* **2009**, *75*, 4093–4100.

227. O'Loughlin, C.T.; Miller, L.C.; Siryaporn, A.; Drescher, K.; Semmelhack, M.F.; Bassler, B.L. A Quorum-Sensing Inhibitor Blocks *Pseudomonas aeruginosa* Virulence and Biofilm Formation. *Proc. Natl. Acad. Sci. USA* **2013**, *110*, 17981–17986.

228. Deep, A.; Chaudhary, U.; Gupta, V. Quorum Sensing and Bacterial Pathogenicity: From Molecules to Disease. *J. Lab. Phys.* **2011**, *3*, 4–11.

7

Antibiotic Resistance Related to Biofilm Formation in *Klebsiella pneumoniae*

Claudia Vuotto [1,3,*], **Francesca Longo** [1], **Maria Pia Balice** [2], **Gianfranco Donelli** [1] **and Pietro E. Varaldo** [3]

[1] Microbial Biofilm Laboratory, IRCCS Fondazione Santa Lucia, Rome 00179, Italy;
E-Mails: f-longo@hotmail.it (F.L.); g.donelli@hsantalucia.it (G.D.)

[2] Clinical Microbiology Laboratory, IRCCS Fondazione Santa Lucia, Rome 00179, Italy;
E-Mail: mp.balice@hsantalucia.it

[3] Department of Biomedical Sciences and Public Health, Section of Microbiology,
Polytechnic University of Marche, Ancona 60126, Italy; E-Mail: pe.varaldo@univpm.it

[*] Author to whom correspondence should be addressed; E-Mail: c.vuotto@hsantalucia.it;

Abstract: The Gram-negative opportunistic pathogen, *Klebsiella pneumoniae*, is responsible for causing a spectrum of community-acquired and nosocomial infections and typically infects patients with indwelling medical devices, especially urinary catheters, on which this microorganism is able to grow as a biofilm. The increasingly frequent acquisition of antibiotic resistance by *K. pneumoniae* strains has given rise to a global spread of this multidrug-resistant pathogen, mostly at the hospital level. This scenario is exacerbated when it is noted that intrinsic resistance to antimicrobial agents dramatically increases when *K. pneumoniae* strains grow as a biofilm. This review will summarize the findings about the antibiotic resistance related to biofilm formation in *K. pneumoniae*.

Keywords: *Klebsiella pneumonia*; biofilm; antibiotic resistance

1. Introduction

Klebsiella pneumoniae was isolated for the first time in 1882 by Friedlander from the lungs of patients who died after pneumonia. This encapsulated bacterium, initially named Friedlander's bacillus, was renamed *Klebsiella* in 1886. Later, it was described as a saprophyte microorganism, not only colonizing the human gastrointestinal tract, skin and nasopharynx, but also able to cause urinary and biliary tract infections, osteomyelitis and bacteremia [1–3].

The virulence factors playing an important role in the severity of *K. pneumoniae* infections are capsular polysaccharides, type 1 and type 3 pili, factors involved in aggregative adhesions and siderophores [3–6], with those studied in greater depth being capsular polysaccharides and type 1 and type 3 pili.

Capsules, whose subunits can be classified into 77 serological types [7], are essential to the virulence of *Klebsiella* [8]. The capsular material, forming fibrillous structures that cover the bacterial surface [9], protects the bacterium from phagocytosis, on the one hand [10], and prevents killing of the bacteria by bactericidal serum factors, on the other [11].

Type 1 and type 3 pili [12] (otherwise known as fimbriae), instead, are non-flagellar, filamentous fimbrial adhesins, often detected on the bacterial surface, that consist of polymeric globular protein subunits (pilin) [13]. On the basis of their ability to agglutinate erythrocytes and depending on whether the reaction is inhibited by D-mannose, these adhesins are designated as mannose-sensitive (MSHA) or mannose-resistant hemagglutinins (MRHA), respectively [14]. Type 1 fimbriae are encoded by an operon (*fim*) containing all of the genes required for the fimbrial structure and assembly, with assembly occurring via the chaperone-usher pathway [15]. Type 1 fimbriae in *K. pneumoniae* are regulated via phase variation in a similar way to the regulation of type 1 fimbriae in *E. coli* [16,17]. Alcántar-Curiel and colleagues demonstrated that the *fim* operon was found in 100% of 69 *K. pneumoniae* isolates and that type 1 fimbriae were detected in 96% of these strains [18]. Conversely, the type 3 fimbriae are encoded by the *mrk* operon and are predicted to be assembled via a chaperone-usher pathway, too, with the *mrk* gene cluster being chromosome or plasmid borne [19–21].

Due to its high pathogenicity, *K. pneumoniae*, in the pre-antibiotic era, was considered as an important causative agent of community-acquired (CA) infections, including a severe form of pneumonia, especially in alcoholics and in diabetic patients. In recent years, while CA pneumonia due to this pathogen has become rare, novel manifestations of *K. pneumoniae* CA infections, including liver abscess complicated by endophthalmitis, different metastatic infections [22], often caused by highly virulent strains of specific serotypes, such as K1 [23], as well as urinary tract infections [24], have been described.

The greater adhesiveness and presumably also the invasiveness of strains may play an important role in the recurrent infections, *K. pneumoniae* strains being able to persist despite appropriate antibiotic treatment [25]. However, unlike the adhesion ability, the invasive capacity of *K. pneumoniae* to cause liver infections [26,27] and urinary tract infections [28] is still controversial and requires further study.

In contrast, starting from the early 1970s, *K. pneumoniae* epidemiology and its spectrum of infections significantly changed when this microorganism was established in the hospital environment and became a leading cause of nosocomial infections, particularly in developed Western countries. In fact, its considerable efficiency of colonization, accompanied by acquired resistance to antibiotics, has enabled *K. pneumoniae* to persist and spread rapidly in healthcare settings, the most common healthcare-associated infections caused by this agent involving the urinary tract, wounds, lungs, abdominal cavity, intra-vascular devices, surgical sites, soft tissues and subsequent bacteremia [3,29–31].

Klebsiella is second only to *Escherichia coli* in nosocomial Gram-negative bacteremia [32], as well as in urinary tract infections (UTIs), affecting catheterized patients (16% and 70%, respectively) [33]. In fact, *K. pneumoniae* has been reported as a prominent cause of infections in individuals with indwelling urinary catheters [34,35].

Of interest, a high incidence of *K. pneumoniae* in UTIs (from 6% to 17%) was reported in previous studies carried out in specific groups of patients at risk, e.g., patients with diabetes mellitus or with neuropathic bladders [36,37].

As concerns the bacteremia associated with intravascular catheters, an epidemiological study on bloodstream infections carried out in Israel revealed that *Staphylococcus aureus* was the most common species (30%), followed by *K. pneumoniae* (10%) [38].

In general, a cohort study indicated that the majority of infections associated with different medical devices, including both urinary and intravascular catheters, was caused by *K. pneumoniae* followed by staphylococcal biofilms, and a high percentage (about 90%) of biofilm-producing bacterial isolates causing infection were multidrug resistant [39].

In 2013, the incidence of *K. pneumoniae* clinical infections was estimated in the United States to be higher in long-term acute care hospitals, compared to short-stay hospital intensive care units [40].

In a prospective study on hospital-acquired infections carried out in Rome in the period January, 2002–December, 2004, *K. pneumoniae* was reported as the second most frequent Gram-negative species (11%) after *Pseudomonas* (25%) [41]. In a countrywide cross-sectional survey carried out in collaboration with twenty-five large clinical microbiology laboratories from 23 Italian cities, Klebsiella pneumoniae carbapenemase (KPC)-producing *K. pneumoniae* (KPC-KP) were revealed to majorly contribute to the epidemic dissemination of carbapenem-resistant *Enterobacteriaceae*, their spreading being mostly sustained by strains of clonal complex 258 (ST-258 producing KPC-2 or KPC-3 and ST-512 producing KPC-3) [42].

In a recent meta-analysis covering studies (2000–2010) on Gram-negative wound infections in hospitalized adult burn patients, *K. pneumoniae* has been reported as one of the most common Gram-negative pathogens, after *P. aeruginosa* [43].

2. Antibiotic Resistance

Although *K. pneumoniae* possesses only moderate amounts of chromosomal penicillinases, it is a well-known "collector" of multidrug resistance plasmids that commonly encoded resistance to aminoglycosides, till the end of 1980s, while, later, encoding extended-spectrum β-lactamases (ESBLs), mostly Temoniera (TEMs) and Sulfhydryl variable (SHVs) active against last generation cephalosporins, as well as a variety of genes conferring resistance to drugs other than β-lactams [3,44].

The acquisition of these plasmids and the occurrence of chromosomal mutations that confer resistance to fluoroquinolones often makes the treatment of *K. pneumoniae* healthcare-associated infections possible only by using carbapenems as "last-line of defense" antibiotics [45–47].

Unfortunately, from the early 2000s, multidrug-resistant (MDR) *K. pneumoniae* strains started to produce also "carbapenemases" encoded by transmissible plasmids and rapidly disseminated within both acute hospitals and long-term care facilities. Later, other enterobacterial species, including *E. coli*, acquired carbapenemase genes, thus suggesting that *K. pneumoniae* may have acted as a pool of β-lactamases [48].

Over the past decade, carbapenemases of Classes A, B and D, which are β-lactamases able to efficiently hydrolyze penicillins, cephalosporins, monobactams, carbapenems and β-lactamase inhibitors, have progressively disseminated among *Enterobacteriaceae* [49]. The Class A KPCs, firstly discovered in the USA in 1996, are the most worrying carbapenemases for their spreading across countries and continents, even if their expansion is dependent on the geographical area [50,51]. Furthermore, the zinc-dependent Class B metallo-β-lactamases (MβLs), mainly represented by the Verona integron-encoded metallo-β-lactamase (VIM), imipenemase metallo-β-lactamase (IMP) and New Delhi metallo-β-lactamase (NDM) types, are encoded on highly transmissible plasmids that spread rapidly between bacteria, rather than relying on clonal proliferation. In particular, NDM-1, originated in Asia, was found in almost every continent within one year from its emergence in India [52]. The picture is completed by the plasmid-expressed Class D carbapenemases of the oxacillinase-48 (OXA-48) type [48,53–55].

KPC enzyme-producing *K. pneumoniae* is generally susceptible to few antibiotics, and it is associated with a high mortality rate among patients with bloodstream infections. In fact, many of these strains are susceptible to colistin, tigecycline and one or more aminoglycosides, but some of them are resistant even to these drugs [56].

3. Biofilm

K. pneumoniae was reported to be able to grow *in vitro* as a biofilm since the end of the 1980s [57], but clear evidence of an *in vivo* biofilm was provided only in 1992 by Reid and coworkers, who investigated by scanning electron microscopy some bladder epithelial cells of a spinal cord injured patient with an asymptomatic urinary tract infection caused by *K. pneumoniae* [58].

Later, *in vitro* studies have demonstrated that about 40% of *K. pneumoniae* isolated not only from urine, but also from sputum, blood and wound swabs, were able to produce biofilm [59], as well as that about 63% of *K. pneumoniae* isolates from urine samples of catheterized patients suffering from UTIs were positive for *in vitro* biofilm production [33]. Recently, also a high rate of *K. pneumoniae* strains isolated from endotracheal tubes (ETT) of patients affected by ventilator-associated pneumonia (VAP) were reported to be able to form an *in vitro* biofilm [39].

Biofilm formation on abiotic surfaces was shown to be more consistent at 40 °C than 35 °C, using atomic force and high-vacuum SEM [60]. The ability of *K. pneumoniae* clinical strains to adhere and form biofilm *in vitro* was recently investigated by field emission scanning electron microscopy (FESEM) [61] and by confocal laser scanning microscopy (Figure 1).

3.1. Virulence and Biofilm Formation

Type 1 or type 3 fimbriae, as well as the capsule and the LPS are the virulence factors mostly involved in the ability of *K. pneumoniae* to grow as biofilm.

Type 3 fimbriae have been demonstrated to be the major appendages that mediate the formation of biofilms on biotic and abiotic surfaces and the attachment to endothelial and bladder epithelial cell lines [62–67]. In particular, growth of *K. pneumoniae* on abiotic surfaces is facilitated by the MrkA type 3 fimbrial protein, whereas growth on surfaces coated with a human extracellular matrix (HECM) requires the presence of the type 3 fimbrial adhesin MrkD [62,64].

Figure 1. Bidimensional (**A**) and three-dimensional (**B**) images of a *K. pneumoniae in vitro* biofilm obtained by Confocal Laser Scanning Microscopy (CLSM) on different areas of a biofilm-covered glass coverslip. SYTO ® 9 green fluorescent nucleic acid stain has been used to detect both live and dead bacteria (Life Technologies, Monza (MB) , Italy).

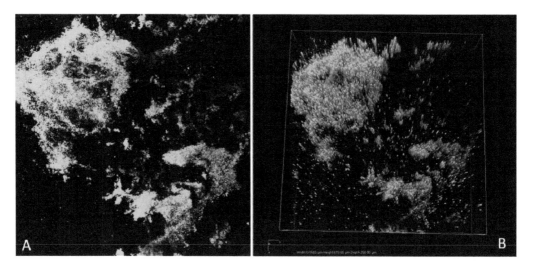

Recent investigations have verified that type 3 fimbrial gene expression is regulated, at least in part, by the intracellular levels of cyclic di-GMP [68].

Type 3 fimbriae have been confirmed by Murphy and colleagues (2013) to be a very important colonization factor in biofilm-mediated infections associated with catheter-associated urinary tract infections (CAUTIs) by obtaining mutants lacking the ability to produce type 1 or type 3 fimbriae or a combined double mutant. These mutants were impaired in colonization and had subsequent persistence under specific experimental conditions [69].

Alcántar-Curiel and colleagues demonstrated that, among the 69 examined *K. pneumoniae* isolates, 55 were able to produce biofilm and all of them contained *mrkA*, but only 57% of them produced MR/K fimbriae [18]. The same group also revealed that 96% of 69 *K. pneumoniae* isolates harbored the *ecpABCDE* operon homolog of the operon encoding the *E. coli* adhesive structure common pilus (ECP), with 94% of them producing ECP during adhesion to cultured epithelial cells and 8% during the formation of biofilms on glass. These results suggest that ECP also seems to be required for biofilm formation, at least *in vitro* [18].

Regarding the involvement of capsule and LPS in *K. pneumoniae* biofilm formation, it has been proven that both of them contribute to the structure of biofilm communities of *K. pneumoniae*. In fact, gene disruption and microscopic analyses showed that LPS is involved in the initial adhesion on abiotic surfaces and that the capsule is necessary for a proper initial coverage of substratum and construction of mature biofilm architecture [70].

Furthermore, *treC* and *sugE* genes have been demonstrated to affect biofilm formation by modulating CPS production [71].

However, conflicting results on the involvement of CPS production in biofilm formation arise from a paper of Huang and coworkers (2014). In fact, the authors found that two knockout mutants, the first one with the entire gene cluster responsible for biosynthesis of the extracellular polysaccharide capsule deleted and the other one with the capsule export subsystem deleted, have lower amounts of capsule, but produce greater amounts of biofilm [72].

3.2. Involvement in Mixed Biofilms

The first investigation of mixed microbial populations including *K. pneumoniae* dates back to 1991. Siebel and colleagues demonstrated the ability of *K. pneumoniae* to form *in vitro* a dual-species biofilm together with *P. aeruginosa*. Authors determined that, although the *K. pneumoniae* specific cellular growth rate was five times that of *P. aeruginosa*, it did not dominate the microbial population, with results indicating that neither the specific cellular product formation rate nor the glucose-oxygen stoichiometric ratio of *K. pneumoniae* or *P. aeruginosa* when grown together were affected by the presence of the other species [73].

Later, *K. pneumoniae* was shown to form a biofilm more successfully in a mixture than in isolation with an increased resistance to disinfection [74].

In the same year, Stickler and colleagues, by using a model of a catheterized bladder, firstly investigated the possible role of *K. pneumoniae* and other uropathogens in the development of crystalline biofilm on catheter surfaces, demonstrating that this microorganism is not able to raise the urinary pH and, thus, to contribute to the crystalline biofilm formation [75].

In 2007, the same research team analyzed 106 biofilms samples developed on urinary catheters, finding that *K. pneumoniae* was able to form a mixed biofilm with *Proteus mirabilis*, when *E. coli*, *Morganella morganii* or *Enterobacter cloacae* were also present [76].

The ability of *K. pneumoniae* to form a mixed-species biofilm *in vitro* with *P. aeruginosa* and *Pseudomonas protegens* was confirmed by adding a fluorescent tag to each species in order to determine the abundance and spatial localization of each of them within the biofilm. The development of the mixed-species biofilm was delayed 1–2 days compared with the single-species biofilms, and the composition and spatial organization of the mixed-species biofilm changed along the flow cell channel. Furthermore, the mixed-species biofilm resulted in being more resistant to sodium dodecyl sulfate and tobramycin with respect to the single-species biofilms [77].

Recent investigations on 35 ETTs obtained from 26 neonates with mechanical ventilation demonstrated that *K. pneumoniae*, together with *Pseudomonas* and *Streptococcus*, was the most common bacteria isolated from ETT-bacterial biofilms, and it was hypothesized that there were interactions among these species in the biofilm [78].

Our recent findings demonstrated that *K. pneumoniae* is able to form a multi-species biofilm together with *Candida albicans* within a urinary catheter removed from a patient hospitalized at the neuromotor rehabilitation hospital, Fondazione Santa Lucia in Rome, Italy (Figure 2).

Figure 2. FESEM micrographs (**a** = 2000×; **b** = 25,000×) of a polymicrobial biofilm grown in the lumen of a urinary catheter removed from a patient recovered at the research hospital for neuromotor rehabilitation, Fondazione Santa Lucia in Rome. The species identified by culture methods were *Klebsiella pneumonia* and *Candida albicans*.

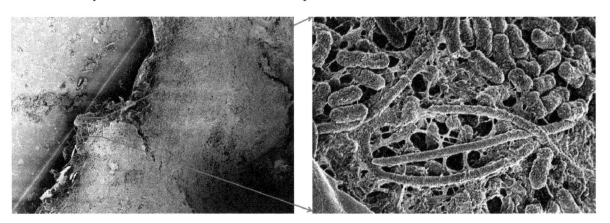

4. Antibiotic Resistance of Biofilm-Growing Strains

The response of *K. pneumoniae* biofilm to different antimicrobial agents has been investigated in several studies in the last decade.

One of the first studies that addressed the issue of the penetration of antimicrobials through *K. pneumoniae* biofilm was in 2000, when Anderl and co-workers used an *in vitro* model system to evaluate the effect of ampicillin and ciprofloxacin on *K. pneumoniae* biofilm developed on microporous membranes with agar nutrient medium. *K. pneumoniae* biofilms resisted killing during prolonged exposure to both antibiotics. The authors directly measured the antibiotics' diffusion, demonstrating that ampicillin did not penetrate wild-type *K. pneumoniae* biofilms, whereas ciprofloxacin and a nonreactive tracer (chloride ion) penetrated the biofilms quickly. Ampicillin was able to penetrate biofilms only when formed by a β-lactamase-deficient mutant, thus demonstrating that the increased resistance of both wild-type and mutant *K. pneumonia* biofilm to ampicillin and ciprofloxacin could not be attributed to slow diffusion [79].

The penetration of ampicillin and ciprofloxacin through *K. pneumoniae* biofilms was then confirmed using transmission electron microscopy (TEM). The authors visualized cells in biofilm after antibiotic exposure, identifying those regions of the biofilm contained on an agar plate that were able to reach 10-fold minimum inhibitory concentration (MIC) with ciprofloxacin or ampicillin [80].

This topic was further addressed one year later by Andrel and colleagues, assuming that the already observed mechanism might be due to the presence, in internal zones of biofilm with nutrient limitations, of stationary-phase bacteria that become tolerant to ampicillin and ciprofloxacin, as observed in free-floating bacteria [81].

A number of other antibiotics, including piperacillin, piperacillin-tazobactam, cefoperazone, ceftazidime, cefepime, meropenem, ciprofloxacin, netilmicin and amikacin, were also evaluated on *K. pneumoniae* biofilm, confirming that adherent bacterial populations exhibited reduced antimicrobial susceptibility with respect to their planktonic counterpart [82].

On the contrary, in 2009, tetracycline and chloramphenicol at a five-fold MIC were demonstrated to affect *K. pneumoniae* biofilms, even if to a different extent ($p < 0.05$ and $p < 0.01$, respectively) [83], and their inhibitory effects could be explained by the fact that both of these antibiotics are protein synthesis inhibitors, which act on the bacterial ribosome [84,85].

The higher resistance of *K. pneumoniae* biofilm to ciprofloxacin, amikacin and piperacillin was confirmed by testing them on different phases relevant for biofilm formation, including planktonic cells at mid-log phase, planktonic cells at stationary phase, adherent monolayers and mature biofilms. *K. pneumoniae* in a biofilm growth mode resulted in being more resistant to all antibiotics. The effect of amikacin and ciprofloxacin on young and older biofilms, at the highest achievable serum concentrations, was also examined, observing that amikacin was able to eradicate the young biofilms, but became completely ineffective when biofilm increased in age. A possible explanation for the increasing resistance during the time of growth was given by calcofluor staining, an enhanced production of exopolysaccharide in older biofilms being observed [86].

Bellifa and coworkers investigated the response of biofilm-growing *K. pneumoniae* strains isolated from medical devices to gentamicin, cefotaxime and ciprofloxacin, detecting that isolates were at least 10–25-times more resistant when grown as a biofilm than in the planktonic form [87].

Recently, differences in the antibiotic resistance of biofilm-growing *K. pneumoniae* strains to gentamicin, depending on the resistance or susceptibility of the planktonic-growing isolates to this antibiotic, have been observed. In fact, gentamicin-resistant isolates dramatically increased their resistance when grown as a biofilm (up to 234-fold), whereas gentamicin-susceptible isolates preserved their susceptibility also in biofilm, thus supporting the use of this antibiotic to successfully treat gentamicin-susceptible biofilm-growing *K. pneumoniae* strains [88].

The efficacy of amikacin has been evaluated also by developing a biofilm model of *K. pneumoniae* B5055, mimicking *in vivo* biofilm system. By using the BacLight viability staining kit, the antibiotic was effective against younger biofilm, but ineffective against older biofilm, possibly due to the heterogeneity and thickness of the biofilm itself [89].

Contrariwise, imipenem recently has shown a potent activity against established *K. pneumoniae* biofilms under both static and flow conditions *in vitro* and *in vivo*, by using a rabbit ear wound model [90].

5. Correlation between Biofilm and Antibiotic Resistance

To date, it has been demonstrated that some correlations exist between antibiotic resistance and the biofilm-forming ability of *K. pneumoniae* strains.

For instance, the ability of 150 *K. pneumoniae* strains, isolated from sputum and urine, to form biofilm exhibited a significant association with their ESBL production. In fact, among the 44.7% biofilm formers, 45.3% of them produced ESBLs [59].

Later, a NDM-1 carrying a *K. pneumoniae* isolate has been demonstrated to be the most virulent in the murine sepsis model and the stronger biofilm producer, as tested with the Calgary device method, with respect to the non-NDM-1 carrying isolates, but there was no clear correlation with *in vitro* virulence factors, such as biofilm formation ability or killing in *Caenorhabditis elegans* [91].

In 2012, a prospective analysis revealed that 80% of the biofilm-producing strains collected from 100 urine samples from catheterized patients with symptoms of UTI over a period of six months, exhibited the MDR phenotype. In particular, biofilm-positive isolates showed 93.3%, 83.3%, 73.3% and 80% resistance to nalidixic acid, ampicillin, cefotaxime and co-trimoxazole, respectively, compared to the 70%, 60%, 35% and 60% resistance shown by biofilm non-producers for the respective antibiotics [92].

Afterwards, Sanchez and coworkers confirmed the propensity of MDR *K. pneumoniae* strains to form a richer biofilm with respect to the susceptible ones, with special reference to those resistant to cephalosporins [93].

The link between antibiotic resistance and biofilm formation has been also examined by growing *K. pneumoniae* strains under antibiotic pressure, mostly with a sub-inhibitory concentration of antimicrobials. Hennequin and colleagues monitored the bactericidal effect of cefotaxime (MIC 516 mg/L) and ofloxacin (MIC 2 mg/L) on CTX-M-15-producing *K. pneumoniae*. While in the presence of sub-MICs of ofloxacin, the biomass decreased in inverse proportion to the antibiotic concentrations; in the presence of cefotaxime at sub-MIC concentrations, the biofilm formation enhanced [94].

Finally, looking more specifically at antibiotic resistance genes responsible for this correlation, *AmpR*, a regulator of *K. pneumoniae* virulence, particularly regulating a cephalosporins resistance gene (*DHA-1*) carried on a plasmid, has been demonstrated to modulate biofilm formation and type 3 fimbrial gene expression, as well as the adhesion to HT-29 intestinal epithelial cells [95].

6. Conclusions

The opportunistic pathogen, *K. pneumoniae*, can give rise to severe diseases, typically nosocomial infections, such as septicemia, pneumonia, UTI and soft tissue infection. *Klebsiella* infections are often considered as a paradigm of hospital-acquired infections. The indiscriminate use of antibiotics has revealed a considerable increase in outbreaks caused by microorganisms resistant to antimicrobial drugs, such as KPC-producing *K. pneumoniae*.

Nosocomial *Klebsiella* infections continue to be a heavy burden on the economy and on the life expectancy of patients in developed countries. Thus, further progress in the prevention of hospital-acquired infections will require new approaches to infection control.

The increasing evidence on the ability of *K. pneumoniae* to form biofilm, mostly on medical devices and the recent data supporting the correlation of such a behavior with the antibiotic resistance acquisition should alert even more regarding the hazard of this pathogen in hospital settings.

The exploration of these virulence factors and the study of new mechanisms to control them could be an important way to counteract *K. pneumoniae* nosocomial infections. In particular, the biofilm mode of growth makes bacteria up to 1,000-times more resistant to antibiotic therapy. In *K. pneumoniae*, many studies were performed in order to better highlight the mechanisms underlying this resistance, demonstrating that the limitation of the penetration of antibiotic molecules through the biofilm matrix is not the main reason for the increasing resistance, but rather the slow growth rate in the center of biofilm is. In any case, other mechanisms are involved, and further studies are requested as a future challenge to elaborate new concepts in the preventive measures against nosocomial *K. pneumoniae* infections.

Acknowledgments

The authors are indebted to Antonino Salvia, Director, and Angelo Rossini, Vice-Director, of the Medical Services of the Fondazione Santa Lucia in Rome for their advice on the clinical issues of this research.

Author Contributions

Claudia Vuotto wrote the manuscript. Francesca Longo selected references and contributed to the manuscript drafting. Maria Pia Balice supplied investigated urinary catheters and *K. pneumoniae* strains. Gianfranco Donelli critically revised the manuscript. Pietro Emanuele Varaldo provided insightful comments.

References

1. Varaldo, P.E.; Biavasco, F.; Mannelli, S.; Pompei, R.; Proietti, A. Distribution and antibiotic susceptibility of extraintestinal clinical isolates of Klebsiella, Enterobacter and Serratia species. *Eur. J. Clin. Microbiol. Infect. Dis.* **1988**, *4*, 495–500

2. Bagley, S.T. Habitat association of *Klebsiella* species. *Infect. Control* **1985**, *6*, 52–58.

3. Podschun, R.; Ullmann, U. *Klebsiella* spp. as nosocomial pathogens: Epidemiology, taxonomy, typing methods, and pathogenicity factors. *Clin. Microbiol. Rev.* **1998**, *11*, 589–603.

4. Arakawa, Y.; Wacharotayankun, R.; Nagatsuka, T.; Ito, H.; Kato, N.; Ohta, M. Genomic organization of the *Klebsiella pneumoniae cps* region responsible for serotype K2 capsular polysaccharide synthesis in virulent strain Chedid. *J. Bacteriol.* **1995**, *177*, 1788–1796.

5. Gerlach, G.F.; Clegg, S.; Allen, B.L. Identification and characterization of the genes encoding the type 3 and type 1 fimbrial adhesins of *Klebsiella pneumoniae*. *J. Clin. Microbiol.* **1989**, *171*, 1262–1270.

6. Martino, P.D.; Bertin, Y.; Girardeau, J.P.; Livrelli, V.; Joly, B.; Darfeuille Michaud, A. Molecular characterization and adhesive properties of CF29K, and adhesion of *Klebsiella pneumoniae* strains involved in nosocomial infections. *Infect. Immun.* **1995**, *63*, 4336–4344.

7. Ørskov, I.; Ørskov, F. Serotyping of *Klebsiella*. *Methods Microbiol.* **1984**, *14*, 143–164.

8. Ehrenwort, L.; Baer, H. The pathogenicity of *Klebsiella pneumoniae* for mice: The relationship to the quantity and rate of production of type-specific capsular polysaccharide. *J. Bacteriol.* **1956**, *72*, 713–717.

9. Amako, K.; Meno, Y.; Takade, A. Fine structures of the capsules of *Klebsiella pneumoniae* and *Escherichia coli* K1. *J. Bacteriol.* **1988**, *170*, 4960–4962.

10. Podschun, R.; Ullmann, U. *Klebsiella* capsular type K7 in relation to toxicity, susceptibility to phagocytosis and resistance to serum. *J. Med Microbiol* **1992** *36*, 250–254.

11. Williams, P.; Lambert, P.A.; Brown, M.R.W.; Jones, R.J. The role of the O and K antigens in determining the resistance of *Klebsiella aerogenes* to serum killing and phagocytosis. *J. Gen. Microbiol.* **1983**, *129*, 2181–2191.

12. Livrelli, V.; de Champs, C.; di Martino, P.; Darfeuille-Michaud, A.; Forestier, C.; Joly, B. Adhesive properties and antibiotic resistance of *Klebsiella*, *Enterobacter*, and *Serratia* clinical isolates involved in nosocomial infections. *J. Clin. Microbiol.* **1996**, *34*, 1963–1969.

13. Jones, G.W.; Isaacson, R.E. Proteinaceous bacterial adhesins and their receptors. *Crit. Rev. Microbiol.* **1983**, *10*, 229–260.

14. Ottow, J.C.G. Ecology, physiology, and genetics of fimbriae and pili. *Annu. Rev. Microbiol.* **1975**, *29*, 79–108.

15. Kline, K.A.; Dodson, K.W.; Caparon, M.G.; Hultgren, S.J. A tale of two pili: Assembly and function of pili in bacteria. *Trends Microbiol.* **2010**, *18*, 224–232.

16. Rosen, D.A.; Pinkner, J.S.; Jones, J.M.; Walker, J.N.; Clegg, S.; Hultgren, S.J. Utilization of an intracellular bacterial community pathway in *Klebsiella pneumoniae* urinary tract infection and the effects of FimK on type 1 pilus expression. *Infect. Immun.* **2008**, *76*, 3337–3345.

17. Struve, C.; Bojer, M.; Krogfelt, K.A. Characterization of *Klebsiella pneumoniae* type 1 fimbriae by detection of phase variation during colonization and infection and impact on virulence. *Infect. Immun.* **2008**, *76*, 4055–4065.

18. Alcántar-Curiel, M.D.; Blackburn, D.; Saldaña, Z.; Gayosso-Vázquez, C.; Iovine, N.M.; de la Cruz, M.A.; Girón, J.A. Multi-functional analysis of *Klebsiella pneumoniae* fimbrial types in adherence and biofilm formation. *Virulence* **2013**, *4*, 129–138.

19. Burmolle, M.; Bahl, M.I.; Jensen, L.B.; Sorensen, S.J.; Hansen, L.H. Type 3 fimbriae, encoded by the conjugative plasmid pOLA52, enhance biofilm formation and transfer frequencies in *Enterobacteriaceae* strains. *Microbiology* **2008**, *154*, 187–195.

20. Ong, C.L.; Ulett, G.C.; Mabbett, A.N.; Beatson, S.A.; Webb, R.I.; Monaghan, W.; Nimmo, G.R.; Looke, D.F.; McEwan, A.G.; Schembri, M.A. Identification of type 3 fimbriae in uropathogenic *Escherichia coli* reveals a role in biofilm formation. *J. Bacteriol.* **2008**, *190*, 1054–1063.

21. Ong, C.L.; Beatson, S.A.; Totsika, M.; Forestier, C.; McEwan, A.G.; Schembri, M.A. Molecular analysis of type 3 fimbrial genes from *Escherichia coli*, *Klebsiella* and *Citrobacter* species. *BMC Microbiol.* **2010**, *10*, 183.

22. Lederman, E.R.; Crum, N.F. Pyogenic liver abscess with a focus on *Klebsiella pneumoniae* as a primary pathogen: An emerging disease with unique clinical characteristics. *Am. J. Gastroenterol.* **2005**, *100*, 322–331.

23. Fung, C.P.; Chang, F.Y.; Lee, S.C.; Hu, B.S.; Kuo, B.I.; Liu, C.Y.; Ho, M.; Siu, L.K. A global emerging disease of *Klebsiella pneumoniae* liver abscess: Is serotype K1 an important factor for complicated endophthalmitis? *Gut* **2002**, *50*, 420–424.

24. Laupland, K.B.; Ross, T.; Pitout, J.D.; Church, D.L.; Gregson, D.B. Community-onset urinary tract infections: A population-based assessment. *Infection* **2007**, *35*, 150–153.

25. Lin, W.H.; Kao, C.Y.; Yang, D.C.; Tseng, C.C.; Wu, A.B.; Teng, C.H.; Wang, M.C.; Wu, J.J. Clinical and microbiological characteristics of *Klebsiella pneumoniae* from community-acquired recurrent urinary tract infections. *Eur. J. Clin. Microbiol. Infect. Dis.* **2014**, *33*, 1533–1539.

26. Tu, Y.C.; Lu, M.C.; Chiang, M.K.; Huang, S.P.; Peng, H.L.; Chang, H.Y.; Jan, M.S.; Lai, Y.C. Genetic requirements for *Klebsiella pneumoniae*-induced liver abscess in an oral infection model. *Infect. Immun.* **2009**, *77*, 2657–2671.

27. Kim, J.K.; Chung, D.R.; Wie, S.H.; Yoo, J.H.; Park, S.W. Risk factor analysis of invasive liver abscess caused by the K1 serotype *Klebsiella pneumoniae*. *Eur. J. Clin. Microbiol. Infect. Dis.* **2009**, *28*, 109–111.

28. Oelschlaeger, T.A.; Tall, B.D. Invasion of cultured human epithelial cells by Klebsiella pneumoniae isolated from the urinary tract. *Infect. Immun.* **1997**, *6*, 2950–2958.

29. Montgomerie, J.Z. Epidemiology of *Klebsiella* and hospital-associated infections. *Rev. Infect. Dis.* **1979**, *1*, 736–753.

30. Gupta, A. Hospital-acquired infections in the neonatal intensive care unit-*Klebsiella pneumoniae*. *Semin. Perinatol.* **2002**, *26*, 340–345.

31. Ko, W.C.; Paterson, D.L.; Sagnimeni, A.J.; Hansen, D.S.; von Gottberg, A.; Mohapatra, S.; Casellas, J.M.; Goossens, H.; Mulazimoglu, L.; Trenholme, G.; *et al.* Community acquired *Klebsiella pneumoniae* bacteremia: Global differences in clinical patterns. *Emerg. Infect. Dis.* **2002**, *8*, 160–166.

32. Yinnon, A.M.; Butnaru, A.; Raveh, D.; Jerassy, Z.; Rudensky, B. *Klebsiella* bacteremia: community *versus* nosocomial infection. *Mon. J. Assoc. Physicians* **1996**, *89*, 933–941.

33. Niveditha, S.; Pramodhini, S.; Umadevi, S.; Kumar, S.; Stephen, S. The isolation and the biofilm formation of uropathogens in the patients with catheter associated urinary tract infections (UTIs). *J. Clin. Diagn. Res.* **2012**, *6*, 1478–1482.

34. Ronald, A. The etiology of urinary tract infection: Traditional and emerging pathogens. *Am. J. Med.* **2002**, *113*, 14S–19S.

35. Frank, D.N.; Wilson, S.S.; St Amand, A.L.; Pace, N.R. Culture independent microbiological analysis of Foley urinary catheter biofilms. *PLoS One* **2009**, *4*, e7811.

36. Lye, W.C.; Chan, R.K.T.; Lee, E.J.C.; Kumarasinghe, G. Urinary tract infections in patients with diabetes mellitus. *J. Infect.* **1992**, *24*, 169–174.

37. Bennett, C.J.; Young, M.N.; Darrington, H. Differences in urinary tract infection in male and female spinal cord injury patients on intermittent catheterization. *Paraplegia* **1995**, *33*, 69–72.

38. Siegman-Igra, Y.; Golan, H.; Schwartz, D.; Cahaner, Y.; de-Mayo, G.; Orni-Wasserlauf, R. Epidemiology of vascular catheter-related bloodstream infections in a large university hospital in Israel. *Scand. J. Infect. Dis.* **2000**, *32*, 411–415.

39. Singhai, M.; Malik, A.; Shahid, M.; Malik, M.A.; Goyal, R. A study on device-related infections with special reference to biofilm production and antibiotic resistance. *J. Glob. Infect. Dis.* **2012**, *4*, 193–198.

40. Lin, M.Y.; Lyles-Banks, R.D.; Lolans, K.; Hines, D.W.; Spear, J.B.; Petrak, R.; Trick, W.E.; Weinstein, R.A.; Hayden, M.K.; Centers for Disease Control and Prevention Epicenters Program. The importance of long-term acute care hospitals in the regional epidemiology of *Klebsiella pneumoniae* carbapenemase-producing *Enterobacteriaceae*. *Clin. Infect. Dis.* **2013**, *57*, 1246–1252.

41. Orsi, G.B.; Scorzolini, L.; Franchi, C.; Mondillo, V.; Rosa, G.; Venditti, M. Hospital-acquired infection surveillance in a neurosurgical intensive care unit. *J. Hosp. Infect.* **2006**, *64*, 23–29.

42. Giani, T.; Pini, B.; Arena, F.; Conte, V.; Bracco, S.; Migliavacca, R.; AMCLI-CRE Survey Participants; Pantosti, A.; Pagani, L.; Luzzaro, F.; *et al.* Epidemic diffusion of KPC carbapenemase-producing *Klebsiella pneumoniae* in Italy: Results of the first countrywide survey, 15 May to 30 June 2011. *Euro Surveill.* **2013**, *30*, 18–22.

43. Azzopardi, E.A.; Azzopardi, E.; Camilleri, L.; Villapalos, J.; Boyce, D.E.; Dziewulski, P.; Dickson, W.A.; Whitaker, I.S. Gram negative wound infection in hospitalised adult burn patients-systematic review and metanalysis. *PLoS One* **2014**, *9*, e95042.

44. Varaldo, P.E.; Nicoletti, G.; Schito, G.C.; Maida, A.; Facinelli, B.; Stefani, S.; Gianrossi, G.; Muresu, E. Circulation in Italy of beta-lactamase-producing strains within the major groups of bacterial pathogens. *Eur. J. Epidemiol.* **1990**, *6*, 287–292.

45. Guérillot, F.; Carret, G.; Flandrois, J.P. A statistical evaluation of the bactericidal effects of ceftibuten in combination with aminoglycosides and ciprofloxacin. *J. Antimicrob. Chemother.* **1993**, *32*, 685–694.

46. Elkhaïli, H.; Kamili, N.; Linger, L.; Levêque, D.; Pompei, D.; Monteil, H.; Jehl, F. *In vitro* time-kill curves of cefepime and cefpirome combined with amikacin, gentamicin or ciprofloxacin against *Klebsiella pneumoniae* producing extended-spectrum beta-lactamase. *Chemotherapy* **1997**, *43*, 245–253.

47. Traub, W.H.; Schwarze, I.; Bauer, D. Nosocomial outbreak of cross-infection due to multiple-antibiotic-resistant *Klebsiella pneumoniae*: Characterization of the strain and antibiotic susceptibility studies. *Chemotherapy* **2000**, *46*, 1–14.

48. Patel, G.; Bonomo, R.A. Status report on carbapenemases: Challenges and prospects. *Expert Rev. Anti Infect. Ther.* **2011**, *9*, 555–570.

49. Voulgari, E.; Poulou, A.; Koumaki, V.; Tsakris, A. Carbapenemase-producing *Enterobacteriaceae*: Now that the storm is finally here, how will timely detection help us fight back? *Future Microbiol.* **2013**, *8*, 27–39.

50. Yigit, H.; Queenan, A.M.; Anderson, G.J.; Domenech-Sanchez, A.; Biddle, J.W.; Steward, C.D.; Alberti, S.; Bush, K.; Tenover, F.C. Novel carbapenem-hydrolyzing beta-lactamase, KPC-1, from a carbapenem-resistant strain of *Klebsiella pneumoniae*. *Antimicrob. Agents Chemother.* **2001**, *45*, 1151–1161.

51. Papp-Wallace, K.M.; Bethel, C.R.; Distler, A.M.; Kasuboski, C.; Taracila, M.; Bonomo, R.A. Inhibitor resistance in the KPC-2 beta-lactamase, a preeminent property of this class A beta-lactamase. *Antimicrob. Agents Chemother.* **2010**, *54*, 890–897.

52. Molton, J.S.; Tambyah, P.A.; Ang, B.S.; Ling, M.L.; Fisher, D.A. The global spread of healthcare-associated multidrug-resistant bacteria: A perspective from Asia. *Clin. Infect. Dis.* **2013**, *56*, 1310–1318.

53. Grundmann, H.; Livermore, D.M.; Giske, C.G.; Canton, R.; Rossolini, G.M.; Campos, J.; Vatopoulos, A.; Gniadkowski, M.; Toth, A.; Pfeifer, Y.; *et al.* CNSE Working Group. Carbapenem-non-susceptible *Enterobacteriaceae* in Europe: Conclusions from a meeting of national experts. *Euro Surveill.* **2010**, *15*, 19711.

54. Miriagou, V.; Cornaglia, G.; Edelstein, M.; Galani, I.; Giske, C.G.; Gniadkowski, M.; Malamou-Lada, E.; Martinez-Martinez, L.; Navarro, F.; Nordmann, P.; *et al.* Acquired carbapenemases in Gram-negative bacterial pathogens: Detection and surveillance issues. *Clin. Microbiol. Infect.* **2010**, *16*, 112–122.

55. Tzouvelekis, L.S.; Markogiannakis, A.; Psichogiou, M.; Tassios, P.T.; Daikos, G.L. Carbapenemases in *Klebsiella pneumoniae* and other *Enterobacteriaceae*: An evolving crisis of global dimensions. *Clin. Microbiol. Rev.* **2012**, *25*, 682–707.

56. Wang, Q.; Li, B.; Tsang, A.K.; Yi, Y.; Woo, P.C.; Liu, C.H. Genotypic analysis of *Klebsiella pneumoniae* isolates in a Beijing Hospital reveals high genetic diversity and clonal population structure of drug-resistant isolates. *PLoS One* **2013**, *8*, e57091.

57. Le Chevallier, M.W.; Cawthon, C.D.; Lee, R.G. Factors promoting survival of bacteria in chlorinated water supplies. *Appl. Environ. Microbiol.* **1988**, *54*, 649–654.

58. Reid, G.; Charbonneau-Smith, R.; Lam, D.; Kang, Y.S.; Lacerte, M.; Hayes, K.C. Bacterial biofilm formation in the urinary bladder of spinal cord injured patients. *Paraplegia* **1992**, *30*, 711–717.

59. Yang, D.; Zhang, Z. Biofilm-forming *Klebsiella pneumoniae* strains have greater likelihood of producing extended-spectrum beta-lactamases. *J. Hosp. Infect.* **2008**, *68*, 369–371.

60. Nicolau Korres, A.M.; Aquije, G.M.; Buss, D.S.; Ventura, J.A.; Fernandes, P.M.; Fernandes, A.A. Comparison of biofilm and attachment mechanisms of a phytopathological and clinical isolate of *Klebsiella pneumoniae* subsp. *pneumoniae*. *Sci. World J.* **2013**, *10*, 925375.

61. Donelli, G.; Vuotto, C. Biofilm-based infections in long-term care facilities. *Future Microbiol.* **2014**, *9*, 175–188.

62. Langstraat, J.; Bohse, M.; Clegg, S. Type 3 fimbrial shaft (MrkA) of *Klebsiella pneumoniae*, but not the fimbrial adhesin (MrkD), facilitates biofilm formation. *Infect. Immun.* **2001**, *69*, 5805–5812.

63. Di Martino, P.; Cafferini, N.; Joly, B.; Darfeuille-Michaud, A. *Klebsiella pneumoniae* type 3 pili facilitate adherence and biofilm formation on abiotic surfaces. *Res. Microbiol.* **2003**, *154*, 9–16.

64. Jagnow, J.; Clegg, S. *Klebsiella pneumoniae* MrkD-mediated biofilm formation on extracellular matrix- and collagen-coated surfaces. *Microbiology* **2003**, *149*, 2397–2405.

65. Lavender, H.F.; Jagnow, J.R.; Clegg, S. Biofilm formation *in vitro* and virulence *in vivo* of mutants of *Klebsiella pneumoniae*. *Infect. Immun.* **2004**, *72*, 4888–4890.

66. Boddicker, J.D.; Anderson, R.A.; Jagnow, J.; Clegg, S. Signature-tagged mutagenesis of *Klebsiella pneumoniae* to identify genes that influence biofilm formation on extracellular matrix material. *Infect. Immun.* **2006**, *74*, 4590–4597.

67. Schroll, C.; Barken, K.B.; Krogfelt, K.A.; Struve, C. Role of type 1 and type 3 fimbriae in *Klebsiella pneumoniae* biofilm formation. *BMC Microbiol.* **2010**, *10*, 179.

68. Johnson, J.G.; Clegg, S. Role of MrkJ, a phosphodiesterase, in type 3 fimbrial expression and biofilm formation in *Klebsiella pneumoniae*. *J. Bacteriol.* **2010**, *192*, 3944–3950.

69. Murphy, C.N.; Mortensen, M.S.; Krogfelt, K.A.; Clegg, S. Role of *Klebsiella pneumoniae* type 1 and type 3 fimbriae in colonizing silicone tubes implanted into the bladders of mice as a model of catheter-associated urinary tract infections. *Infect. Immun.* **2013**, *81*, 3009–3017.

70. Balestrino, D.; Ghigo, J.M.; Charbonnel, N.; Haagensen, J.A.; Forestier, C. The characterization of functions involved in the establishment and maturation of *Klebsiella pneumoniae in vitro* biofilm reveals dual roles for surface exopolysaccharides. *Environ. Microbiol.* **2008**, *10*, 685–701.

71. Wu, M.C.; Lin, T.L.; Hsieh, P.F.; Yang, H.C.; Wang, J.T. Isolation of genes involved in biofilm formation of a Klebsiella pneumoniae strain causing pyogenic liver abscess. *PLoS One* **2011**, *6*, e23500.

72. Huang, T.W.; Lam, I.; Chang, H.Y.; Tsai, S.F.; Palsson, B.O.; Charusanti, P. Capsule deletion via a λ-Red knockout system perturbs biofilm formation and fimbriae expression in *Klebsiella pneumoniae* MGH 78578. *BMC Res. Notes* **2014**, *8*, 7–13.

73. Siebel, M.A.; Characklis, W.G. Observations of binary population biofilms. *Biotechnol. Bioeng.* **1991**, *37*, 778–789.

74. Skillman, L.C.; Sutherland, I.W.; Jones, M.V. The role of exopolysaccharides in dual species biofilm development. *J. Appl. Microbiol.* **1998**, *85*, 13S–18S.

75. Stickler, D.; Morris, N.; Moreno, M.C.; Sabbuba, N. Studies on the formation of crystalline bacterial biofilms on urethral catheters. *Eur. J. Clin. Microbiol. Infect. Dis.* **1998**, *17*, 649–652.

76. Macleod, S.M.; Stickler, D.J. Species interactions in mixed-community crystalline biofilms on urinary catheters. *J. Med. Microbiol.* **2007**, *56*, 1549–1557.

77. Lee, K.W.; Periasamy, S.; Mukherjee, M.; Xie, C.; Kjelleberg, S.; Rice, S.A. Biofilm development and enhanced stress resistance of a model, mixed-species community biofilm. *ISME J.* **2014**, *8*, 894–907.

78. Chen, B.M.; Yu, J.L.; Liu, G.X.; Hu, L.Y.; Li, L.Q.; Li, F.; Yang, H. Electron microscopic analysis of biofilm on tracheal tubes removed from intubated neonates and the relationship between bilofilm and lower respiratory infection. *Zhonghua Er Ke Za Zhi.* **2007**, *45*, 655–660.

79. Anderl, J.N.; Franklin, M.J.; Stewart, P.S. Role of antibiotic penetration limitation in *Klebsiella pneumoniae* biofilm resistance to ampicillin and ciprofloxacin. *Antimicrob. Agents Chemother.* **2000**, *44*, 1818–1824.

80. Zahller, J.; Stewart, P.S. A transmission electron microscopic study of antibiotic action on *Klebsiella pneumoniae* biofilm. *Antimicrob. Agents Chemother.* **2002**, *46*, 2679–2683.

81. Anderl, J.N.; Zahller, J.; Roe, F.; Stewart, P.S. Role of nutrient limitation and stationary-phase existence in *Klebsiella pneumoniae* biofilm resistance to ampicillin and ciprofloxacin. *Antimicrob. Agents Chemother.* **2003**, *47*, 1251–1256.

82. Cernohorská, L.; Votava, M. Determination of minimal regrowth concentration (MRC) in clinical isolates of various biofilm-forming bacteria. *Folia Microbiol. (Praha)* **2004**, *49*, 75–78.

83. Liaqat, I.; Sumbal, F.; Sabri, A.N. Tetracycline and chloramphenicol efficiency against selected biofilm forming bacteria. *Curr. Microbiol.* **2009**, *59*, 212–220.

84. Fonseca, A.P.; Extremina, C.; Fonseca, A.F.; Sousa, J.C. Effect of subinhibitory concentration of piperacillin/tazobactam on *Pseudomonas aeruginosa*. *J. Med. Microbiol.* **2004**, *53*, 903–910.

85. Rachid, S.; Ohlsen, K.; Witte, W.; Hacker, J.; Ziebuhr, W. Effect of subinhibitory antibiotic concentrations on polysaccharide intercellular adhesion expression in biofilm forming *Staphylococcus epidermidis*. *Antimicrob. Agents Chemother.* **2000**, *44*, 3357–3363.

86. Singla, S.; Harjai, K.; Chhibber, S. Susceptibility of different phases of biofilm of *Klebsiella pneumoniae* to three different antibiotics. *J. Antibiot. (Tokyo)* **2013**, *66*, 61–66.

87. Bellifa, S.; Hassaine, H.; Balestrino, D.; Charbonnel, N.; M'hamedi, I.; Terki, I.K.; Lachachi, M.; Didi, W.; Forestier, C. Evaluation of biofilm formation of *K. pneumoniae* isolated from medical devices at the University Hospital of Tlemcen, Algeria. *Afr. J. Microbiol. Res.* **2013**, *7*, 5558–5564.

88. Naparstek, L.; Carmeli, Y.; Navon-Venezia, S.; Banin, E. Biofilm formation and susceptibility to gentamicin and colistin of extremely drug-resistant KPC-producing *Klebsiella pneumoniae*. *J. Antimicrob. Chemother.* **2014**, *69*, 1027–1034.

89. Singla, S.; Harjai, K.; Chhibber, S. Artificial *Klebsiella pneumoniae* biofilm model mimicking *in vivo* system: Altered morphological characteristics and antibiotic resistance. *J. Antibiot. (Tokyo)* **2014**, *67*, 305–309.

90. Chen, P.; Seth, A.K.; Abercrombie, J.J.; Mustoe, T.A.; Leung, K.P. Activity of imipenem against *Klebsiella pneumoniae* biofilms *in vitro* and *in vivo*. *Antimicrob. Agents Chemother.* **2014**, *58*, 1208–1213.

91. Fuursted, K.; Schøler, L.; Hansen, F.; Dam, K.; Bojer, M.S.; Hammerum, A.M.; Dagnæs-Hansen, F.; Olsen, A.; Jasemian, Y.; Struve, C. Virulence of a *Klebsiella pneumoniae* strain carrying the New Delhi metallo-beta-lactamase-1 (NDM-1). *Microbes Infect.* **2012**, *14*, 155–158.

92. Subramanian, P.; Shanmugam, N.; Sivaraman, U.; Kumar, S.; Selvaraj, S. Antiobiotic resistance pattern of biofilm-forming uropathogens isolated from catheterized patients in Pondicherry, India. *Australas. Med. J.* **2012**, *5*, 344–348.

93. Sanchez, C.J., Jr.; Mende, K.; Beckius, M.L.; Akers, K.S.; Romano, D.R.; Wenke, J.C.; Murray, C.K. Biofilm formation by clinical isolates and the implications in chronic infections. *BMC Infect. Dis.* **2013**, *29*, 13–47.

94. Hennequin, C.; Aumeran, C.; Robin, F.; Traore, O.; Forestier, C. Antibiotic resistance and plasmid transfer capacity in biofilm formed with a CTX-M-15-producing *Klebsiella pneumoniae* isolate. *J. Antimicrob. Chemother.* **2012**, *67*, 2123–2130.

95. Hennequin, C.; Robin, F.; Cabrolier, N.; Bonnet, R.; Forestier, C. Characterization of a DHA-1-producing *Klebsiella pneumoniae* strain involved in an outbreak and role of the AmpR regulator in virulence. *Antimicrob. Agents Chemother.* **2012**, *56*, 288–294.

8

Biofilms in Infections of the Eye

Paulo J. M. Bispo, Wolfgang Haas and Michael S. Gilmore *

Departments of Ophthalmology, Microbiology and Immunology, Massachusetts Eye and Ear Infirmary, Harvard Medical School, Boston, MA, 02114 USA

* Author to whom correspondence should be addressed;
 E-Mail: michael_gilmore@meei.harvard.edu

Academic Editor: Gianfranco Donelli

Abstract: The ability to form biofilms in a variety of environments is a common trait of bacteria, and may represent one of the earliest defenses against predation. Biofilms are multicellular communities usually held together by a polymeric matrix, ranging from capsular material to cell lysate. In a structure that imposes diffusion limits, environmental microgradients arise to which individual bacteria adapt their physiologies, resulting in the gamut of physiological diversity. Additionally, the proximity of cells within the biofilm creates the opportunity for coordinated behaviors through cell–cell communication using diffusible signals, the most well documented being quorum sensing. Biofilms form on abiotic or biotic surfaces, and because of that are associated with a large proportion of human infections. Biofilm formation imposes a limitation on the uses and design of ocular devices, such as intraocular lenses, posterior contact lenses, scleral buckles, conjunctival plugs, lacrimal intubation devices and orbital implants. In the absence of abiotic materials, biofilms have been observed on the capsule, and in the corneal stroma. As the evidence for the involvement of microbial biofilms in many ocular infections has become compelling, developing new strategies to prevent their formation or to eradicate them at the site of infection, has become a priority.

Keywords: biofilm; eye; ocular infections, postoperative ocular infections; device-related ocular infections

1. Introduction

Ever since Robert Koch and Louis Pasteur in the 1860's established the modern field of bacteriology, studies employing pure bacterial cultures, often grown in liquid media (planktonic growth), have shaped our understanding of bacterial physiology and behavior. Pure cultures were required to establish microbial causes of disease, and growth in liquid media ensured that all cells were exposed to similar conditions and behaved in the same manner. As a result, most of the measures to control pathogenic bacteria (e.g., vaccines and antimicrobial agents) have been developed based on knowledge of bacteria grown as planktonic cells.

An appreciation for the fact that in nature, bacteria adhere to many abiotic or biotic surfaces and form communities of differentiated, interacting communities known as "biofilms", emerged over the past few decades [1], and this concept was enthusiastically promoted by William (Bill) Costerton among others. Evidence of biofilm formation has been found in the analysis of microbial fossils including those from deep-sea hydrothermal sediments. This suggests that the ability to form biofilm is an ancient adaptation that dates back more than 3 billion years [2,3]. Biofilm formation conferred to individual bacteria the ability to collaborate and to adapt to a range of harsh environmental conditions, perhaps most of all, to evade predation by phagocytic microbes. The formation of a biofilm provides a microbe with a small measure of control over the local environment, including fluctuations in temperatures, pH, ultraviolet light, starvation, and exposure to toxic agents [4,5].

The ubiquity of biofilm formation in natural ecosystems, industrial systems, and medical settings has accelerated the pace of biofilm research. Advances in medical biofilm research have led to an understanding that biofilms represent the prevalent form of bacterial life during tissue colonization, and may occur in over 80% of microbial infections in the body [6]. Biofilms play important roles in human infections including native valve endocarditis, otitis media, chronic bacterial prostatitis, lung infections in patients with cystic fibrosis and periodontitis [7,8]. In addition, biofilms form on indwelling devices including prosthetic heart valves, coronary stents, intravascular catheters, urinary catheters, intrauterine devices, ventricular assist devices, neurosurgical ventricular shunts, prosthetic joint, cochlear implants, intraocular and contact lenses [7,8]. Due to their medical importance, development of anti-biofilm compounds for clinical use are of vital interest [9].

2. Microbial Biofilms

The very first description of a biofilm dates back to the 17th century when Anthony van Leeuwenhoek examined his own teeth scrapings with one of the first microscopes and found a large amount of small living "animalcules" in his dental plaque matter. He concluded in his report to the Royal Society of London in 1684 that the thick white material found between his teeth protected the bacteria embedded in this substance against the action of the vinegar that he used to wash his mouth [10]. At the time, miasmatic and humoral theories of disease were dominant, and it took an additional 200 years until the germ theory of disease was advanced by Robert Koch before a connection between microbes and disease was made.

Today, biofilms are generally defined as a community of sessile microbes held together by a polymeric extracellular matrix, adherent to a surface, interface or to other cells that are phenotypically distinct from their planktonic counterparts [8]. This definition, although reflective of many biofilms, is in our view restrictive, as there is no particular requirement that microbes be held together by an extracellular matrix as opposed to any other adherence principle (surface charge, a network of surface attached proteins, *etc.*), or that they even adhere to a surface (as a raft consisting of only microbes could achieve all of the behaviors usually ascribed to a biofilm, e.g., microbes transiting the lumen of the colon).

Members of a biofilm community, which can be of the same or multiple species, show varying stages of differentiation and exchange information, metabolites, and genes with each other. As a result, members of the biofilm community are in a diversity of physiologies influenced by the unequal sharing of nutrients and metabolic byproducts, which results in subpopulations with increased tolerance to antimicrobials and environmental stresses, the host immune system, and predatory microorganisms [8,11–14].

Canonically, biofilm development has been grouped into five stages that are reflective of conditions in many, but not all biofilms: (1) reversible aggregation of planktonic cells on a surface; (2) irreversible adhesion; (3) formation of microcolonies; (4) biofilm maturation; and (5) detachment and dispersion of cells [11,15]. The events that are of special significance for ocular infections and the treatment of biofilm infections will be discussed in greater detail below, while the reader is referred to several excellent reviews for details on other biofilm-related subjects [8,11–16].

In the established view of biofilm formation, planktonic cells initially adhere to a surface in a reversible, non-specific manner due to electrostatic interactions between the bacterial cell and the surface. Water contact angle measurements on bacterial cell lawns have shown that the surface of *P. aeruginosa* is highly hydrophobic, while *S. aureus* is highly hydrophilic [17]. Therefore, surface properties of a solid object can favor colonization by one microorganism over another.

Surfaces exposed to liquid solutions are generally coated with a conditioning layer consisting of molecules present in the solution. Antimicrobial agents that are present in multipurpose solutions, for example, bind non-specifically to the contact lenses [18]. Once the lens is placed on the surface of the eye, the disinfectant diffuses off the lens and is replaced by lipids and proteins present in the tear fluid [17,19,20]. The lens material plays an important role in this interaction, as it has been shown that hydrophilic contact lenses preferentially adsorb lysozyme from the tear film, while hydrophobic contact lenses accumulate more lipocalin and lactoferrin [17].

In addition to determining the local antimicrobial properties, this unique conditioning layer also provides specific anchor points for bacterial adhesion. Microbial adhesion to surfaces coated by proteins and other biomolecules is often accomplished by a class of molecules termed Microbial Surface Components Recognizing Adhesive Matrix Molecules (MSCRAMM), as well as other adhesive surface proteins [21]. As an example of the latter, in *S. epidermidis* and other staphylococci the bifunctional autolysin/adhesion protein AtlE, an abundant surface protein, mediates first attachment to abiotic surfaces and also matrix protein-covered devices [22].

In a moving suspension, cells are exposed to fairly uniform conditions. However, following attachment, the individual experience of a cell begins to differ from its neighbors (*i.e.*, a cell in the middle of a group will experience more excreted products and fewer factors from the environment than a cell on the periphery of a population), and as a result, cells begin to differentiate [23]. Many biofilms involve production of an extracellular matrix (ECM) that encases the cells, and in some cases, binds the cells together and that can be composed of polysaccharides, lipopolysaccharides, proteins, or extracellular DNA [24]. This process may be active or passive, in that cells on the surface of an adherent colony that are lysed by the ejection of neutrophil antimicrobial factors may encase and protect siblings below in a matrix consisting simply of cell lysate. Whatever the nature of the matrix, its chemical and physical properties contribute to the differentiation of cells within the encased population, a process that can protect the bacteria from the action of antimicrobial agents, host immune responses, bacteriophages and phagocytic amoeba [8]. In staphylococci, it appears that polysaccharide intercellular adhesin (PIA, encoded by the *icaADBC* locus), matrix proteins including the accumulation-associated protein (Aap) [25], and possibly the biofilm-associated homologue protein (Bhp, termed Bap in *S. aureus*) contribute to this matrix [26]. Commensal isolates of *S. epidermidis* and other coagulase-negative staphylococci (CoNS) recovered from healthy conjunctiva carry most of the genes related to biofilm maturation, suggesting that the ability to form biofilms is an integral part of their life-style [27–29].

As the microcolony grows through cell division or recruitment of more planktonic cells, the biofilm grows and takes on a three-dimensional structure that often includes open water channels [8,23]. Growing biofilms on various types of contact lenses have shown differences in cell densities and three-dimensional structures *in vitro*, suggesting an effect of the substrate on the development of the biofilm [30]. However, while several studies have measured biofilm thickness on various contact lens materials, with the underlying assumption that thicker biofilms are more likely to result in disease, the biological significance of these results remains unclear. In one experiment, Tam *et al.* [31] grew *P. aeruginosa* biofilms on custom contact lenses and tested them in a rat model of contact lens-associated keratitis [31]. Biofilms grown *in vitro* to low and to high cell densities both caused disease symptoms within 7–8 days, indicating that initial biofilm thickness did not matter [31]. In contrast, contaminated contact lenses that were transferred from one rat to a different healthy animal resulted in keratitis symptoms within 2 days [31]. These results suggest that adaptation to the host environment is a critical step in the pathogenesis of biofilm-related infections.

The three-dimensional organization of the biofilm causes gradients of oxygen, pH, and nutrients, resulting in the development of different microniches [32,33]. The cell's individual physiological adaptations to these microniches results in physiological heterogeneity [13]. Cells near the surface of the biofilm will be exposed to more nutrients and oxygen and are therefore more metabolically active, while cells in the deep regions will be less active or even dormant. This heterogeneity results in a range of responses to antimicrobial agents, with metabolically active cells at the surface being rapidly killed while more internal, dormant cells are comparatively unaffected [32]. This, together with potential effects on diffusion of antimicrobial molecules within the biofilm, causes some cells in a biofilm to be recalcitrant to antimicrobial treatment, with antibiotic susceptibilities reduced by 10 to 1000-fold compared to planktonic counterparts [32].

The high local concentration of cells in a biofilm creates an ideal environment for information exchange through cell-to-cell communication and lateral gene transfer. Cell signaling mediated by secreted, accumulating messenger molecules, known as quorum sensing, allows bacteria to sense and respond to their environment and couple cell-density and other environmental cues with gene expression in ways that allow adaptive phenotypic responses. Quorum sensing has been shown to be involved in the control of biofilm formation and production of virulence and colonization factors in a variety of organisms of medical importance [34]. Cell-to-cell signaling is also involved in biofilm dispersion, which is of general and medical interest [35].

Bacterial cells can leave or be shed from the biofilm and revert to a planktonic life-style, often by degrading the ECM that holds the cells together [35]. For example, thermonuclease is a bacterial enzyme that degrades the extracellular DNA that holds *S. aureus* biofilms together, while alginate lyase degrades the alginate matrix important for *P. aeruginosa* biofilms [36,37]. These processes are coordinated by small signaling molecules that induce the expression of genes for biofilm dispersal. For example, *N*-butanoyl-L-homoserine lactone (C4HSL) belongs to the family of cell-density dependent autoinducers and has been implicated in the dispersal of *P. aeruginosa* biofilms [38]. Other small molecules implicated in biofilm dispersal include the *Pseudomonas* quinolone signal PQS, the furanosylborate autoinducer AI-2 from *Vibrio cholerae*, and the staphylococcal peptides δ-toxin and AIP-I [35].

3. Ocular Infections

The two leading causes of vision impairment worldwide are uncorrected refractive errors and cataract [39]. Measures to manage those eye abnormalities frequently include the use of contact lenses and the placement of intraocular lenses, and have enhanced the quality of life of millions of patients. Although use of such devices is of the utmost importance for correction of a variety of visual aberrations, they also provide a new surface on which many microbial pathogens can form biofilms (Table 1). As a result, device-related ocular infections are an important limitation of the success of such procedures. Moreover, many infections progress to secondary permanent sequelae that may lead to poor visual outcomes and occasionally loss of sight, such as acute bacterial endophthalmitis or corneal ulceration.

Table 1. Biofilm-associated infections of the eye.

Disease	Main Causative Agents of Infection and/or Found in the Biofilms	Biofilm Localization
Endophthalmitis	Coagulase negative staphylococci and *Propionibacterium acnes*	Intraocular lens
		Posterior capsule
Keratitis	*Staphylococcus aureus* and other staphylococcal species, *Pseudomonas aeruginosa* and *Serratia* spp. Fungi and *Acanthamoeba* less frequently	Contact lens
	Viridans group streptococci. Gram negative bacilli and yeasts less frequently	Corneal stroma (crystalline keratophaty)
Scleral buckle infection	Gram positive cocci and nontuberculous *Mycobacterium* [1]	Scleral buckles
Lacrimal system infections	*Staphylococcus* spp., *P. aeruginosa* and *M. chelonae*	Lacrimal intubation devices
	Staphylococcus spp [2]	Punctual plugs
Periorbital infections	*Staphylococcus* spp. and mixed species biofilms	Sockets and orbital plates

[1] Common causative agents of buckle-associated infections. Scleritis resulting of scleral extension of corneal infections are mainly caused by *P. aeruginosa* and other common agents of infectious keratitis;

[2] The presence of biofilms has not been demonstrated on plugs recovered from symptomatic eyes presenting with dacryocystitis and canaliculitis. However, clinical features of these infections are compatible with biofilm-associated infections such as the late onset, and difficulty to treat with antimicrobial therapy alone.

4. Biofilms in Endophthalmitis

Endophthalmitis is a rare but severe intraocular inflammation that results from the introduction of a microbial pathogen into the posterior segment of the eye. Organisms may gain access to the intraocular tissues exogenously after trauma caused to the ocular globe following intraocular surgery, intravitreal injections, penetrating open globe injury, and in cases of keratitis progressing to corneal perforation. Endogenous endophthalmitis may occur in patients with bacteremia by seeding the eye with bacteria from a distal site of infection [40].

Endophthalmitis Following Cataract Surgery

Postoperative endophthalmitis is the most common presentation and is frequently associated with cataract surgery [41,42]. It is estimated that 17.2% of the population older than 40 years in the United States suffers from cataracts. This prevalence increases with age, being more than 35% for patients between 70–74 and almost 50% for patients between 75–79 years of age [43]. As a result, cataract extraction with replacement of the crystalline lens by an artificial intraocular lens (IOL) represents the most frequent surgery procedure performed by ophthalmologists, with more than 1 million procedures performed each year in United Stated [44]. Postoperative endophthalmitis is the leading blinding complication of cataract surgery. Its overall incidence varies according to the technique and region of the world, ranging from 0.028% to 0.2% [45–47]. Despite the low overall incidence, given the large number of cataract surgeries performed annually, a substantial number of patients are affected by this sight-threatening infection.

Post-cataract endophthalmitis is caused predominantly by Gram positive organisms originating from the ocular surface microbiota. Coagulase-negative staphylococci (CoNS), especially *Staphylococcus epidermidis*, are the most frequently encountered microbes from culture-proven acute endophthalmitis [41,42,48]. Delayed-onset endophthalmitis is mainly caused by *Propionibacterium acnes*, which usually presents with a more indolent and persistent infection, with lower frequency of hypopyon and better final visual outcome compared to acute cases [49]. Both pathogens, *S. epidermidis* and *P. acnes,* are able to adhere to, and form biofilms on intraocular lenses. Some evidences suggest that they can also adhere to and form biofilms in the posterior capsular bag [50–58]. Commensal organisms colonizing the ocular surface and periocular tissues are the primary source of bacteria that cause postoperative endophthalmitis. In the large Endophthalmitis Vitrectomy Study, 67.7% of paired CoNS isolates from the eyelid and intraocular fluids were indistinguishable by pulsed field gel electrophoresis [59].

The ocular surface is often colonized by Gram positive organisms, with CoNS being most commonly associated with healthy conjunctiva, lids and tears, followed by *Propionibacterium acnes*, *Corynebacterium* spp. and *S. aureus* [60]. Rates of contamination of the anterior chamber after uneventful cataract surgery range from 2% to 46%, and are due to the most common Gram positive commensal organisms found on the ocular surface, most frequently *S. epidermidis* [61–64]. Rates of anterior chamber contamination are much higher than the incidence of postoperative intraocular infection. This suggests that in most cases, the anterior chamber is capable of clearing the bacterial inoculum without progressing to endophthalmitis, likely due in part to the rapid turnover of the aqueous humor [65]. However, most of the organisms found in the ocular microbiota are able to attach to the IOL and posterior lens capsule, and often become well established if they reach the posterior chamber. In comparison to aqueous humor, vitreous is relatively static and constitutes a good environment for establishment of an infection. Intraocular lenses, such as those constructed from polymethylmethacrylate (PMMA) may become contaminated with commensal conjunctival bacteria (mainly *S. epidermidis*) during insertion, and carry the organisms from the ocular surface to the posterior chamber [66,67]. The ability of commensal bacteria to form biofilms on the surface of IOLs prevents their clearance, and likely represents an important mechanism in the pathogenesis of post-cataract endophthalmitis. The occurrence of microbes in biofilms is consistent with the low rates of culture positivity for aqueous and vitreous samples [68].

As described above, the *ica* locus and other genes play an integral part in staphylococcal biofilm formation. One report from Japan found a prevalence of 60% and 69.4% for *ica*A positive strains of *S. epidermidis* isolated from the conjunctiva of healthy volunteers and patients undergoing cataract surgery, respectively. Most of these isolates (approximately 40%) tested positive for slime production on Congo red agar [29]. Among a collection of *S. epidermidis* isolates from Mexico, 17% of commensal conjunctival isolates were able to form biofilms under conditions used *in vitro,* and 26.7% were positive for the *ica*A and/or *ica*D genes [27]. The frequency of *ica* genes was observed to be 36% for CoNS species other than *S. epidermidis* recovered from the normal conjunctiva of student and staff eyes at an institute in India [28]. For *S. epidermidis* recovered from intraocular fluids of patients with endophthalmitis, the distribution of *ica*A and *ica*D genes seemed to be group specific. Among strains isolated from endophthalmitis cases in South Florida, *ica*AD genes were present (86%) only among isolates that possess the accessory gene regulator locus (*agr*) type I. The frequency of *aap* and *bhp* genes among all isolates was 78.5% and 43.1%, respectively, with *bhp* being more prevalent among *agr* type II isolates [69].

Previous reports have demonstrated the ability of *S. epidermidis* to form biofilms on IOLs (Figure 1) using different *in vitro* conditions [53–55,57], and in a model that resembles the intraocular environment [51,52]. The degree of biofilm formation is affected by the material used to manufacture the IOL and also by the genomic content of each *S. epidermidis* lineage tested. Strains of *S. epidermidis* carrying the *ica* locus are able to form stronger biofilms on different IOL surfaces compared to strains lacking this locus [53,55,57]. In one study [55], using various hydrophobic IOLs, the ability of *S. epidermidis* strains ATCC 12228 (*ica* negative) and ATCC 35984 (*ica* positive) to form biofilms was significantly higher on acrylic lenses followed by PMMA and MPC (2-methacryloyloxyethyl phosphorylcholine) surface-modified acrylic. Weaker biofilms were found on silicone IOLs. Interestingly, modification of the acrylic IOL surface by treatment with MPC decreased biofilm formation [55] and this may be associated with an increase in the hydrophilicity [70]. The same effect has been demonstrated for MPC-modified silicone IOL [71]. Other reports [51,53,72,73], however, have found different results for each IOL material and that was also affected by the strains tested. Foldable IOLs made with silicone supported greater *S. epidermidis* biofilm formation compared to PMMA IOL for strain ATCC 35984, but the same was not seen for the strain ATCC 12228 [53]. In the same study, variations of up to two orders of magnitude in the degree of biofilm formation, as determined by CFU counting, were observed for the same IOL material depending on different models and manufacturers. Acrylic lenses were again the most prone to form stronger biofilms and fluorine-treated

PMMA the least. The presence of polypropylene haptics in the PMMA IOL increased the biofilm quantity compared to single-piece PMMA IOL [53]. In agreement, it has been demonstrated that polypropylene haptics represents a significant risk factor for post-cataract surgery endophthalmitis [72], and increases *in vitro* adhesion of *S. epidermidis* compared to single- and three-piece PMMA IOL [73]. In a model using a bioreactor with flow conditions similar to the anterior chamber, *S. epidermidis* was able to form biofilms on different IOL materials, which significantly increased as a function of time [52]. Silicone was more permissive to biofilm formation in this model, followed by hydrophobic acrylic and PMMA, with the fewest attached cells found on hydrophilic acrylic.

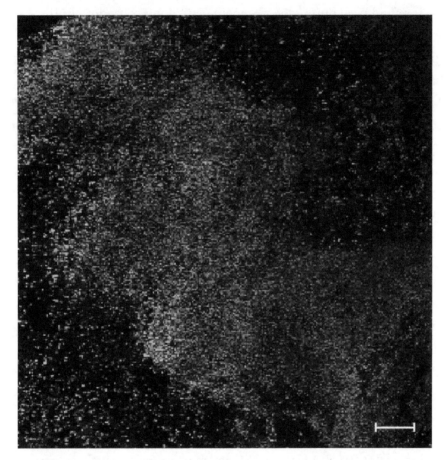

Figure 1. Confocal laser scanning micrograph of a 24 h biofilm. The biofilm of *Staphylococcus epidermidis* RP62A was grown *in vitro* on hydrophilic acrylic intraocular lens, and was visualized after staining using the live/dead viability stain, which contains SYTO9 (green fluorescence, live cells) and propidium iodine (red fluorescence, bacterial cells that have a defective cell membrane, which is indicative of dead cells). Magnification X 400, scale bar is 20 μm.

Despite the variations within each study, hydrophobicity is consistently observed to be an important determinant of biofilm formation. Modification of the surface to make it more hydrophilic may reduce initial binding and development of robust staphylococcal biofilms. The initial adherence of *S. epidermidis* to the IOL surface, an important initial step for subsequent colony expansion and biofilm maturation, has been demonstrated to be decreased by IOLs with hydrophilic surfaces [74,75]. Surface modifications that increase an IOL's water content have been made using different agents including MPC, fluorine and heparin. While MPC and fluorine have been demonstrated to decrease the density of biofilms formed on PMMA and silicone IOLs [53,55,71], data for heparin-modified lenses are mixed. Initial adhesion of *S. epidermidis*, *S. aureus* and *P. aeruginosa* to heparin-surface-modified (HSM) PMMA IOL has been shown to be reduced compared to non-treated PMMA IOLs [76,77]. However, biofilm formation on HSM PMMA IOLs seems not to be affected, and in fact biomass measures were higher compared to non-treated PMMA [53]. In addition, although the anti-adhesive effect of soluble heparin in the media has been demonstrated *in vitro* using *S. epidermidis* and PMMA IOLs [78], this protective effect was not demonstrated *in vivo* by the addition of low molecular weight heparin to the infusion fluid used during the phacoemulsification procedure [79].

Although infrequent, enterococcal endophthalmitis may occur after cataract surgery and is associated with poor visual outcomes even after appropriate clinical and surgical management [80]. *In vitro* studies have demonstrated that *Enterococcus faecalis* is able to form robust biofilms on IOLs, especially on PMMA and hydrophobic acrylic IOLs after 48 h and 72 h of incubation, while less biomass was observed on silicone IOLs [81]. Recurrent cases of post-cataract endophthalmitis caused by *E. faecalis* have been associated with bacteria attached to the capsular bag and acrylic IOL [82,83].

While acrylic IOLs have demonstrated to be the most permissive material for biofilm formation of Gram positive pathogens, as described above, this material seems to be less susceptible to adherence and biofilm formation of *Pseudomonas aeruginosa*, compared to PMMA and silicone [84]. This is consistent with the finding that the surface of *P. aeruginosa* is highly hydrophobic, while that of staphylococci is highly hydrophilic [17]. Although *P. aeruginosa* does not represent an important organism associated with endophthalmitis after uneventful cataract surgery, it has been associated with multiple outbreaks of post-cataract surgery endophthalmitis, usually due to environmental contamination including the internal tubes of phacoemulsification machines and contaminated solutions used during the surgery [85]. In a recent outbreak of *P. aeruginosa* endophthalmitis following cataract surgery, a thorough investigation identified the hydrophilic acrylic IOL implanted in the patients and the preservative solution as the source of the contamination. The *P. aeruginosa* isolates from the IOL and the preservative solution had the same genetic profile as the isolates from the patients' aqueous and vitreous fluids, as demonstrated by ERIC-PCR [86]. In the context of *P. aeruginosa* endophthalmitis outbreaks after cataract surgery, biofilm formation has not been directly associated in the pathogenesis of these infections, but it likely plays a role as a reservoir for contamination. Biofilms found in the hospital environment have been demonstrated to be a common source of *P. aeruginosa* associated with outbreaks in intensive care units [87,88]. *P. aeruginosa* evolved to form biofilms on surfaces in contact with water, including sinks, water pipes and other natural interfaces [89], and this property is undoubtedly central to its ability to colonize the surgical equipment and irrigation fluids that have been linked to endophthalmitis outbreaks.

5. Biofilms in Keratitis

Microbial keratitis is an infection of the cornea that can lead to loss of vision if not carefully managed [90]. Decades ago, most cases were associated with ocular surface disease and trauma. However, the widespread of contact lenses has made them the most common predisposing risk factor for infectious keratitis [91,92]. The type of organisms causing keratitis varies by geography because of differences in climate, environment and occupational risk [93]. Bacterial keratitis, especially contact lens-associated infection, is caused by both Gram negative pathogens, such as *P. aeruginosa* and *Serratia* spp., and Gram positive organisms, such as *S. aureus* [94,95] and other staphylococcal species [93,96,97]. Risk factors for fungal keratitis include tropical or subtropical climate, agricultural work, and corneal trauma [93,98]. In the United States, the prevalence of fungal keratitis is much lower than bacterial keratitis [99], and the primary predisposing factor is unambiguously contact lens wear [100,101]. When it does occur, *Fusarium* spp. usually accounts for the majority of fungal keratitis cases [101]. Additionally, *Acanthamoeba* are protozoa that cause a rare but aggressive form of infectious keratitis that is also frequently associated with contact lens wear [102].

5.1. Contact Lens-Associated Keratitis

Contact lens use represents the main risk factor for the development of microbial keratitis in developed countries, where it is associated with bacterial, fungal and amoebic keratitis [91,92,100–103]. In the United States, previous estimates of microbial keratitis suggested more than 30,000 cases per year [104]. Other estimates of ulcerative keratitis in northern California found an incidence of 27.6 cases per 100,000 person/year [103]. This incidence was higher than observed previously, and was thought to be associated with increasing contact lens wear, since the rate of keratitis was half of that for non-contact lens wearers [103].

The incidence of contact lens-associated microbial keratitis has been shown to be impacted by the contact lens material, and also by the wear schedule. Early epidemiological studies reported a higher risk for daily wear soft contact lenses compared to daily wear rigid gas permeable lenses. The risk was further increased for extended wear (overnight wear) soft contact lenses [95,105]. More recently introduced daily disposable and silicone hydrogel contact lenses have also been associated with a higher incidence of keratitis compared to rigid gas permeable contact lenses [106,107].

The increased risk for the development of microbial keratitis in contact lens wearers has been associated with the ability of the lens to induce modification of the corneal epithelium, to carry organisms to the ocular surface that otherwise would not be found in this niche, and to limit natural clearance mechanisms [108,109]. The close interaction between the lens and the corneal epithelium induces local alterations, including hypoxia and hypercapnia, which affect the ability of the epithelium to respond to damage. Tear fluid exchange may be compromised between the anterior and posterior sides of the lens, altering the composition of the tear fluid on the ocular surface and limiting its antimicrobial properties [108]. In addition, contact lenses provide a surface where microorganisms may attach and colonize the surface as a biofilm, which represents a source for microorganisms to spread to a previously damaged corneal epithelium [109]. It has been demonstrated that poor hygiene and infrequent replacement of the contact lens storage cases were independent risk factors for moderate and sever keratitis [110]. However, not all individuals with poor contact lens hygiene will experience keratitis, while others with good cleaning routines also suffered infections, suggesting that other factors play a role as well [111].

Corneal damage promotes colonization and infection by commensal and environmental organisms. The high prevalence of Gram negative organisms among contact lens-associated keratitis isolates, which are usually not found as commensals on the ocular surface, is likely due to their ubiquitous presence in the environment and their ability to adhere and subsequently form biofilms on the surface of contact lenses and storage cases. *P. aeruginosa* has a repertoire of genes that allow its adaptation and survival under different stress conditions [112]. Its ability to adhere to different contact lens materials has been demonstrated *in vitro* [113] and is mainly driven by surface hydrophobicity [17,114]. Development of mature biofilms in the posterior surface of the contact lens has been associated with *P. aeruginosa* keratitis in humans [115] and in animal models [31].

In addition to bacteria, fungi and *Acanthamoeba spp.* are also able of causing contact lens associated keratitis. Some of these cases were linked to specific multipurpose contact lens cleaning solutions (MPS), which led to the removal of these products from the market. The first case involved the fungus *Fusarium solani*, which was associated with keratitis in patients that used ReNu with MoistureLoc. This finding came as a surprise because all MPS have to pass antimicrobial efficacy testing against several microorganisms, including *F. solani*. An investigation [116] found that planktonic *Fusarium* strains were susceptible to MoistureLoc as expected, but *Fusarium* biofilms showed reduced susceptibility. In addition, *F. solani* ATCC 36031, the reference strain recommended for antimicrobial efficacy testing, was shown to be incapable of forming biofilms under the conditions tested [116]. This case highlights the need to consider the physiological state of microbes and the strains used in establishing testing standards—standards largely developed using planktonic cells. The second case involves Complete MoisturePlus and protozoa of the genus *Acanthamoeba*. These amoebae are ubiquitous in water and are able to survive harsh conditions, including chemical treatment, by differentiating into dormant cysts that can resume growth once favorable conditions return. Bacterial biofilm formation on contact lenses is a risk factor for contact lens-associated keratitis by *Acanthamoeba* because these organisms graze on the biofilm [117–119]. Complete MoisturePlus was recalled because, rather than killing all cells, it resulted in the encystment of *Acanthamoeba*, which then went on to cause keratitis [120]. Prior to this recall, antimicrobial efficacy testing that included *Acanthamoeba* was not required [121].

5.2. Infectious Crystalline Keratopathy

Crystalline keratopathy is a disease associated with crystalline deposits in the corneal epithelium and stroma, which may be a result of multiple conditions that ultimately lead to the accumulation of metabolic products in the affected corneal tissue. Among the causes of such deposits are corneal infections and systemic diseases [122]. Infectious crystalline keratopathy (ICK) is a chronic and difficult to treat infection of the cornea characterized by the presence of branching crystalline opacities associated with minimum inflammatory response [123,124]. It may occur in normal or diseased corneas and is often associated with corneal surgery, especially penetrating keratoplasty, and the topical use of steroids [122,124,125]. Viridans streptococci are the main pathogens associated with ICK, but other bacterial and fungal species, as well as *Acanthamoeba*, may cause this infection [125–128].

Because of the indolent clinical evolution of this disease, and the relative lack of immune response and recalcitrance to antimicrobial therapy, it was first hypothesized that ICK resulted from organisms associated with a biofilm in the corneal tissue. This was supported by analysis of corneal samples collected by biopsy or penetrating keratoplasty from patients with ICK [129–131]. Transmission electron microscopy examination of corneal samples fixed with ruthenium red found *Candida albicans* and also bacteria surrounded by an extracellular matrix consistent with a biofilm [129,130]. Microscopic evidence of bacterial biofilms growing on the corneal tissue was also found for 3 patients diagnosed with ICK, but for 5 other cases of chronic bacterial and fungal keratitis. This indicates that *in vivo* biofilm formation in the corneal stroma is fairly specific for ICK [130]. The intensity of the periodic acid-Schiff stain of the corneal samples from ICK [130] is indicative of high concentrations of polysaccharides, often a main factor associated with the ability of bacteria to form a strong and well organized multicellular structure. The presence of extracellular polysaccharides in abundant amounts also has been observed in a histologic analysis of corneal sections from rabbits with crystalline lesions induced by a *Streptococcus sanguis* type II strain, but were absent in the eyes that developed suppurative stromal lesion [132]. Interestingly, this study showed that *S. sanguis* grown in medium supplemented with sucrose produced exopolysaccharides, resulting in a mucoid phenotype and a crystalline lesion similar to ICK in 71% of the corneas inoculated. In contrast, strains grown without sucrose showed a rough phenotype, caused crystalline lesions in only 25% of the eyes, and were more frequently associated with suppurative infiltrates [132].

It is unclear what cues induce microbes to grow as planktonic cells or invade tissues and form a biofilm in ICK. Prolonged topical corticosteroid therapy and/or prior penetrating keratoplasty have been identified as risk factors for the development of ICK in the vast majority of patients [123–126,128–131]. Anatomical modification from the keratoplasty procedure, often resulting in inflammation and altered local immune activity, appears to predispose microbes to grow in a biofilm, but the underlying mechanism has not been thoroughly explored.

As for other biofilm-related infections, antimicrobial treatment of ICK is challenging in that it is usually prolonged and the disease is often unresponsive. Physical means have been explored for improving the success of ICK treatment, including the use of laser disruption of biofilms [133,134]. In this case, Nd:YAG (neodymium-doped yttrium aluminum garnet) laser photocoagulation was used to disrupt the crystalline deposits in the cornea of patients unsuccessfully treated with antibiotics. In all cases, laser disruption with further antimicrobial therapy resolved ICK within weeks, and no recurrence was observed.

6. Biofilms Associated with Other Implant-Related Ocular Infections

6.1. Scleral Buckles

The placement of permanent scleral buckles between the conjunctiva and sclera is a common surgical treatment for rhegmatogenous retinal detachment. The bands encircling the sclera are commonly made of silicone and may have a solid or sponge form. One of the main complications associated with this surgery is the extrusion of the bands, which is frequently associated with an infection. Scleral buckle-associated infections are frequently caused by Gram positive cocci, especially coagulase-negative staphylococci, and nontuberculous *Mycobacterium* [135,136]. These infections often have a delayed onset and are usually refractory to antimicrobial therapy, requiring removal of the bands for complete resolution [135]. Due to the chronic evolution of this infection, the presence of a biofilm in the explanted material has been assumed to play an important role in its pathogenesis. Biofilms have been demonstrated by scanning electron microscopy for 65% of scleral buckles (solid and sponge forms) removed for infection and extrusion [137]. Gram positive bacteria, and less frequently *Mycobacterium chelonae* and *Proteus mirabilis,* were cultured from these buckle elements [137]. Buckle materials removed from patients because of conjunctival erosion and infection, or due to technical reasons at the time of revision surgery, contained demonstrable bacterial biofilms in 5 out 28 cases examined by scanning electron microscopy following fixation with ruthenium red [138]. Of those five, one was removed due to extrusion, and one was associated with a diagnosed infection. The three remaining buckles were removed for other reasons from patients lacking signs of infection. It seems likely that at the time of surgery, bacteria attach to the buckle material and form biofilms that lead to indolent infections, or infections lacking any overt signs.

6.2. Conjunctival Plug

Punctual plugs are frequently used to treat ocular surface dryness unresponsive to topical medication, by occluding the lacrimal ducts and blocking tear drainage. Plugs are made of silicone, hydrophobic acrylic, collagen and hydrogel. However, secondary complications may occur following implantation, including canaliculitis, dacryocystitis and acute conjunctivitis [139,140]. Although the presence of biofilms has not been demonstrated on plugs recovered from patients with dacryocystitis and canaliculitis, these infections typically have a late onset and are usually not responsive to antimicrobial treatment alone, requiring additional intervention, as is typical for biofilm-related infections [141,142]. Examination of punctual plugs removed from patients without clinical signs of infection revealed the presence of bacterial biofilms in 53% of the samples assessed by electron microscopy [143]. However, since the patients were asymptomatic with respect to infection, the causal association between the biofilms growing on punctual plugs and progress to an eye infection remains speculative. A single case of conjunctivitis has been associated with biofilm formation on a punctual plug [140]. That patient presented with acute conjunctivitis in the same eye that had received a punctual plug five and half months earlier. A whitish material that was culture positive for *S. haemolyticus* and *Candida tropicalis* was present in the top of the plug. Analysis of this plug by scanning electron microscopy demonstrated the presence of a bacterial biofilm. The plug was removed and the patient resolved the infection after 1 month of topical antimicrobial treatment [140].

6.3. Lacrimal Intubation Devices and Orbital Implants

Lacrimal intubation devices including lacrimal stents and Jones tubes are commonly used during the dacryocystorhinostomy procedure to treat nasolacrimal duct obstruction, a common cause of epiphora. As for other biomaterials implanted in the eyes, both lacrimal stents and Jones tube may provide with a surface for biofilm formation [144–146]. Biofilm formation on polyurethane nasolacrimal stents has been associated with delayed failure of the device [145]. In a study undertaken to identify the rates of biofilm colonization on silicone stents inserted during dacryocystorhinostomy, 90% of stent fragments removed 8 weeks after surgery revealed the presence of coccoid and/or rod-shaped bacteria encased in a biofilm matrix [144]. All patients included in this last study had received postoperative antibiotics for 1 week (oral) and 3 weeks (topical) and the silicone tubes were collected at the 8th week post-surgery. Most of these silicone stents were culture positive for *S. epidermidis* and *P. aeruginosa* [144].

A report of 2 cases of nasolacrimal infection following placement of a lacrimal silicone and a Jones tube described recalcitrant culture-negative infections associated with the presence of bacterial biofilms in the lacrimal intubation devices [147]. Evaluation of both silicone stent and Jones tube by scanning electron microscopy revealed the presence of a polymicrobial biofilm. Interestingly, the authors were able to identify a variety of cell morphologies in the silicone stent biofilms, including short rods, spirochetes, fusiforms and cocci. Analysis of the internal surfaces of the silicone stent by confocal laser scanning microscopy revealed the presence of viable biofilms along the tube [147].

In a series of cases with recalcitrant infections associated with silicone stents ($n = 10$) and Jones tube implants ($n = 2$), a high prevalence of *Mycobacterium chelonae* (90%) was found associated with the silicone stents, sometimes along with other bacterial organisms [146]. In this same study, the authors evaluated the culture results and presence of biofilms in other periorbital biomaterials, including orbital plates ($n = 5$) and anophthalmic socket sphere implants ($n = 4$) [146]. Cultures were positive for *S. aureus* in all orbital spheres, in addition to one isolate of *M. chelonae* and one *Pantoea agglomerans* that were found in polymicrobial cases. Culture results of orbital plates demonstrated more species diversity with the isolation of yeasts (*Candida* spp., and *Trichosporon* spp.), *Staphylococcus* spp., *M. chelonae* and Gram negative bacilli (*Achromobacter xylosoxidans* and *P. aeruginosa*). Scanning electron microscopy analysis of selected samples also demonstrated the presence of mixed species biofilms on porous polyethylene orbital floor implant, metal screws from orbital plate implant and on orbital sphere implants [146].

7. Perspectives on Agents for Prevention and Treatment of Biofilms

Since biofilms have been recognized for their great medical importance, efforts have been made to either prevent their formation, or to remove them once they have formed. The colonization of surfaces can be prevented by covalently attaching biocidal molecules, slowly releasing antibiotics, or modifying the surface topology to interfere with microbial adhesion. While the first two approaches would be practically easier to achieve as it depends basically on coating current ocular devices with available molecules, the last may be more challenging as modifications in the topology of the material may alter its optical clarity. However, both approaches have their advantages and disadvantages. As an example for prevention of surface colonization using biocides, in a previous study authors have demonstrated a 100-fold reduction in cell counts when *S. aureus*, *S. epidermidis*, *E. coli*, or *P. aeruginosa* were sprayed onto glass slides that were coated with covalently attached poly(4-vinyl-*N*-alkylpyridinium bromide) or *N*-hexylated poly(4-vinylpyridine) [148]. Surface coatings that slowly release antibiotics, such as rifampin, clarithromycin and doxycycline, were able to prevent biofilm formation for up to three weeks *in vitro* [149]. An IOL designed to release norfloxacin to prevent postoperative bacterial infection after cataract surgery has been tested *in vitro* and in a rabbit model, and might soon become commercially available [150]. Antimicrobial peptides have also been used successfully to prevent biofilm formation and have the added advantage that they are active against antibiotic-resistant strains [151]. Other molecules that can prevent the formation of biofilms, such as gallium nitrate or silver, have also shown potential [151]. While molecules that are slowly released from a surface to prevent biofilm formation show great promise for some applications, questions remain regarding their use in medical devices. The concentration of the antimicrobial agent would have to remain sufficiently high as long as colonization and infection is a risk, and not select for resistant strains. In addition, lack of toxicity and long-term compatibility with surrounding tissues is important [152]. The advantages of using ocular devices that slowly release antimicrobial agents is that tissue toxicity, penetration and half-life is already known for a number of antibiotics routinely used in ophthalmology. On the other hand, long-term exposure to these drugs may favor selection of spontaneous resistant mutants and perturbs the ocular surface microbiome.

Modifying the surface structure of ocular devices to make it less adhesive for bacteria attempting to colonize is a tempting approach since it would potentially eliminate the need for coating with antimicrobial or biocide agents that could be reserved for treatment and perioperative prophylaxis. However, alterations in the material topology that results in material opacities may limit its use for optical correction. Polymers, such polyacrylamide, dextran, or polyethylene glycol, can form linear, star-shaped, or 'bottle brush' shaped surface nanostructures that interfere with the microbe's ability to adhere to the substrate [153,154]. Nanopores, nanotubes, and nanopillars made of anodized aluminum, titanium dioxide, or polymethylmethacrylate have also been investigated to reduce microbial adhesion to coated surfaces [152]. Even low-fouling substrates may eventually become colonized due to degradation or erosion of the anti-adhesive surface [154], so this will have to be explored. Furthermore, some medical devices require the firm binding of the implant to the surrounding tissue for optimal biointegration, which may limit the use of this strategy in some cases. Other devices, such as contact lenses, may be difficult to modify this way without negatively affecting critical properties, such as optical clarity.

An alternative strategy for the removal of microbial biofilms is to stimulate the reversion of microbes to planktonic physiology. While the enzymes that degrade the ECM or the substratum might be too large and costly to be of practical clinical value, small signaling molecules that induce expression of factors that stimulate the dissimilation of biofilms might be a viable alternative. Cell signaling molecules, such as C4HSL, PQS, AI-2, and AIP-I or their derivatives, may be of great therapeutic value [35,38].

While typical antibiotics work well against growing planktonic cells and are less active, or inactive, against the dormant cells in a biofilm, they may still have a use in combination therapies. The acyldepsipeptide antibiotic, ADEP4, was shown to bind to the ClpP protease of *S. aureus* and convert it into a nonspecific protease that degrades over 400 proteins, killing growing as well as dormant cells [155]. Treatment with ADEP4 resulted in the emergence of ADEP4-resistant *clpP* mutants, but those were highly susceptible to killing by various antibiotics. Using a deep-seated mouse biofilm infection model, the authors showed that ADEP4 in combination with rifampicin was able to reduce the number of *S. aureus* below detectable limits, while neither rifampicin, vancomycin, nor ADEP4 by themselves were able to do so [155]. The use of bacteriophage endolysins as well as engineered phages expressing anti-biofilm enzymes may also be promising options for eradication of bacterial biofilms in the site of infection [156,157]. Evolutionary distinct bacteriophage endolysins have shown to be effective in killing planktonic cells as well biofilms of *S. aureus* and prevented death of 100% of mice inoculated intraperitoneally with lethal doses of MRSA [157]. A T7 bacteriophage engineered to express dispersin B (DspB), an enzyme that hydrolyzes β-1,6-*N*-acetyl-D-glucosamine, has been successfully used to simultaneously infect and kill the bacterial cells in the biofilm, in this case *E. coli*, and also attack the extracellular polymeric biofilm matrix [156].

The field of biofilm dispersal and eradication is an area of very active research and the next five years will see a substantial increase in our understanding of the physiological states associated with biofilms. It is hoped that this will lead to the development of new agents that will pass clinical trials and serve as new treatments for microbial infections caused by cells in a biofilm state.

8. Conclusions

Our understanding of biofilms has advanced substantially since early descriptions more than three decades ago. As medical interventions rely increasingly on medical devices and prosthesis, the need to prevent, reduce, or eliminate microbial biofilms is becoming an important constraint. In the eye care field, contact lenses and IOLs have had a great impact on restoring and improving vision, but their use is limited by ocular infection. Strategies, such as anti-biofilm surface coatings and developing biofilm-active therapeutics, are exciting avenues of future research to reduce the risk of biofilm-associated ocular infection.

Acknowledgments

Portions of this project were supported by NIH grants EY024285, Molecular Basis for Ocular Surface Tropism in Conjunctivitis, and by the Harvard-wide Program on Antibiotic Resistance, AI083214. P.J.M.B was supported by a grant from the Coordenação de Aperfeiçoamento de Pessoal de Nível Superior, Brazil (CAPES #9775-13-7).

References

1. Costerton, J.W.; Geesey, G.G.; Cheng, K.J. How bacteria stick. *Sci. Am.* **1978**, *238*, 86–95.
2. Rasmussen, B. Filamentous microfossils in a 3235-million-year-old volcanogenic massive sulphide deposit. *Nature* **2000**, *405*, 676–679.
3. Westall, F.; Witb, M.J.; Dannb, J.; van der Gaastc, S.; de Ronded, C.E.J.; Gernekee, D. Early archean fossil bacteria and biofilms in hydrothermally-influenced sediments from the barberton greenstone belt, south africa. *Precambrian Res.* **2001**, *106*, 93–116.
4. Hall-Stoodley, L.; Costerton, J.W.; Stoodley, P. Bacterial biofilms: From the natural environment to infectious diseases. *Nat. Rev. Microbiol.* **2004**, *2*, 95–108.
5. Harrison, J.J.; Ceri, H.; Turner, R.J. Multimetal resistance and tolerance in microbial biofilms. *Nat. Rev. Microbiol.* **2007**, *5*, 928–938.
6. National Institute of Health. Research on microbial biofilms (PA-03-047). Available online: http://grants.nih.gov/grants/guide/pa-files/PA-03-047.html. 20 December, 2002. (accessed on 10 January 2015).
7. Costerton, J.W.; Montanaro, L.; Arciola, C.R. Biofilm in implant infections: Its production and regulation. *Int. J. Artif. Organs* **2005**, *28*, 1062–1068.

8. Donlan, R.M.; Costerton, J.W. Biofilms: Survival mechanisms of clinically relevant microorganisms. *Clin. Microbiol. Rev.* **2002**, *15*, 167–193.

9. Romero, D.; Kolter, R. Will biofilm disassembly agents make it to market? *Trends Microbiol.* **2011**, *19*, 304–306.

10. Van Leeuwenhoek, A. Microscopical observations about animals in the scurf of the teeth. *Philos. Trans.* **1684**, *1684*, 568–574.

11. Annous, B.A.; Fratamico, P.M.; Smith, J.L. Scientific status summary. *J. Food Sci.* **2009**, *74*, R24–R37.

12. Hooshangi, S.; Bentley, W.E. From unicellular properties to multicellular behavior: Bacteria quorum sensing circuitry and applications. *Curr. Opin. Biotechnol.* **2008**, *19*, 550–555.

13. Stewart, P.S.; Franklin, M.J. Physiological heterogeneity in biofilms. *Nat. Rev. Microbiol.* **2008**, *6*, 199–210.

14. Watnick, P.; Kolter, R. Biofilm, city of microbes. *J. Bacteriol.* **2000**, *182*, 2675–2679.

15. Behlau, I.; Gilmore, M.S. Microbial biofilms in ophthalmology and infectious disease. *Arch. Ophthalmol.* **2008**, *126*, 1572–1581.

16. Costerton, J.W.; Stewart, P.S. Battling biofilms. *Sci. Am.* **2001**, *285*, 74–81.

17. Bruinsma, G.M.; van der Mei, H.C.; Busscher, H.J. Bacterial adhesion to surface hydrophilic and hydrophobic contact lenses. *Biomaterials* **2001**, *22*, 3217–3224.

18. Powell, C.H.; Lally, J.M.; Hoong, L.D.; Huth, S.W. Lipophilic *versus* hydrodynamic modes of uptake and release by contact lenses of active entities used in multipurpose solutions. *Contact Lens Anterior Eye* **2010**, *33*, 9–18.

19. Baguet, J.; Sommer, F.; Claudon-Eyl, V.; Duc, T.M. Characterization of lacrymal component accumulation on worn soft contact lens surfaces by atomic force microscopy. *Biomaterials* **1995**, *16*, 3–9.

20. Bright, F.V.; Merchea, M.M.; Kraut, N.D.; Maziarz, E.P.; Liu, X.M.; Awasthi, A.K. A preservative-and-fluorescein interaction model for benign multipurpose solution-associated transient corneal hyperfluorescence. *Cornea* **2012**, *31*, 1480–1488.

21. Patti, J.M.; Allen, B.L.; McGavin, M.J.; Hook, M. Mscramm-mediated adherence of microorganisms to host tissues. *Annu. Rev. Microbiol.* **1994**, *48*, 585–617.

22. Heilmann, C.; Hussain, M.; Peters, G.; Gotz, F. Evidence for autolysin-mediated primary attachment of *Staphylococcus epidermidis* to a polystyrene surface. *Mol. Microbiol.* **1997**, *24*, 1013–1024.

23. Sauer, K.; Camper, A.K.; Ehrlich, G.D.; Costerton, J.W.; Davies, D.G. *Pseudomonas aeruginosa* displays multiple phenotypes during development as a biofilm. *J. Bacteriol.* **2002**, *184*, 1140–1154.

24. Flemming, H.C.; Wingender, J. The biofilm matrix. *Nat. Rev. Microbiol.* **2010**, *8*, 623–633.

25. Rohde, H.; Burandt, E.C.; Siemssen, N.; Frommelt, L.; Burdelski, C.; Wurster, S.; Scherpe, S.; Davies, A.P.; Harris, L.G.; Horstkotte, M.A.; *et al.* Polysaccharide intercellular adhesin or protein factors in biofilm accumulation of *Staphylococcus epidermidis* and *Staphylococcus aureus* isolated from prosthetic hip and knee joint infections. *Biomaterials* **2007**, *28*, 1711–1720.

26. Lasa, I.; Penades, J.R. Bap: A family of surface proteins involved in biofilm formation. *Res. Microbiol.* **2006**, *157*, 99–107.

27. Juarez-Verdayes, M.A.; Ramon-Perez, M.L.; Flores-Paez, L.A.; Camarillo-Marquez, O.; Zenteno, J.C.; Jan-Roblero, J.; Cancino-Diaz, M.E.; Cancino-Diaz, J.C. Staphylococcus epidermidis with the icaa(−)/icad(−)/is256(−) genotype and protein or protein/extracellular-DNA biofilm is frequent in ocular infections. *J. Med. Microbiol.* **2013**, *62*, 1579–1587.

28. Makki, A.R.; Sharma, S.; Duggirala, A.; Prashanth, K.; Garg, P.; Das, T. Phenotypic and genotypic characterization of coagulase negative staphylococci (CoNS) other than *Staphylococcus epidermidis* isolated from ocular infections. *Investig. Ophthalmol. Vis. Sci.* **2011**, *52*, 9018–9022.

29. Suzuki, T.; Kawamura, Y.; Uno, T.; Ohashi, Y.; Ezaki, T. Prevalence of *Staphylococcus epidermidis* strains with biofilm-forming ability in isolates from conjunctiva and facial skin. *Am. J. Ophthalmol.* **2005**, *140*, 844–850.

30. Randler, C.; Matthes, R.; McBain, A.J.; Giese, B.; Fraunholz, M.; Sietmann, R.; Kohlmann, T.; Hubner, N.O.; Kramer, A. A three-phase *in vitro* system for studying *Pseudomonas aeruginosa* adhesion and biofilm formation upon hydrogel contact lenses. *BMC Microbiol.* **2010**, *10*, 282, doi:10.1186/1471-2180-10-282.

31. Tam, C.; Mun, J.J.; Evans, D.J.; Fleiszig, S.M. The impact of inoculation parameters on the pathogenesis of contact lens-related infectious keratitis. *Investig. Ophthalmol. Vis. Sci.* **2010**, *51*, 3100–3106.

32. Davies, D. Understanding biofilm resistance to antibacterial agents. *Nat. Rev. Drug Discov.* **2003**, *2*, 114–122.

33. Hall-Stoodley, L.; Stoodley, P. Evolving concepts in biofilm infections. *Cell. Microbiol.* **2009**, *11*, 1034–1043.

34. Spoering, A.L.; Gilmore, M.S. Quorum sensing and DNA release in bacterial biofilms. *Curr. Opin. Microbiol.* **2006**, *9*, 133–137.

35. Kaplan, J.B. Biofilm dispersal: Mechanisms, clinical implications, and potential therapeutic uses. *J. Dent. Res.* **2010**, *89*, 205–218.

36. Boyd, A.; Chakrabarty, A.M. Role of alginate lyase in cell detachment of *Pseudomonas aeruginosa*. *Appl. Environ. Microbiol.* **1994**, *60*, 2355–2359.

37. Mann, E.E.; Rice, K.C.; Boles, B.R.; Endres, J.L.; Ranjit, D.; Chandramohan, L.; Tsang, L.H.; Smeltzer, M.S.; Horswill, A.R.; Bayles, K.W.; *et al*. Modulation of eDNA release and degradation affects *Staphylococcus aureus* biofilm maturation. *PLoS One* **2009**, *4*, e5822.

38. Dong, Y.H.; Zhang, X.F.; An, S.W.; Xu, J.L.; Zhang, L.H. A novel two-component system BqsS-BqsR modulates quorum sensing-dependent biofilm decay in *Pseudomonas aeruginosa*. *Commun. Integr. Biol.* **2008**, *1*, 88–96.

39. Pascolini, D.; Mariotti, S.P. Global estimates of visual impairment: 2010. *Br. J. Ophthalmol.* **2012**, *96*, 614–618.

40. Sadaka, A.; Durand, M.L.; Gilmore, M.S. Bacterial endophthalmitis in the age of outpatient intravitreal therapies and cataract surgeries: Host-microbe interactions in intraocular infection. *Prog. Retin. Eye Res.* **2012**, *31*, 316–331.

41. Han, D.P.; Wisniewski, S.R.; Wilson, L.A.; Barza, M.; Vine, A.K.; Doft, B.H.; Kelsey, S.F. Spectrum and susceptibilities of microbiologic isolates in the endophthalmitis vitrectomy study. *Am. J. Ophthalmol.* **1996**, *122*, 1–17.

42. Benz, M.S.; Scott, I.U.; Flynn, H.W., Jr.; Unonius, N.; Miller, D. Endophthalmitis isolates and antibiotic sensitivities: A 6-year review of culture-proven cases. *Am. J. Ophthalmol.* **2004**, *137*, 38–42.

43. Klein, R.; Klein, B.E. The prevalence of age-related eye diseases and visual impairment in aging: Current estimates. *Investig. Ophthalmol. Vis. Sci.* **2013**, *54*, ORSF5–ORSF13.

44. Prevent Blindness America. Vision problems in the U.S. Prevalence of adult vision impairment and age-related eye disease in america. Available online: http://www.preventblindness.net/site/DocServer/VPUS_2008_update.pdf. 2008. (accessed 10 January 2015).

45. Taban, M.; Behrens, A.; Newcomb, R.L.; Nobe, M.Y.; Saedi, G.; Sweet, P.M.; McDonnell, P.J. Acute endophthalmitis following cataract surgery: A systematic review of the literature. *Arch. Ophthalmol.* **2005**, *123*, 613–620.

46. Wykoff, C.C.; Parrott, M.B.; Flynn, H.W., Jr.; Shi, W.; Miller, D.; Alfonso, E.C. Nosocomial acute-onset postoperative endophthalmitis at a university teaching hospital (2002–2009). *Am. J. Ophthalmol.* **2010**, *150*, 392–398.e2.

47. West, E.S.; Behrens, A.; McDonnell, P.J.; Tielsch, J.M.; Schein, O.D. The incidence of endophthalmitis after cataract surgery among the U.S. Medicare population increased between 1994 and 2001. *Ophthalmology* **2005**, *112*, 1388–1394.

48. Schimel, A.M.; Miller, D.; Flynn, H.W., Jr. Endophthalmitis isolates and antibiotic susceptibilities: A 10-year review of culture-proven cases. *Am. J. Ophthalmol.* **2013**, *156*, 50–52.e1.

49. Shirodkar, A.R.; Pathengay, A.; Flynn, H.W., Jr.; Albini, T.A.; Berrocal, A.M.; Davis, J.L.; Lalwani, G.A.; Murray, T.G.; Smiddy, W.E.; Miller, D.; *et al.* Delayed- *versus* acute-onset endophthalmitis after cataract surgery. *Am. J. Ophthalmol.* **2012**, *153*, 391–398.e392.

50. Adan, A.; Casaroli-Marano, R.P.; Gris, O.; Navarro, R.; Bitrian, E.; Pelegrin, L.; Sanchez-Dalmau, B. Pathological findings in the lens capsules and intraocular lens in chronic pseudophakic endophthalmitis: An electron microscopy study. *Eye* **2008**, *22*, 113–119.

51. Baillif, S.; Casoli, E.; Marion, K.; Roques, C.; Pellon, G.; Hartmann, D.J.; Freney, J.; Burillon, C.; Kodjikian, L. A novel *in vitro* model to study staphylococcal biofilm formation on intraocular lenses under hydrodynamic conditions. *Investig. Ophthalmol. Vis. Sci.* **2006**, *47*, 3410–3416.

52. Baillif, S.; Ecochard, R.; Casoli, E.; Freney, J.; Burillon, C.; Kodjikian, L. Adherence and kinetics of biofilm formation of *Staphylococcus epidermidis* to different types of intraocular lenses under dynamic flow conditions. *J. Cataract Refract. Surg.* **2008**, *34*, 153–158.

53. Garcia-Saenz, M.C.; Arias-Puente, A.; Fresnadillo-Martinez, M.J.; Matilla-Rodriguez, A. *In vitro* adhesion of *Staphylococcus epidermidis* to intraocular lenses. *J. Cataract Refract. Surg.* **2000**, *26*, 1673–1679.

54. Griffiths, P.G.; Elliot, T.S.; McTaggart, L. Adherence of *Staphylococcus epidermidis* to intraocular lenses. *Br. J. Ophthalmol.* **1989**, *73*, 402–406.

55. Okajima, Y.; Kobayakawa, S.; Tsuji, A.; Tochikubo, T. Biofilm formation by *Staphylococcus epidermidis* on intraocular lens material. *Investig. Ophthalmol. Vis. Sci.* **2006**, *47*, 2971–2975.

56. Sawusch, M.R.; Michels, R.G.; Stark, W.J.; Bruner, W.E.; Annable, W.L.; Green, W.R. Endophthalmitis due to *Propionibacterium acnes* sequestered between iol optic and posterior capsule. *Ophthalmic Surg.* **1989**, *20*, 90–92.

57. Shimizu, K.; Kobayakawa, S.; Tsuji, A.; Tochikubo, T. Biofilm formation on hydrophilic intraocular lens material. *Curr. Eye Res.* **2006**, *31*, 989–997.

58. Teichmann, K.D. *Propionibacterium acnes* endophthalmitis requiring intraocular lens removal after failure of medical therapy. *J. Cataract Refract. Surg.* **2000**, *26*, 1085–1088.

59. Bannerman, T.L.; Rhoden, D.L.; McAllister, S.K.; Miller, J.M.; Wilson, L.A. The source of coagulase-negative staphylococci in the endophthalmitis vitrectomy study. A comparison of eyelid and intraocular isolates using pulsed-field gel electrophoresis. *Arch. Ophthalmol.* **1997**, *115*, 357–361.

60. Willcox, M.D. Characterization of the normal microbiota of the ocular surface. *Exp. Eye Res.* **2013**, *117*, 99–105.

61. Bausz, M.; Fodor, E.; Resch, M.D.; Kristof, K. Bacterial contamination in the anterior chamber after povidone-iodine application and the effect of the lens implantation device. *J. Cataract Refract. Surg.* **2006**, *32*, 1691–1695.

62. Mistlberger, A.; Ruckhofer, J.; Raithel, E.; Muller, M.; Alzner, E.; Egger, S.F.; Grabner, G. Anterior chamber contamination during cataract surgery with intraocular lens implantation. *J. Cataract Refract. Surg.* **1997**, *23*, 1064–1069.

63. Samad, A.; Solomon, L.D.; Miller, M.A.; Mendelson, J. Anterior chamber contamination after uncomplicated phacoemulsification and intraocular lens implantation. *Am. J. Ophthalmol.* **1995**, *120*, 143–150.

64. Srinivasan, R.; Tiroumal, S.; Kanungo, R.; Natarajan, M.K. Microbial contamination of the anterior chamber during phacoemulsification. *J. Cataract Refract. Surg.* **2002**, *28*, 2173–2176.

65. Durand, M.L. Endophthalmitis. *Clin. Microbiol. Infect.* **2013**, 19, 227–234.

66. Vafidis, G.C.; Marsh, R.J.; Stacey, A.R. Bacterial contamination of intraocular lens surgery. *Br. J. Ophthalmol.* **1984**, *68*, 520–523.

67. Doyle, A.; Beigi, B.; Early, A.; Blake, A.; Eustace, P.; Hone, R. Adherence of bacteria to intraocular lenses: A prospective study. *Br. J. Ophthalmol.* **1995**, *79*, 347–349.

68. Melo, G.B.; Bispo, P.J.; Yu, M.C.; Pignatari, A.C.; Hofling-Lima, A.L. Microbial profile and antibiotic susceptibility of culture-positive bacterial endophthalmitis. *Eye* **2011**, *25*, 382–387.

69. Bispo, P.J.; Miller, D. Distinct frequency of biofilm (bf)-related genes among ciprofloxacin (cip) susceptible and resistant *S. epidermidis* (sepi) agr types i (ti) and ii (tii) isolates from endophthalmitis (end). In Proceedings of the Interscience Conference on Antimicrobial Agents and Chemotherapy, San Francisco, CA, USA, 9–12 September 2012.

70. Hirota, K.; Murakami, K.; Nemoto, K.; Miyake, Y. Coating of a surface with 2-methacryloyloxyethyl phosphorylcholine (mpc) co-polymer significantly reduces retention of human pathogenic microorganisms. *FEMS Microbiol. Lett.* **2005**, *248*, 37–45.

71. Huang, X.D.; Yao, K.; Zhang, H.; Huang, X.J.; Xu, Z.K. Surface modification of silicone intraocular lens by 2-methacryloyloxyethyl phosphoryl-choline binding to reduce *Staphylococcus epidermidis* adherence. *Clin. Exp. Ophthalmol.* **2007**, *35*, 462–467.

72. Menikoff, J.A.; Speaker, M.G.; Marmor, M.; Raskin, E.M. A case-control study of risk factors for postoperative endophthalmitis. *Ophthalmology* **1991**, *98*, 1761–1768.

73. Raskin, E.M.; Speaker, M.G.; McCormick, S.A.; Wong, D.; Menikoff, J.A.; Pelton-Henrion, K. Influence of haptic materials on the adherence of staphylococci to intraocular lenses. *Arch. Ophthalmol.* **1993**, *111*, 250–253.

74. Kodjikian, L.; Burillon, C.; Roques, C.; Pellon, G.; Freney, J.; Renaud, F.N. Bacterial adherence of *Staphylococcus epidermidis* to intraocular lenses: A bioluminescence and scanning electron microscopy study. *Investig. Ophthalmol. Vis. Sci.* **2003**, *44*, 4388–4394.

75. Schauersberger, J.; Amon, M.; Aichinger, D.; Georgopoulos, A. Bacterial adhesion to rigid and foldable posterior chamber intraocular lenses: *In vitro* study. *J. Cataract Refract. Surg.* **2003**, *29*, 361–366.

76. Portoles, M.; Refojo, M.F.; Leong, F.L. Reduced bacterial adhesion to heparin-surface-modified intraocular lenses. *J. Cataract Refract. Surg.* **1993**, *19*, 755–759.

77. Abu el-Asrar, A.M.; Shibl, A.M.; Tabbara, K.F.; al-Kharashi, S.A. Heparin and heparin-surface-modification reduce *Staphylococcus epidermidis* adhesion to intraocular lenses. *Int. Ophthalmol.* **1997**, *21*, 71–74.

78. Kadry, A.A.; Fouda, S.I.; Shibl, A.M.; Abu El-Asrar, A.A. Impact of slime dispersants and anti-adhesives on *in vitro* biofilm formation of *Staphylococcus epidermidis* on intraocular lenses and on antibiotic activities. *J. Antimicrob. Chemother.* **2009**, *63*, 480–484.

79. Manners, T.D.; Turner, D.P.; Galloway, P.H.; Glenn, A.M. Heparinised intraocular infusion and bacterial contamination in cataract surgery. *Br. J. Ophthalmol.* **1997**, *81*, 949–952.

80. Scott, I.U.; Loo, R.H.; Flynn, H.W., Jr.; Miller, D. Endophthalmitis caused by *Enterococcus faecalis*: Antibiotic selection and treatment outcomes. *Ophthalmology* **2003**, *110*, 1573–1577.

81. Kobayakawa, S.; Jett, B.D.; Gilmore, M.S. Biofilm formation by *Enterococcus faecalis* on intraocular lens material. *Curr. Eye Res.* **2005**, *30*, 741–745.

82. Teoh, S.C.; Lee, J.J.; Chee, C.K.; Au Eong, K.G. Recurrent *Enterococcus faecalis* endophthalmitis after phacoemulsification. *J. Cataract Refract. Surg.* **2005**, *31*, 622–626.

83. Miller, K.V.; Eisley, K.M.; Shanks, R.M.; Lahr, R.M.; Lathrop, K.L.; Kowalski, R.P.; Noecker, R.J. Recurrent enterococcal endophthalmitis seeded by an intraocular lens biofilm. *J. Cataract Refract. Surg.* **2011**, *37*, 1355–1359.

84. Gabriel, M.M.; Ahearn, D.G.; Chan, K.Y.; Patel, A.S. *In vitro* adherence of *Pseudomonas aeruginosa* to four intraocular lenses. *J. Cataract Refract. Surg.* **1998**, *24*, 124–129.

85. Pathengay, A.; Flynn, H.W., Jr.; Isom, R.F.; Miller, D. Endophthalmitis outbreaks following cataract surgery: Causative organisms, etiologies, and visual acuity outcomes. *J. Cataract Refract. Surg.* **2012**, *38*, 1278–1282.

86. Ramappa, M.; Majji, A.B.; Murthy, S.I.; Balne, P.K.; Nalamada, S.; Garudadri, C.; Mathai, A.; Gopinathan, U.; Garg, P. An outbreak of acute post-cataract surgery *Pseudomonas* sp. endophthalmitis caused by contaminated hydrophilic intraocular lens solution. *Ophthalmology* **2012**, *119*, 564–570.

87. Yakupogullari, Y.; Otlu, B.; Dogukan, M.; Gursoy, C.; Korkmaz, E.; Kizirgil, A.; Ozden, M.; Durmaz, R. Investigation of a nosocomial outbreak by alginate-producing pan-antibiotic-resistant *Pseudomonas aeruginosa*. *Am. J. Infect. Control* **2008**, *36*, e13–e18.

88. Hota, S.; Hirji, Z.; Stockton, K.; Lemieux, C.; Dedier, H.; Wolfaardt, G.; Gardam, M.A. Outbreak of multidrug-resistant *Pseudomonas aeruginosa* colonization and infection secondary to imperfect intensive care unit room design. *Infect. Control Hosp. Epidemiol.* **2009**, *30*, 25–33.

89. Elabed, H.; Maatallah, M.; Hamza, R.; Chakroun, I.; Bakhrouf, A.; Gaddour, K. Effect of long-term starvation in salty microcosm on biofilm formation and motility in *Pseudomonas aeruginosa*. *World J. Microbiol. Biotechnol.* **2013**, *29*, 657–665.

90. Vajpayee, R.B.; Dada, T.; Saxena, R.; Vajpayee, M.; Taylor, H.R.; Venkatesh, P.; Sharma, N. Study of the first contact management profile of cases of infectious keratitis: A hospital-based study. *Cornea* **2000**, *19*, 52–56.

91. Bourcier, T.; Thomas, F.; Borderie, V.; Chaumeil, C.; Laroche, L. Bacterial keratitis: Predisposing factors, clinical and microbiological review of 300 cases. *Br. J. Ophthalmol.* **2003**, *87*, 834–838.

92. Keay, L.; Edwards, K.; Naduvilath, T.; Taylor, H.R.; Snibson, G.R.; Forde, K.; Stapleton, F. Microbial keratitis predisposing factors and morbidity. *Ophthalmology* **2006**, *113*, 109–116.

93. Shah, A.; Sachdev, A.; Coggon, D.; Hossain, P. Geographic variations in microbial keratitis: An analysis of the peer-reviewed literature. *Br. J. Ophthalmol.* **2011**, *95*, 762–767.

94. Alexandrakis, G.; Alfonso, E.C.; Miller, D. Shifting trends in bacterial keratitis in South Florida and emerging resistance to fluoroquinolones. *Ophthalmology* **2000**, *107*, 1497–1502.

95. Cheng, K.H.; Leung, S.L.; Hoekman, H.W.; Beekhuis, W.H.; Mulder, P.G.; Geerards, A.J.; Kijlstra, A. Incidence of contact-lens-associated microbial keratitis and its related morbidity. *Lancet* **1999**, *354*, 181–185.

96. Passos, R.M.; Cariello, A.J.; Yu, M.C.; Hofling-Lima, A.L. Microbial keratitis in the elderly: A 32-year review. *Arq. Bras. Oftalmol.* **2010**, *73*, 315–319.

97. Lichtinger, A.; Yeung, S.N.; Kim, P.; Amiran, M.D.; Iovieno, A.; Elbaz, U.; Ku, J.Y.; Wolff, R.; Rootman, D.S.; Slomovic, A.R.; *et al.* Shifting trends in bacterial keratitis in toronto: An 11-year review. *Ophthalmology* **2012**, *119*, 1785–1790.

98. Bharathi, M.J.; Ramakrishnan, R.; Meenakshi, R.; Padmavathy, S.; Shivakumar, C.; Srinivasan, M. Microbial keratitis in south india: Influence of risk factors, climate, and geographical variation. *Ophthalmic Epidemiol.* **2007**, *14*, 61–69.

99. Ritterband, D.C.; Seedor, J.A.; Shah, M.K.; Koplin, R.S.; McCormick, S.A. Fungal keratitis at the New York eye and ear infirmary. *Cornea* **2006**, *25*, 264–267.

100. Oechsler, R.A.; Feilmeier, M.R.; Miller, D.; Shi, W.; Hofling-Lima, A.L.; Alfonso, E.C. *Fusarium* keratitis: Genotyping, *in vitro* susceptibility and clinical outcomes. *Cornea* **2013**, *32*, 667–673.

101. Keay, L.J.; Gower, E.W.; Iovieno, A.; Oechsler, R.A.; Alfonso, E.C.; Matoba, A.; Colby, K.; Tuli, S.S.; Hammersmith, K.; Cavanagh, D.; *et al.* Clinical and microbiological characteristics of fungal keratitis in the united states, 2001–2007: A multicenter study. *Ophthalmology* **2011**, *118*, 920–926.

102. Hammersmith, K.M. Diagnosis and management of *Acanthamoeba* keratitis. *Curr. Opin. Ophthalmol.* **2006**, *17*, 327–331.

103. Jeng, B.H.; Gritz, D.C.; Kumar, A.B.; Holsclaw, D.S.; Porco, T.C.; Smith, S.D.; Whitcher, J.P.; Margolis, T.P.; Wong, I.G. Epidemiology of ulcerative keratitis in Northern California. *Arch. Ophthalmol.* **2010**, *128*, 1022–1028.

104. Pepose, J.S.; Wilhelmus, K.R. Divergent approaches to the management of corneal ulcers. *Am. J. Ophthalmol.* **1992**, *114*, 630–632.

105. Dart, J.K.; Stapleton, F.; Minassian, D. Contact lenses and other risk factors in microbial keratitis. *Lancet* **1991**, *338*, 650–653.

106. Dart, J.K.; Radford, C.F.; Minassian, D.; Verma, S.; Stapleton, F. Risk factors for microbial keratitis with contemporary contact lenses: A case-control study. *Ophthalmology* **2008**, *115*, 1647–1654.e3.

107. Stapleton, F.; Keay, L.; Edwards, K.; Naduvilath, T.; Dart, J.K.; Brian, G.; Holden, B.A. The incidence of contact lens-related microbial keratitis in australia. *Ophthalmology* **2008**, *115*, 1655–1662.

108. Fleiszig, S.M.; Evans, D.J. Pathogenesis of contact lens-associated microbial keratitis. *Optom. Vis. Sci.* **2010**, *87*, 225–232.

109. Willcox, M.D.; Carnt, N.; Diec, J.; Naduvilath, T.; Evans, V.; Stapleton, F.; Iskandar, S.; Harmis, N.; de la Jara, P.L.; Holden, B.A.; *et al.* Contact lens case contamination during daily wear of silicone hydrogels. *Optom. Vis. Sci.* **2010**, *87*, 456–464.

110. Stapleton, F.; Edwards, K.; Keay, L.; Naduvilath, T.; Dart, J.K.; Brian, G.; Holden, B. Risk factors for moderate and severe microbial keratitis in daily wear contact lens users. *Ophthalmology* **2012**, *119*, 1516–1521.

111. McLaughlin-Borlace, L.; Stapleton, F.; Matheson, M.; Dart, J.K. Bacterial biofilm on contact lenses and lens storage cases in wearers with microbial keratitis. *J. Appl. Microbiol.* **1998**, *84*, 827–838.

112. Stover, C.K.; Pham, X.Q.; Erwin, A.L.; Mizoguchi, S.D.; Warrener, P.; Hickey, M.J.; Brinkman, F.S.; Hufnagle, W.O.; Kowalik, D.J.; Lagrou, M.; *et al.* Complete genome sequence of *Pseudomonas aeruginosa* PAO1, an opportunistic pathogen. *Nature* **2000**, *406*, 959–964.

113. Dutta, D.; Cole, N.; Willcox, M. Factors influencing bacterial adhesion to contact lenses. *Mol. Vis.* **2012**, *18*, 14–21.

114. Klotz, S.A.; Butrus, S.I.; Misra, R.P.; Osato, M.S. The contribution of bacterial surface hydrophobicity to the process of adherence of *Pseudomonas aeruginosa* to hydrophilic contact lenses. *Curr. Eye Res.* **1989**, *8*, 195–202.

115. Stapleton, F.; Dart, J. Pseudomonas keratitis associated with biofilm formation on a disposable soft contact lens. *Br. J. Ophthalmol.* **1995**, *79*, 864–865.

116. Imamura, Y.; Chandra, J.; Mukherjee, P.K.; Lattif, A.A.; Szczotka-Flynn, L.B.; Pearlman, E.; Lass, J.H.; O'Donnell, K.; Ghannoum, M.A. *Fusarium* and *Candida albicans* biofilms on soft contact lenses: Model development, influence of lens type, and susceptibility to lens care solutions. *Antimicrob. Agents Chemother.* **2008**, *52*, 171–182.

117. Khan, N.A. Pathogenesis of Acanthamoeba infections. *Microb. Pathog.* **2003**, *34*, 277–285.

118. Khan, N.A. *Acanthamoeba*: Biology and increasing importance in human health. *FEMS Microbiol. Rev.* **2006**, *30*, 564–595.

119. Niederkorn, J.Y.; Alizadeh, H.; Leher, H.; McCulley, J.P. The pathogenesis of Acanthamoeba keratitis. *Microbes Infect./Inst. Pasteur* **1999**, *1*, 437–443.

120. Kilvington, S.; Heaselgrave, W.; Lally, J.M.; Ambrus, K.; Powell, H. Encystment of *Acanthamoeba* during incubation in multipurpose contact lens disinfectant solutions and experimental formulations. *Eye Contact Lens* **2008**, *34*, 133–139.

121. Anger, C.; Lally, J.M. *Acanthamoeba*: A review of its potential to cause keratitis, current lens care solution disinfection standards and methodologies, and strategies to reduce patient risk. *Eye Contact Lens* **2008**, *34*, 247–253.

122. Scheie, H.G.; Grayson, M.C. Ocular manifestations of systemic diseases. *Disease-a-Month DM* **1971**, *17*, 1–51.

123. Meisler, D.M.; Langston, R.H.; Naab, T.J.; Aaby, A.A.; McMahon, J.T.; Tubbs, R.R. Infectious crystalline keratopathy. *Am. J. Ophthalmol.* **1984**, *97*, 337–343.

124. Reiss, G.R.; Campbell, R.J.; Bourne, W.M. Infectious crystalline keratopathy. *Surv. Ophthalmol.* **1986**, *31*, 69–72.

125. Osakabe, Y.; Yaguchi, C.; Miyai, T.; Miyata, K.; Mineo, S.; Nakamura, M.; Amano, S. Detection of *Streptococcus* species by polymerase chain reaction in infectious crystalline keratopathy. *Cornea* **2006**, *25*, 1227–1230.

126. Ainbinder, D.J.; Parmley, V.C.; Mader, T.H.; Nelson, M.L. Infectious crystalline keratopathy caused by *Candida guilliermondii. Am. J. Ophthalmol.* **1998**, *125*, 723–725.

127. Khater, T.T.; Jones, D.B.; Wilhelmus, K.R. Infectious crystalline keratopathy caused by gram-negative bacteria. *Am. J. Ophthalmol.* **1997**, *124*, 19–23.

128. Rhem, M.N.; Wilhelmus, K.R.; Font, R.L. Infectious crystalline keratopathy caused by *Candida parapsilosis. Cornea* **1996**, *15*, 543–545.

129. Elder, M.J.; Matheson, M.; Stapleton, F.; Dart, J.K. Biofilm formation in infectious crystalline keratopathy due to *Candida albicans. Cornea* **1996**, *15*, 301–304.

130. Fulcher, T.P.; Dart, J.K.; McLaughlin-Borlace, L.; Howes, R.; Matheson, M.; Cree, I. Demonstration of biofilm in infectious crystalline keratopathy using ruthenium red and electron microscopy. *Ophthalmology* **2001**, *108*, 1088–1092.

131. Georgiou, T.; Qureshi, S.H.; Chakrabarty, A.; Noble, B.A. Biofilm formation and coccal organisms in infectious crystalline keratopathy. *Eye* **2002**, *16*, 89–92.

132. Hunts, J.H.; Matoba, A.Y.; Osato, M.S.; Font, R.L. Infectious crystalline keratopathy. The role of bacterial exopolysaccharide. *Arch. Ophthalmol.* **1993**, *111*, 528–530.

133. Daneshvar, H.; MacInnis, B.; Hodge, W.G. Nd:Yag laser corneal disruption as adjuvant treatment for infectious crystalline keratopathy. *Am. J. Ophthalmol.* **2000**, *129*, 800–801.

134. Masselos, K.; Tsang, H.H.; Ooi, J.L.; Sharma, N.S.; Coroneo, M.T. Laser corneal biofilm disruption for infectious crystalline keratopathy. *Clin. Exp. Ophthalmol.* **2009**, *37*, 177–180.

135. Smiddy, W.E.; Miller, D.; Flynn, H.W., Jr. Scleral buckle removal following retinal reattachment surgery: Clinical and microbiologic aspects. *Ophthalmic Surg.* **1993**, *24*, 440–445.

136. Pathengay, A.; Karosekar, S.; Raju, B.; Sharma, S.; Das, T. Hyderabad Endophthalmitis Research Group. Microbiologic spectrum and susceptibility of isolates in scleral buckle infection in india. *Am. J. Ophthalmol.* **2004**, *138*, 663–664.

137. Holland, S.P.; Pulido, J.S.; Miller, D.; Ellis, B.; Alfonso, E.; Scott, M.; Costerton, J.W. Biofilm and scleral buckle-associated infections. A mechanism for persistence. *Ophthalmology* **1991**, *98*, 933–938.

138. Asaria, R.H.; Downie, J.A.; McLauglin-Borlace, L.; Morlet, N.; Munro, P.; Charteris, D.G. Biofilm on scleral explants with and without clinical infection. *Retina* **1999**, *19*, 447–450.

139. Bourkiza, R.; Lee, V. A review of the complications of lacrimal occlusion with punctal and canalicular plugs. *Orbit* **2012**, *31*, 86–93.

140. Yokoi, N.; Okada, K.; Sugita, J.; Kinoshita, S. Acute conjunctivitis associated with biofilm formation on a punctal plug. *Jpn. J. Ophthalmol.* **2000**, *44*, 559–560.

141. Joganathan, V.; Mehta, P.; Murray, A.; Durrani, O.M. Complications of intracanalicular plugs: A case series. *Orbit* **2010**, *29*, 271–273.

142. SmartPlug Study, G. Management of complications after insertion of the smartplug punctal plug: A study of 28 patients. *Ophthalmology* **2006**, *113*, 1859–1862.e2.

143. Sugita, J.; Yokoi, N.; Fullwood, N.J.; Quantock, A.J.; Takada, Y.; Nakamura, Y.; Kinoshita, S. The detection of bacteria and bacterial biofilms in punctal plug holes. *Cornea* **2001**, *20*, 362–365.

144. Balikoglu-Yilmaz, M.; Yilmaz, T.; Cetinel, S.; Taskin, U.; Banu Esen, A.; Taskapili, M.; Kose, T. Comparison of scanning electron microscopy findings regarding biofilm colonization with microbiological results in nasolacrimal stents for external, endoscopic and transcanalicular dacryocystorhinostomy. *Int. J. Ophthalmol.* **2014**, *7*, 534–540.

145. Ibanez, A.; Trinidad, A.; Garcia-Berrocal, J.R.; Gomez, D.; San Roman, J.; Ramirez-Camacho, R. Biofilm colonisation in nasolacrimal stents. *B-Ent* **2011**, *7*, 7–10.

146. Samimi, D.B.; Bielory, B.P.; Miller, D.; Johnson, T.E. Microbiologic trends and biofilm growth on explanted periorbital biomaterials: A 30-year review. *Ophthalmic Plast. Reconstr. Surg.* **2013**, *29*, 376–381.

147. Parsa, K.; Schaudinn, C.; Gorur, A.; Sedghizadeh, P.P.; Johnson, T.; Tse, D.T.; Costerton, J.W. Demonstration of bacterial biofilms in culture-negative silicone stent and jones tube. *Ophthalmic Plast. Reconstr. Surg.* **2010**, *26*, 426–430.

148. Tiller, J.C.; Liao, C.J.; Lewis, K.; Klibanov, A.M. Designing surfaces that kill bacteria on contact. *Proc. Natl. Acad. Sci. USA* **2001**, *98*, 5981–5985.

149. Rose, W.E.; Otto, D.P.; Aucamp, M.E.; Miller, Z.; de Villiers, M.M. Prevention of biofilm formation by methacrylate-based copolymer films loaded with rifampin, clarithromycin, doxycycline alone or in combination. *Pharm. Res.* **2014**, *32*, 61–73.

150. Garty, S.; Shirakawa, R.; Warsen, A.; Anderson, E.M.; Noble, M.L.; Bryers, J.D.; Ratner, B.D.; Shen, T.T. Sustained antibiotic release from an intraocular lens-hydrogel assembly for cataract surgery. *Investig. Ophthalmol. Vis. Sci.* **2011**, *52*, 6109–6116.

151. Kazemzadeh-Narbat, M.; Lai, B.F.; Ding, C.; Kizhakkedathu, J.N.; Hancock, R.E.; Wang, R. Multilayered coating on titanium for controlled release of antimicrobial peptides for the prevention of implant-associated infections. *Biomaterials* **2013**, *34*, 5969–5977.

152. Desrousseaux, C.; Sautou, V.; Descamps, S.; Traore, O. Modification of the surfaces of medical devices to prevent microbial adhesion and biofilm formation. *J. Hosp. Infect.* **2013**, *85*, 87–93.

153. May, R.M.; Hoffman, M.G.; Sogo, M.J.; Parker, A.E.; O'Toole, G.A.; Brennan, A.B.; Reddy, S.T. Micro-patterned surfaces reduce bacterial colonization and biofilm formation

in vitro: Potential for enhancing endotracheal tube designs. *Clin. Transl. Med.* **2014**, *3*, 8, doi:10.1186/2001-1326-3-8.

154. Salwiczek, M.; Qu, Y.; Gardiner, J.; Strugnell, R.A.; Lithgow, T.; McLean, K.M.; Thissen, H. Emerging rules for effective antimicrobial coatings. *Trends Biotechnol.* **2014**, *32*, 82–90.

155. Conlon, B.P.; Nakayasu, E.S.; Fleck, L.E.; LaFleur, M.D.; Isabella, V.M.; Coleman, K.; Leonard, S.N.; Smith, R.D.; Adkins, J.N.; Lewis, K.; *et al.* Activated ClpP kills persisters and eradicates a chronic biofilm infection. *Nature* **2013**, *503*, 365–370.

156. Lu, T.K.; Collins, J.J. Dispersing biofilms with engineered enzymatic bacteriophage. *Proc. Natl. Acad. Sci. USA* **2007**, *104*, 11197–11202.

157. Schmelcher, M.; Shen, Y.; Nelson, D.C.; Eugster, M.R.; Eichenseher, F.; Hanke, D.C.; Loessner, M.J.; Dong, S.; Pritchard, D.G.; Lee, J.C.; *et al.* Evolutionarily distinct bacteriophage endolysins featuring conserved peptidoglycan cleavage sites protect mice from mrsa infection. *J. Antimicrob. Chemother.* **2015**, in press.

9

Antibiofilm Effect of Octenidine Hydrochloride on *Staphylococcus aureus*, MRSA and VRSA

Mary Anne Roshni Amalaradjou * and Kumar Venkitanarayanan

Department of Animal Science, University of Connecticut, 3636 Horse Barn Hill Road Ext., Unit 4040, Storrs, CT 06269, USA; E-Mail: kumar.venkitanarayanan@uconn.edu

* Author to whom correspondence should be addressed; E-Mail: mary_anne.amalaradjou@uconn.edu;

Abstract: Millions of indwelling devices are implanted in patients every year, and staphylococci (*S. aureus*, MRSA and vancomycin-resistant *S. aureus* (VRSA)) are responsible for a majority of infections associated with these devices, thereby leading to treatment failures. Once established, staphylococcal biofilms become resistant to antimicrobial treatment and host response, thereby serving as the etiological agent for recurrent infections. This study investigated the efficacy of octenidine hydrochloride (OH) for inhibiting biofilm synthesis and inactivating fully-formed staphylococcal biofilm on different matrices in the presence and absence of serum protein. Polystyrene plates and stainless steel coupons inoculated with *S. aureus*, MRSA or VRSA were treated with OH (zero, 0.5, one, 2 mM) at 37 °C for the prevention of biofilm formation. Additionally, the antibiofilm effect of OH (zero, 2.5, five, 10 mM) on fully-formed staphylococcal biofilms on polystyrene plates, stainless steel coupons and urinary catheters was investigated. OH was effective in rapidly inactivating planktonic and biofilm cells of *S. aureus*, MRSA and VRSA on polystyrene plates, stainless steel coupons and urinary catheters in the presence and absence of serum proteins. The use of two and 10 mM OH completely inactivated *S. aureus* planktonic cells and biofilm (>6.0 log reduction) on all matrices tested immediately upon exposure. Further, confocal imaging revealed the presence of dead cells and loss in biofilm architecture in the OH-treated samples when compared to intact live biofilm in the control. Results suggest that OH could be applied as an effective antimicrobial to control biofilms of *S. aureus*, MRSA and VRSA on appropriate hospital surfaces and indwelling devices.

Keywords: biofilm; inactivation; *S. aureus*; MRSA; VRSA; octenidine hydrochloride

1. Introduction

The Nosocomial Infections Surveillance System recognizes *Staphylococcus aureus* as the most frequently isolated nosocomial pathogen from patients [1]. Additionally, a high percentage of these isolates were found to be methicillin resistant (89% of identified *S. aureus* isolates). Methicillin-resistant *S. aureus* (MRSA) is the most commonly identified antibiotic resistant pathogen [2]. It is responsible for causing complicated skin and skin-structure infections and serious hospital-acquired infections [3]. Vancomycin has long been used as the antimicrobial agent for the treatment of MRSA infections in patients. However, this has led to the emergence of vancomycin-resistant *S. aureus* [4] (VRSA). It is estimated that staphylococci normally colonize 20%–25% of healthy adults permanently and 75%–80% transiently [5]. Millions of indwelling devices are implanted in patients every year, and staphylococci are responsible for a majority of infections and treatment failures linked to these devices [6]. Indwelling devices become coated with host-derived extracellular matrix proteins that provide a rich surface for bacterial attachment [7]. This ability to bind proteins facilitates pathogen attachment to plastic surfaces and other matrices [8]. Once established, staphylococcal biofilms are resistant to antimicrobial treatment and host response, besides serving as the etiological agent for recurrent infections [9]. Biofilm-associated staphylococci can lead to several diseases, including osteomyelitis, chronic wound infection endocarditis, polymicrobial biofilm infections and indwelling medical device infections [10].

The most commonly followed approach in the management of such infections is the removal and replacement of the contaminated devices [10]. An alternative to this is the use of antimicrobials or other technologies to prevent and control bacterial biofilms on indwelling devices. A variety of antimicrobials, including plant essential oils, phages, EDTA, nitric oxide, quorum sensing inhibitors and biofilm dispersants, such as oxidizing biocides, have been evaluated for controlling staphylococcal biofilms [10,11]. Although these approaches have shown promise in the control of staphylococcal biofilms, it is essential that these compounds maintain their efficacy in the presence of host proteins.

Octenidine hydrochloride (OH) is a positively-charged bispyridinamine exhibiting antimicrobial activity against plaque-producing organisms, such as *Streptococcus mutans* and *S. sanguis* [12]. Recent studies have also demonstrated its antimicrobial effect against *E. coli* O157:H7, *Salmonella* Enteritidis, *Acinetobacter baumannii*, *Candida albicans* and *Fusobacterium nucleatum*, *S. aureus* and *Pseudomonas aeruginosa* [13–17]. Toxicity studies in a variety of species have shown that OH is not absorbed through the mucous membrane and gastrointestinal tract, with no reported carcinogenicity, genotoxicity or mutagenicity [18].

The objective of this study was to investigate the efficacy of OH for inhibiting biofilm formation by *S. aureus*, MRSA and VRSA and inactivating pre-formed *S. aureus*, MRSA and VRSA biofilms at 37 °C in the presence and absence of serum proteins on polystyrene matrix, stainless steel coupons and urinary catheters.

2. Results and Discussion

OH was found to be equally effective against *S. aureus*, MRSA and VRSA biofilms. No significant differences were observed between the different isolates ($p < 0.05$). Therefore, the results obtained with one representative isolate of *S. aureus* (ATCC 35556), VRSA (VRS 8) and MRSA (NRS 123) are provided here. OH was found not only to be effective at killing planktonic cells and preventing biofilm formation, but also at inactivated fully established staphylococcal biofilms.

2.1. Prevention of Biofilm Formation

The efficacy of OH in preventing biofilm formation on polystyrene and stainless steel coupons is depicted in Figures 1 and 2. OH was effective in rapidly inactivating planktonic staphylococci cells, thereby preventing the establishment of biofilms on polystyrene and stainless steel surfaces. With planktonic cells, 2 mM of OH completely inactivated staphylococcal populations immediately upon exposure, whereas 1 mM of OH reduced bacterial counts by greater than 3.0 log CFU/mL on contact (Figures 1 and 2). As expected, staphylococcal populations in negative control samples remained the same throughout the sampling period. A set of samples were also assayed after 24 h to investigate biofilm formation. It was observed that the negative control samples had a fully formed biofilm, while the treated samples did not have any surviving population at 24 h (data not shown). When the efficacy of OH was tested for its ability to prevent biofilm formation in the presence of serum protein, OH retained its antimicrobial efficacy and resulted in a similar antibiofilm effect, as observed in the absence of protein (data not shown).

Figure 1. Inhibition of *S. aureus* (ATCC 35556), vancomycin-resistant *S. aureus* (VRSA) (VRS 8) and MRSA (NRS 123) biofilm formation on polystyrene by octenidine hydrochloride (OH). Duplicate samples were used for each treatment, and the experiment was replicated three times. Data are represented as the mean ± SEM.

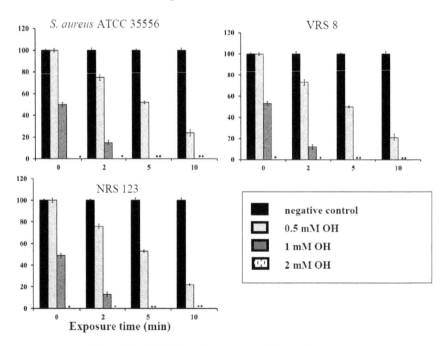

Note: Y-axis, Biofilm (Percentage of control)

Figure 2. Inhibition of *S. aureus* (ATCC 35556), VRSA (VRS 8) and MRSA (NRS 123) biofilm on stainless steel by octenidine hydrochloride. Duplicate samples were used for each treatment, and the experiment was replicated three times. Data are represented as the mean ± SEM (Standard Error of Mean).

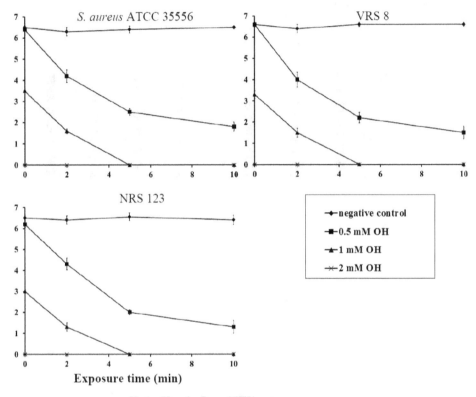

Note: Y-axis, Log CFU/coupon.

2.2. Inactivation of Established Biofilm

OH was also effective at killing fully formed biofilms of *S. aureus*, MRSA and VRSA on polystyrene and stainless steel ($p < 0.05$). Staphylococcus has been demonstrated to form biofilms on stainless steel implants, such as screws and fragment implants [19]. Therefore, the antibiofilm effect of OH was also investigated on a stainless steel matrix. At 10- and 5-mM levels, OH completely inactivated the biofilm immediately after addition (0 min) and 5 min of exposure, respectively (Figures 3 and 4). As observed with planktonic cells, the biofilm inactivation by OH was not affected by the presence of serum albumin (data not shown). A similar reduction in biofilm populations was observed by Junka and others [16], who tested the antimicrobial efficacy of octenisept, a commercially available antiseptic that contains octenidine dihydrochloride. They observed a complete inactivation of the *S. aureus* biofilm on polystyrene discs within 1 min of contact time. Another study by Sennhenn-Kirchner [20] evaluated the antimicrobial efficacy of OH on biofilm formed by aerobic oral bacteria on rough titanium surfaces. Their study revealed that rinsing with OH for 8 min reduced the biofilm by 99.8%. However, our study demonstrates that exposure of the biofilm to 10 mM OH completely inactivated it immediately after addition. Besides biofilm inactivation, it is also interesting to note that the antibiofilm effect of OH was irrespective of the strains employed. It was equally effective on the antibiotic-resistant strains (MRSA and VRSA), especially in light of their association with nosocomial and community-acquired infections.

Figure 3. Inactivation of *S. aureus* (ATCC 35556), VRSA (VRS 8) and MRSA (NRS 123) biofilm on polystyrene by octenidine hydrochloride. Duplicate samples were used for each treatment, and the experiment was replicated three times. Data are represented as the mean ± SEM (Standard Error of Mean).

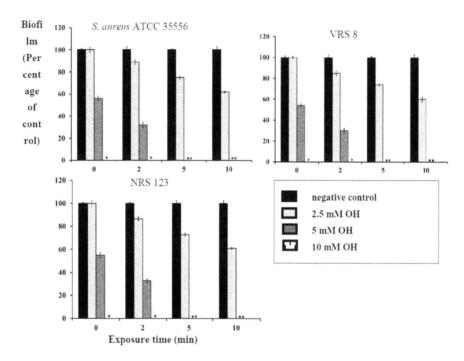

Figure 4. Inactivation of *S. aureus* (ATCC 35556), VRSA (VRS 8) and MRSA (NRS 123) biofilm on stainless steel by octenidine hydrochloride. Duplicate samples were used for each treatment, and the experiment was replicated three times. Data are represented as the mean ± SEM (Standard Error of Mean).

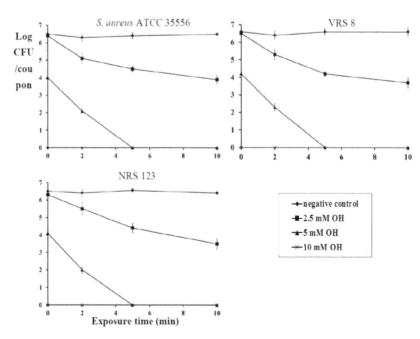

Staphylococci have been shown to infect and form biofilms on orthopedic implants, stents, intravenous catheters, infusion pumps, mechanical heart valves, pacemakers and cosmetic surgical implants [19]. Treatment of these foreign-body-associated infections caused by MRSA and VRSA are difficult because of the limited availability of antibiotic options that are effective against bacterial biofilms [21]. The current treatment protocol against MRSA involves the use of vancomycin (plus rifampin when the bacteria are susceptible) [22]. However, the increase in the MICs of vancomycin and rifampicin needed for the treatment against MRSA and VRSA is of significant concern [23]. Chaudhury and others [24] investigated the ability of ethanol for the eradication of MRSA biofilms. They observed that the use of ethanol at a 40% concentration could inactivate the biofilms in 1 h. Although efficacious, there are several concerns regarding ethanol use. These include concerns about systemic exposure to ethanol, an increase in catheter dysfunction [25] and the effect of prolonged exposure to ethanol on catheter integrity, which have limited the widespread use of ethanol locks. Besides ethanol, recent study by Rosenblatt and others [26] demonstrated that the use of lock solution containing 7% citrate, 20% ethanol and 0.01% glyceryl trinitrate was able to inactivate MRSA biofilm in 2 h of exposure. Although these approaches have shown promise in the control of MRSA biofilms, it is essential that these compounds maintain their efficacy in the presence of host proteins. A study by Zumbotel and others [17] evaluated the ability of OH to prevent or delay *S. aureus* biofilm formation in OH-coated tracheostomy tubes. This study demonstrated that OH-coated tubes reduced the biofilm associated *S. aureus* population by 2 log compared to the negative control. However, reprocessing of the OH-coated tubes did not result in any significant reduction in biofilm formation. Therefore, in this present study, we investigated the antibiofilm effect of OH as a lock solution using urinary catheters as a model for indwelling devices. Inoculation of catheters with *S. aureus*, MRSA or VRSA resulted in a mature biofilm by the fifth day of incubation at 37 °C. A fully-formed staphylococcal biofilm was recovered from negative control catheters even after 24 h of incubation, whereas no biofilm was detected on catheters within 15 min of exposure to 10 mM of OH (Figure 5). After 60 min of exposure, 5 mM of OH also completely eliminated staphylococcal biofilms (Figure 5). However, staphylococcal biofilm counts on negative control catheters remained at 6.0 log CFU/mL throughout the experiment (Figure 5). A similar antibiofilm effect of OH was also observed in the presence of serum albumin. The ability of OH to retain its antibiofilm efficacy in the presence of serum albumin is of significance, since the presence of host proteins on the indwelling devices enhances the ability of pathogens to attach and form biofilms [1]. The antibiofilm effect of OH was compared with that of tetrasodium EDTA at a concentration of 40 mg/mL [11]. No significant decrease in staphylococcus populations in the biofilm was observed, even after an exposure time of 60 min to the EDTA (data not shown).

OH exerts its antimicrobial effect by binding to the negatively charged bacterial cell envelope, thereby disrupting the vital functions of the cell membrane and killing the cell [27]. It has a high affinity towards cardiolipin, a prominent lipid in bacterial cell membranes, making it selectively lethal to bacterial cells without adversely affecting eukaryotic cells [21]. In addition, Al-Doori and coworkers [28] reported that repeated exposure of *S. aureus* to OH for up to three months did not induce resistance to the compound.

Figure 5. Inactivation of *S. aureus* (ATCC 35556), VRSA (VRS 8) and MRSA (NRS 123) biofilm on urinary catheters by octenidine hydrochloride. Duplicate samples were used for each treatment, and the experiment was replicated three times. Data are represented as the mean ± SEM (Standard Error of Mean).

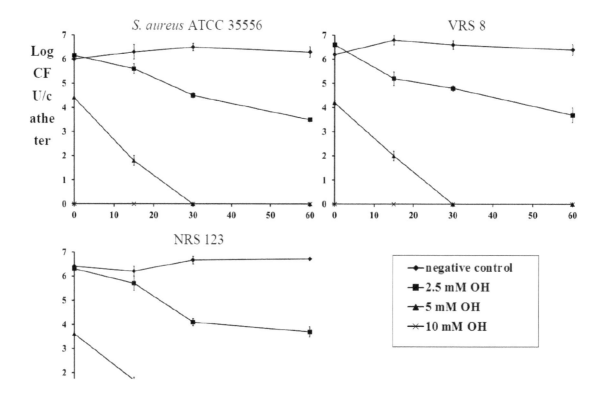

2.3. Confocal Microscopy

To investigate the effect of OH on biofilm structure, staphylococcus biofilms formed on glass coverslips were analyzed by confocal microscopy. Positive staining using SYTO® (Green fluorescent nucleic acid stain) and propidium iodide (PI) was used for the imaging. The confocal images of the negative control biofilm (Figure 6A) with no added OH revealed the formation of dense biofilm (average thickness 15 µm) viewed as green cells (live) stained by the SYTO dye, while the image of OH-treated samples (Figure 6B) revealed patchy breaks in biofilm due to the loss of cells and the disruption of organization, viewed as red cells (dead) stained by PI. The average thickness of OH-treated biofilms was 1 µm. These data collectively indicate that OH was effective at preventing biofilm formation by *S. aureus*, MRSA and VRSA, as well as rapidly inactivating pre-formed biofilms on polystyrene, stainless steel and urinary catheters.

Figure 6. Confocal microscopy of MRSA (NRS 385) biofilm without treatment (**A**) and after treatment with octenidine hydrochloride (**B**).

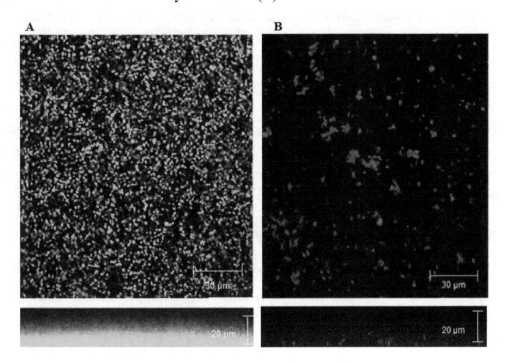

3. Experimental Section

3.1. Culture Preparation

All bacteriological media were purchased from Difco (Becton Dickinson, Sparks, MD, USA). The antibiofilm effect of OH was investigated on *S. aureus* (ATCC 35556, and ATCC 12600), methicillin-resistant *S. aureus* (MRSA; NRS 123, NRS 385, NRS 194) and vancomycin-resistant *S. aureus* (VRSA; VRS 8, VRS 9, VRS 10). MRSA and VRSA strains were obtained from the Network on Antibiotic Resistant *Staphylococcus aureus* (NARSA, Chantilly, VI, USA). Stock cultures were stored at −80 °C in brain heart infusion broth (BHI) with 50% glycerol. Prior to each experiment, a loopful of culture was grown in 10 mL of BHI with incubation at 37 °C for 24 h. The culture was sedimented by centrifugation ($3600\times$ g, 12 min, at 4 °C), washed and resuspended in phosphate buffered saline ($1\times$ PBS pH 7.2 consisting of 137 mM NaCl, 2.7 mM KCl, 10 mM Na_2HPO_4 and 2 mM KH_2PO_4) and used as the inoculum. The bacterial count of the inoculum was determined by plating on BHI agar plates and incubation at 37 °C for 24 h.

3.2. Octenidine Hydrochloride

OH (>99%) was obtained from Dishman USA, Middlesex, NJ, USA.

3.3. Prevention of Biofilm Formation by S. aureus, MRSA and VRSA on Polystyrene by OH

The efficacy of OH in inhibiting *S. aureus*, MRSA and VRSA biofilm production was investigated according to the method of Amalaradjou *et al.* [29]. Briefly, *S. aureus*, MRSA and VRSA strains were separately grown overnight in BHI at 37 °C. Following incubation, the cultures were sedimented by centrifugation (3,600× g for 15 min), washed twice with PBS and resuspended in 10 mL of BHI. Two hundred microliters of the washed culture were used as the inoculum (~6.0 log CFU). Sterile 96-well polystyrene tissue culture plates (Falcon, Franklin lakes, NJ) were inoculated with 200 μL of bacterial suspension, followed by the addition of 0 (negative control), 0.5 (0.25 μL), 1 (0.5 μL) or 2 (1 μL) mM OH (dissolved in 95% ethanol). The plates were incubated at 37 °C. Following 0, 2, 5 and 10 min of OH exposure, the surviving bacterial populations were enumerated by serial dilution (1:10 in PBS) and plating on duplicate BHI plates. When *S. aureus* was not detected by direct plating, samples were tested for surviving cells by enrichment at 37 °C for 24 h in 100 mL of BHI, followed by streak plating on mannitol salt agar (MSA). Representative colonies on BHI were confirmed as staphylococci based on colony morphology on MSA. Triplicate samples were included for each treatment, and the experiment was replicated three times.

3.4. Inactivation of S. aureus, MRSA and VRSA Biofilms Formed on Polystyrene by OH

The antibiofilm effect of OH was determined by microtiter plate assay [29]. Sterile 96-well polystyrene tissue culture plates (Costar, Corning Incorporated, Corning, NY, USA) were inoculated with 200 μL of the each bacterial cell suspension (~6.0 logCFU) and incubated at 37 °C for 24 h without agitation for biofilm production. Following biofilm formation, the effect of OH was tested at 0 (negative control), 2.5 (1.5 μL), 5 (2.5 μL) and 10 (5 μL) mM concentrations with an exposure time of 0, 2, 5 and 10 min. After exposure to OH for the specified time, the wells were washed three times with 200 μL of sterile PBS, dried at room temperature and finally stained with 1% crystal violet for 15 min. After rinsing three times with sterile distilled water and subsequent destaining with 95% ethanol, the absorbance of the adherent biofilm was measured at 570 nm in a microplate reader (Model 550, Bio-Rad, Hercules, CA, USA). Uninoculated wells containing BHI were used as blanks. Blank-corrected absorbance values were used for reporting biofilm production. Five replicate wells were included for each treatment, and the assay was repeated three times.

3.5. Enumeration of Bacterial Counts in Biofilm

In addition to the microtiter plate assay, the antibiofilm effect of OH was also assayed by enumerating surviving bacterial populations in the biofilm using the viable plate count method [29]. Following exposure to OH, the wells were washed three times with PBS, and the adherent biofilm was scraped and plated directly or after serial dilution in PBS on BHI plates. The plates were incubated at 37 °C for 24 h before enumerating the bacterial colonies.

3.6. Biofilm Assay on Stainless Steel Matrix

Stainless steel (type 304 with a 4b finish) was used for making coupons (diameter: 1 cm) [30]. Stainless steel coupons were washed and cleaned prior to use, as described by Amalaradjou *et al.* [27].

3.6.1. Biofilm Assay

S. aureus, MRSA and VRSA cells were grown and diluted 1:40, as described before. Two hundred microliters of the inoculum were then dispensed onto the stainless steel coupons submerged in a

24-well plate (Falcon, Becton Dickson Labware, Franklin Lakes, NJ, USA). Biofilm was formed at 37 °C, as before, and treated with 0 (negative control), 2.5, 5 and 10 mM of OH for an exposure time of 0, 2, 5 or 10 min. A procedure described by Ayebah and coworkers [30] was used to remove, disperse and enumerate the cells in biofilm. Duplicate coupons were included for each treatment, and the experiment was replicated three times.

3.7. Biofilm Assay on Catheters

The efficacy of OH for inactivating fully-formed *S. aureus*, MRSA and VRSA biofilms on catheters was determined according to a previously described protocol [29]. A latex 12 F Foley urinary tract catheter (AtHomeMedical) was cut into 3-cm pieces. Each catheter piece was sealed at one end, filled with 1 mL of bacterial culture (~6.0 log CFU) and sealed at the other end. The catheter pieces were then incubated at 37 °C for 5 days to facilitate biofilm formation onto the catheter lumen surface. After 5 days, each catheter piece was washed with sterile saline to remove unattached cells, sealed at one end, filled with 1 mL of sterile normal saline (negative control) or saline containing 2.5, 5 and 10 mM of OH, sealed at the other end and incubated at 37 °C. The biofilm-associated bacterial population was determined following OH exposure (0, 15, 30 and 60 min) by enumerating bacteria after dislodging the biofilm from the catheter surface. This was achieved by vortexing the catheter pieces in separate tubes containing 10 mL of PBS for 1 minute, followed by sonication at 40 KHz for 5 min in a bath sonicator (Branson, North Olmstead, OH, USA). After sonication, viable bacterial counts in PBS from each tube were enumerated after serial dilution (1:10 in PBS) and plating on duplicate BHI plates. Three catheter pieces were included, and the experiment was repeated three times.

3.8. Antibiofilm Effect of OH in the Presence of Serum Protein

The efficacy of OH for inhibiting and inactivating the biofilm of *S. aureus*, MRSA and VRSA in the presence of serum protein was determined according to the method of Edmiston and others [31]. Rehydrated bovine serum albumin (20%) was used to simulate the presence of proteins on indwelling devices. To determine the efficacy of OH in preventing *S. aureus*, MRSA and VRSA biofilm from planktonic cells in the presence of serum proteins, bovine serum albumin was added to each well/stainless steel coupon prior to microbial challenge followed by OH addition (0 (negative control), 0.5, 1 or 2 mM) for 0, 1, 2 and 5 min at 37 °C. Following exposure to OH, the surviving population of bacteria was enumerated by the viable plate count, as described previously. Three samples were included for each treatment, and the assay was replicated three times. For determining the efficacy of OH for killing established bacterial biofilms in the presence of proteins, biofilms were grown in the presence of bovine serum albumin on the different matrices tested and exposed to OH (0 (negative control), 2.5, 5 and 10 mM)| for 0, 2, 5 and 10 min on polystyrene and stainless steel and 0, 15, 30 and 60 min on catheters. The biofilms were assayed, as described before. This study was done at 37 °C. Five replicate wells were included for each treatment, and the assay was repeated three times.

3.9. Confocal Microscopy

To obtain depth-selective information on the three-dimensional structure of the biofilm, *in situ* confocal laser scanning microscopy was performed. For microscopic assessment, biofilms were grown at 37 °C in BHI on a Lab-Tech 8-chambered #1 borosilicate cover glass system (Lab-Tek, Nalge Nunc International, Rochester, NY, USA). The microscopy was performed according to the method reported by Amalaradjou *et al.* [29]. The biofilms formed on cover slips were treated with OH (10 mM), and the live and dead cells were imaged after staining with 2.5 μM SYTO (Molecular probes, OR) and 5 μM propidium iodide (PI, Molecular probes, OR). Biofilms not exposed to OH (negative control) were also imaged to view the normal architecture of *S. aureus*, MRSA and VRSA biofilm. Samples were examined under a Leica true confocal scanner SP2 microscope using the water immersion lens. A krypton-argon mixed gas laser with a PMT2 (Photomultiplier tube 2) filter served as the excitation source.

3.10. Statistical Analysis

Duplicate samples were used for each treatment, and each experiment was replicated three times. For each treatment and the control, the data from independent replicate trials were pooled and analyzed using the proc mixed sub-routine of the statistical analysis software. The model included the treatment concentrations and time as the major effects. A least significant difference test was used to determine significant differences ($p < 0.05$) due to treatment concentrations and time on bacterial counts.

4. Conclusions

In conclusion, our study demonstrates that OH was effective in preventing biofilm formation by *S. aureus*, MRSA and VRSA and rapidly inactivating pre-formed biofilms on polystyrene, stainless steel and urinary catheters. In addition, OH was equally effective against biofilms in the presence and absence of serum proteins. These results suggest that OH can be potentially used as a sanitizer for hospital surfaces. Since *S. aureus*, MRSA and VRSA have the ability to persist in the hospital environment and form biofilms on a wide variety of fomite surfaces, OH can be used as a potential antimicrobial lock solution in both treatment and prophylactic modalities. However, further experiments are needed to further evaluate the efficacy of OH in comparison with other anti-MRSA therapies *in vitro* and *in vivo*. Along with improvements in catheter design and coating, the universal adoption of strict aseptic techniques and the appropriate use of novel catheter lock solutions, such as OH, that minimize catheter-related infections may help to decrease the morbidity and mortality associated with foreign-body-associated infections.

Author Contributions

Kumar Venkitanarayanan and Mary Anne Roshni Amalaradjou conceived of the idea of, designed the experiments for and wrote the manuscript. Mary Anne Roshni Amalaradjou performed the experiments and analyzed the data.

References

1. Otto, M. Staphylococcal biofilms. *Curr. Top. Microbiol. Immunol.* **2008**, *322*, 207–228.

2. Ippolito, G.; Leone, S.; Lauria, F.N.; Nicastri, E.; Wenzel, R.P. Methicillin-resistant *Staphylococcus aureus*: The superbug. *Int. J. Infect. Dis.* **2010**, *14*, S7–S11.

3. Gould, I.M.; David, M.Z.; Esposito, S. New insights into meticillin-resistant *Staphylococcus aureus* (MRSA) pathogenesis, treatment and resistance. *Int. J. Antimicrob. Agents* **2012**, *39*, 96.

4. Gould, I.M. Treatment of bacteremia: Methicillin-resistant *Staphylococcus aureus* (MRSA) to vancomycin-resistant *S. aureus* (VRSA). *Int. J. Antimicrob. Agents* **2013**, *42*, S17–S21.

5. Archer, N.K.; Mazaitis, M.J.; Costerton, J.W. *Staphylococcus aureus* biofilms: Properties, regulation, and roles in human disease.*Virulence* **2011**, *2*, 445–459.

6. Baldoni, D.; Haschke, M.; Rajacic, Z. Linezolid alone or combined with rifampin against methicillin-resistant *Staphylococcus aureus* in experimental foreign-body infection. *Antimicrob. Agents Chemother.* **2009**, *53*, 1142–1148.

7. Herrmann, M.; Vaudaux, P.E.; Pittet, D.; Auckenthaler, R.; Lew, P.D.; Schumacher-Perdreau, F.; Peters, G.; Waldvogel, F.A. Fibronectin, fibrinogen, and laminin act as mediators of adherence of clinical staphylococcal isolates to foreign material. *J. Infect. Dis.* **1988**, *158*, 693–701.

8. Marraffini, L.A.; DeDent, A.C.; Schneewind, O. Sortases and the art of anchoring proteins to the envelopes of gram-positive bacteria. *Microbiol. Mol. Biol. Rev.* **2006**, *70*, 192–221.

9. Jones, S.M.; Morgan, M.; Humphrey, T.J. Effect of vancomycin and rifampicin on meticillin-resistant *Staphylococcus aureus* biofilms. *Lancet* **2001**, *357*, 40–41.

10. Kiedrowski, M.R.; Horswill, A.R. New approaches for treating staphylococcal biofilm infections. *Ann. N. Y. Acad. Sci.* **2011**, *1241*, 104–121.

11. Percival, S.L.; Kite, P.; Eastwood, K. Tetrasodium EDTA as a novel central venous catheter lock solution against biofilm. *Infect. Control Hosp. Epidemiol.* **2005**, doi: 10.1086/502577.

12. Bailey, D.M.; DeGrazia, C.G.; Hoff, S.J. Bispyridinamines: A new class of topical antimicrobial agents as inhibitors of dental plaque. *J. Med. Chem.* **1984**, *27*, 1457–1464.

13. Baskaran, S.A.; Upadhyay, A.; Upadhyaya, I.; Bhattaram, V.; Venkitanarayanan, K. Efficacy of octenidine hydrochloride for reducing *Escherichia coli* O157:H7, *Salmonella* spp., and *Listeria monocytogenes* on cattle hides. *Appl. Environ. Microbiol.* **2012**, *78*, 4538–4541.

14. Selçuk, C.T.; Durgun, M.; Ozalp, B. Comparison of the antibacterial effect of silver sulfadiazine 1%, mupirocin 2%, Acticoat and octenidine dihydrochloride in a full-thickness rat burn model contaminated with multi drug resistant *Acinetobacter Baumannii*. *Burns* **2012**, *38*, 1204–1209.

15. Rohrer, N.; Widmer, A.F.; Waltimo, T. Antimicrobial efficacy of 3 oral antiseptics containing octenidine, polyhexamethylene biguanide, or Citroxx: Can chlorhexidine be replaced? *Infect. Control Hosp. Epidemiol.* **2010**, doi:10.1086/653822.

16. Junka, A.; Bartoszewicz, M.; Smutnicka, D.; Secewicz, A.; Szymczyk, P. Efficacy of antiseptics containing povidone-iodine, octenidine dihydrochloride and ethacridine lactate against biofilm formed by *Pseudomonas aeruginosa* and *Staphylococcus aureus* measured with the novel biofilm-oriented antisepotics test. *Int. Wound J.* **2013**, doi:10.1111/iwj.12057.

17. Zumbotel, M.; Assadian, O.; Leonhar, M.; Stadler, M.; Schneider, B. The antimicrobial efficacy of Octenidine-dihydrochloride coated polymer tracheotomy tubes on *Staphylococcus aureus* and *Pseudomonas aeruginosa* colonization. *BMC Microbiol.* **2009**, *9*, 150.

18. Hirsch, T.; Jacobsen, F.; Rittig, A. A comparative *in vitro* study of cell toxity of clinically used antiseptics. *Hautarzt* **2009**, *60*, 984–991.

19. Costerton, J.W.; Montanaro, L.; Arciola, C.R. Biofilm in implant infections: Its production and regulation. *Int. J. Artif. Organs* **2005**, *28*, 1062–1068.

20. Sennhenn-Kirchner, S.; Nadine, W.; Klaue, S.; Mergeryan, H.; Zepelin, M. Decontamination efficacy of antiseptic agents on *in vivo* grown biofilms on rough titanium surfaces. *Quintessence Int.* **2009**, *10*, e80–e88.

21. Stewart, P.S.; Costerton, J.W. Antibiotic resistance of bacteria in biofilms. *Lancet* **2001**, *358*, 135–138.

22. Liu, C.; Bayer, A.; Cosgrove, S.E. Clinical practice guidelines by the infectious diseases society of america for the treatment of methicillin-resistant *Staphylococcus aureus* infections in adults and children: Executive summary. *Clin. Infect. Dis.* **2011**, *52*, e18–e55.

23. Garrigós, C.; Murillo, O.; Lora-Tamayo, J. RNAIII inhibiting peptide against foreign-body infection by methicillin-resistant *Staphylococcus aureus*. *J. Infect.* **2012**, *65*, 586.

24. Kayton, M.L.; Garmey, E.G.; Ishill, N.M.; Cheung, N.K.; Kushner, B.H.; Kramer, K.; Modak, S.; Rossetto, C.; Henelly, C.; Doyle, M.P.; *et al.* Preliminary results of a phase I trial of prophylactic ethanol-lock administration to prevent mediport catheter-related bloodstream infections. *J. Pediatr. Surg.* **2010**, *45*, 1961–1966.

25. Rosenblatt, J.; Reitzel, R.; Dvorak, T.; Jiang, Y.; Hachem, R.Y.; Raad II. Glyceryl trinitrate complements citrate and ethanol in a novel antimicrobial catheter lock solution to eradicate biofilm organisms. *Antimicrob. Agents Chemother.* **2013**, *57*, doi: 10.1128/AAC.00229-13.

26. Chaudhury, A.; Rangineni, J.B.V. Catheter lock technique: *In* vitro efficacy of ethanol for eradication of methicillin-resistant staphylococcal biofilm compared with other agents. *FEMS Immunol. Med. Microbiol.* **2012**, *65*, 305–308.

27. Brill, F.; Goroncy-Bermes, P.; Sand, W. Influence of growth media on the sensitivity of *Staphylococcus aureus* and *Pseudomonas aeruginosa* to cationic biocides. *Int. J. Hyg. Environ. Health.* **2006**, *209*, 89–95.

28. Al-Doori, Z.; Goroncy-Bermes, P.; Gemmell, C.G. Low-level exposure of MRSA to octenidine dihydrochloride does not select for resistance. *J. Antimicrob. Chemother.* **2007**, *59*, 1280–1282.

29. Amalaradjou, M.A.; Narayanan, A.; Baskaran, S.; Venkitanarayanan, K. Antibiofilm effect of trans-cinnamaldehyde on uropathogenic *Escherichia coli*. *J. Urol.* **2010**, *184*, 358–363.

30. Ayebah, B.; Hung, Y.C.; Frank, J.F. Enhancing the bactericidal effect of electrolyzed water on *Listeria. monocytogenes* biofilms formed on stainless steel. *J. Food Prot.* **2005**, *68*, 1375–1380.

31. Edmiston, C.E., Jr.; Goheen, M.P.; Seabrook, G.R. Impact of selective antimicrobial agents on staphylococcal adherence to biomedical devices. *Am. J. Surg.* **2006**, *192*, 344–354.

10

Pseudomonas aeruginosa Diversification during Infection Development in Cystic Fibrosis Lungs

Ana Margarida Sousa and Maria Olívia Pereira *

CEB—Centre of Biological Engineering, LIBRO—Laboratório de Investigação em Biofilmes Rosário
Oliveira, University of Minho, Campus de Gualtar, 4710-057 Braga, Portugal;
E-Mail: anamargaridasousa@deb.uminho.pt

* Author to whom correspondence should be addressed; E-Mail: mopereira@deb.uminho.pt;

Abstract: *Pseudomonas aeruginosa* is the most prevalent pathogen of cystic fibrosis (CF) lung disease. Its long persistence in CF airways is associated with sophisticated mechanisms of adaptation, including biofilm formation, resistance to antibiotics, hypermutability and customized pathogenicity in which virulence factors are expressed according the infection stage. CF adaptation is triggered by high selective pressure of inflamed CF lungs and by antibiotic treatments. Bacteria undergo genetic, phenotypic, and physiological variations that are fastened by the repeating interplay of mutation and selection. During CF infection development, *P. aeruginosa* gradually shifts from an acute virulent pathogen of early infection to a host-adapted pathogen of chronic infection. This paper reviews the most common changes undergone by *P. aeruginosa* at each stage of infection development in CF lungs. The comprehensive understanding of the adaptation process of *P. aeruginosa* may help to design more effective antimicrobial treatments and to identify new targets for future drugs to prevent the progression of infection to chronic stages.

Keywords: *Pseudomonas aeruginosa*; cystic fibrosis; clonal diversification; phenotypic variation; mucoid phenotype

1. Introduction

Cystic fibrosis (CF) is an autosomal recessive disease caused by a defect in the cystic fibrosis conductance regulator (CFTR) gene located in human on chromosome 7 that mainly affects lungs, digestive and reproductive systems, but also the secretory glands, such as the endocrine and sweat glands [1]. Although CF is a multi-system disorder causing several complications on the human body, its effects on lungs are the best studied so far due to the severe symptoms that patients suffer and high mortality rate associated to poor lung function.

It is generally accepted that CFTR acts as a channel that pumps chloride from the intracellular to extracellular space through the membrane of the epithelial cells that produce sputum. Several hypotheses have been formulated attempting to explain the relationship between CFTR deficiency and sputum accumulation. It has been considered that the transport of chloride partially controls water movement and consequently influences the production of thin and flowing sputum, fundamental to keeping the lungs protected [1,2]. The CFTR lacks causes, thus, a defective chloride secretion creating an osmotic gradient that, consequently, provokes water hyper-reabsorption and abnormal thick and sticky sputum [1,3]. This sputum with altered pH interfere with, reducing or even inhibiting the activity of epithelial antimicrobial molecules of innate immune system and ciliary functions, both crucial for homeostasis.

Other functions are also associated with CTFR, including inhibition of sodium absorption, of which loss causes excessive sodium (and water) absorption, regulation of HCO_3^- and some proteins transport through epithelial cell membranes [3,4]. The relevance of the latter mechanisms in CF airway is unclear, however, it is believed that reduced chloride secretion or sodium hyper-absorption can occur. Both mechanisms lead to airway-surface-liquid depletion and sputum viscosity increase, causing impaired cilia beats and accumulation of thick dehydrated airway sputum, which profoundly accounts for the typical symptoms suffered by CF patients [4,5]. The defective mucociliary transport and the compromised immune defenses predispose CF patients to the establishment of recurrent bronchopulmonary infections. Sputum retention leads to infection and consequently to inflammation, and this circle perpetuates itself since inflammatory products, such as elastase released by neutrophils, stimulate sputum secretion and breakdown [3,6]. The accumulated sputum is rich in nutrients being, thus, a good environment for microbial colonization [7,8]. CF lungs are infected with a complex microbial flora, mainly composed by bacteria, provoking acute and chronic infections that result in decline of the lung function, respiratory failure, and premature death of patients. Once bacterial infections are established, their eradication by antibiotic treatment is hardly ever achieved [9,10].

Some progress was made in this field extending the life expectancy of CF patients, however, it remains very reduced, around 37 years, mainly because of bacterial infections [11]. In the last decades, new therapies have emerged, based on the knowledge of CFTR dysfunction and airway CF microbiome, such as targeting CFTR replacement, stimulation of alternative chloride channels, inhibition of sodium absorption, and airway rehydration, in order to avoid sputum accumulation and, consequently, the establishment of bacterial infections [3–5,12]. None of these strategies has sufficient potential to stop CF infections development thus far. The actual and more effective approach to fight CF-associated infections relies on antimicrobial treatment. Currently, there is no consensual antimicrobial treatment to eradicate bacterial infection from CF lungs [13,14]. Treatments vary among clinics, countries, and even continents. Numerous strategies have been used varying in route of antibiotic administration (systemic, oral, inhaled antibiotics, or routes combination), classes of antibiotics, and treatment duration. Inhaled antibiotics, mainly aminoglycosides, have high success rates in bacteria eradication, in particular against *Pseudomonas aeruginosa*, due to the direct delivery of high-dose of antibiotic to the bronchial lumen space with limited systemic toxicity. For instance, a tobramycin inhalation solution has been used to treat long-term and chronic bacterial infection with significant benefits for lung function delaying re-infection and reduce mortality [15–17]. Oral and intravenous antibiotics have also attracted interest and currently quinolones, in particular ciprofloxacin, are the most used. However, ciprofloxacin usage is somewhat limited due to the rapid emergence of resistance. As a solution, ciprofloxacin is frequently combined with other antibiotics through other routes of administration. Combination of inhaled colistin or inhaled tobramycin with oral ciprofloxacin has been used successfully [13]. Some authors had suggested the still used broad-spectrum penicillins and cephalosporins in efforts to improve outcomes for CF patients infected with *P. aeruginosa* [18].

Other antibiotics have been introduced and used as alternative agents, such as inhaled amikacin, aztreonam lysine, and the combination of fosfomycin and tobramycin [12–14]. However, it has assisted to the failure of these antibiotic courses, making urgent the comprehension of the mechanisms underlying antibiotic resistance to rapidly define effective strategies to eradicate those infections.

2. *Pseudomonas aeruginosa*

The microbial community resident in CF lungs is known to be complex and it has considerably changed, mainly due to alterations in antibiotic regimens. Nevertheless, *P. aeruginosa* is still the most common pathogen isolated from CF sputum, being more prevalent in adults [2,10,19].

P. aeruginosa is a versatile microorganism, ubiquitously distributed in different environments, including terrestrial, aquatic, animal, human, and plant. It is a Gram-negative opportunist pathogen in hospitalized or immune-compromised patients, causing infections, such as pneumonia, burn, wound, urinary tract and gastrointestinal infections, otitis media, and keratitis [19,20]. Its versatility arises from its large genome, with nearly 6000 genes that enclose, for instance, genes associated with diverse metabolic pathways, virulence factors, transport, efflux, and chemotaxis, conferring to *P. aeruginosa* great adaptive ability. Moreover, this bacterium is able to coordinate metabolic pathways, optimize nutritional and reproductive potential according to the surrounding conditions and resources and, thus, it can survive, grow and cause infection in different environments [20,21].

The presence of *P. aeruginosa* in CF airways is highly associated with poor lung function, morbidity and mortality of patients. Despite the inflammatory response and the long-term and intensive antibiotic treatments, infections caused by *P. aeruginosa* persist in CF lungs. Once entering in CF airways, *P. aeruginosa* is virtually impossible to eradicate due to its remarkable genome plasticity that allows it to rapidly adapt to the greatly stressful CF environment [2,22,23]. After *P. aeruginosa* colonization, patients may suffer of successive episodes of re-colonization until resulting in a chronic infection that can persist from years to decades, or even never eradicated [23,24]. Several factors can influence the infection course in CF airways and, unfortunately, there is limited knowledge about the characteristics of this microorganism that have impact on the severity of infection. Until now, it is just known that during CF infection development, *P. aeruginosa* switch from an acute environment virulent pathogen, characteristic from early infection stages, to a CF-adapted pathogen, typical of chronic infection stages [6,21,25]. This review aimed to provide an overview of the successive adaptations that *P. aeruginosa* undergo, and to describe their impact on long-term persistence in the airways. The identification of the genetic background, interactions, and strategies, used by *P. aeruginosa* are crucial, and a prerequisite to develop new approaches for effectively eradicate lung infections.

3. Sources of Phenotypic Diversification

The long-term persistence of *P. aeruginosa* infections in CF lung is associated with clonal diversification, or expansion, into specialized phenotypes (Figure 1). Driven by the challenging selective pressures imposed by the typical CF conditions, e.g., interspecies competition, deficient oxygen availability, biofilm growth, the immune system action, oxidative stress, and antibiotic treatment, *P. aeruginosa* progressively generates phenotypes specially adapted to CF airways conditions [2,9,26,27]. The CF selection forces are evident when clinical isolates of *P. aeruginosa* are frequently mucoid and highly resistant to antibiotics. Indeed, mucoid variants are rarely isolated from non-CF environments, suggesting the existence of specific CF selective pressure [2,23]. For this reason, *P. aeruginosa* conversion from non- to mucoid form is considered the hallmark of CF airway.

Figure 1. Time course of *P. aeruginosa* infection development. (**a**) Sputum colonization stage - *P. aeruginosa* equipped with full virulence factors enter in CF sputum; (**b**) Early infection stage—*P. aeruginosa*, which exhibit the environmental or wild-phenotypes species characteristics, starts its adaptation to CF environmental conditions; (**c**) Chronic infection stage—*P. aeruginosa* is full adapted to CF environment. At this stage, there is high phenotypic and genotypic diversity and formation of biofilms.

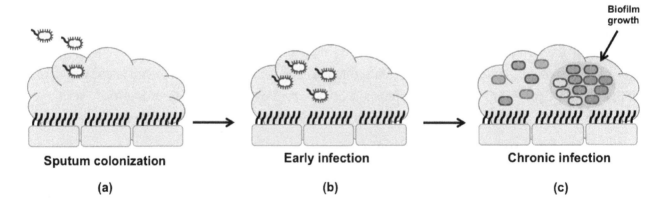

However, other phenotypic features of clonal variants adapted to CF airways have been frequently observed, including small colony variants (SCV), non-pigmented variants, increased antibiotic resistance, altered metabolic pathways, and attenuated virulence potential [3,22,27]. This phenotypic variation occurs for adaptation to the different niches in CF airways. The repeated occurrence of these particular phenotypic features and/or gene expression in chronic isolates, sampled from different patients and clinical settings, suggests the existence of a parallel evolution of *P. aeruginosa* in CF airways [28,29]. This topic is discussed in detail in Section 4.2.

The biofilm-lifestyle represents a reservoir of high phenotypic diversity and it is considered one of the most important adaptive mechanisms of *P. aeruginosa* within CF sputum (Figure 1c) [22,30,31]. Worlitzsch *et al.* (2002) [32] have shown that in the conductive zone, the region from the trachea to the terminal bronchiolus, *P. aeruginosa* grows mainly in biofilms, whereas very few bacteria are localized at the epithelial surface of the bronchi. Biofilms are microbial communities encased in self-produced matrix composed of exopolysaccharides, proteins and DNA [33–35]. Nowadays, biofilms are recognized as an important issue in human disease management due to their notoriously resistance, achieving 10- to 1000-fold higher tolerance to antimicrobial agents than corresponding planktonic bacteria [35,36]. Biofilm resistance has multifactorial nature resulting from the combination of several mechanisms, including restricted penetration of antimicrobials through the exopolysaccharide matrix, slow growth of bacteria within biofilms caused by nutrient and oxygen restriction, and accumulated metabolic wastes, and quorum-sensing (QS) molecules [37–40]. The limited penetration of antibiotics and immune defenses through the exopolysaccharide matrix is definitely a great contributor for their ineffective action and *P. aeruginosa* persistence. Alginate is the major component of CF biofilm matrix providing structure and protection to bacteria from the stressful environmental conditions of CF lungs. Augmented levels of alginate are generally observed in CF patients chronically infected and it is associated with poor prognosis because alginate triggers a vigorous antibody response [41,42].

Airway CF biofilms are genetic, proteomic and physiologic different of surface-attached biofilms formed, for instance, on indwelling devices (catheters, prostheses, pacemakers, stents), and medical and clinical equipment. Instead of the direct surface colonization, clearly observed in device-associated infections, bacteria in the CF lungs preferentially form multicellular clusters or macrocolonies within the sputum and not on the surface epithelium in the bronchi and non-respiratory bronchioles as initially supposed [31,32,43,44]. Additionally, the environment in which CF-associated biofilms are formed is considered to be microaerophilic or anaerobic. Bacteria enter and colonize CF sputum, consume oxygen via respiration, and generate steep oxygen gradients within the sputum [9,30,44]. The limited oxygen availability to potentially anaerobic environments in CF sputum was confirmed by direct *in situ* oxygen measurements using a microelectrode [32]. The oxygen-limited and anaerobic growth conditions significantly increase antibiotic resistance of biofilm-forming bacteria [45].

Until now, it is not clear what time bacteria after CF airway colonization switch to sessile lifestyle, but it is known that biofilm formation enables bacteria to successfully establish chronic infections. Presumably, *P. aeruginosa* form biofilms in response to stressful conditions including microaerophily and/or antibiotic treatments [23,46].

To switch from planktonic to biofilm mode of growth, bacteria undergo a number of complex physiological, metabolic, and phenotypic differentiations. For instance, biofilm-growing bacteria undertake specific changes in protein regulation, especially those related with proteins involved in resistance to oxidative damage, exopolysaccharide production, phospholipid synthesis, and membrane transport [47–49]. Global gene expression analyses of mature *P. aeruginosa* biofilms have revealed 1% of differential gene expression between the planktonic and biofilm mode of growth, with 0.5% of the genes being activated and about 0.5% being repressed [50]. Among the transcription factors, repression of flagellar and pili genes and stress response regulator genes, such as *rpoS*, hyperexpression of genes for ribosomal proteins and metabolism and transport functions were the most identified. Interestingly, in the same study, QS-regulated genes were not identified. QS is a cell-cell communication system used by bacteria to regulate gene expression in response to fluctuations in cell-population density and it has being reported to play a role in early and later stages of biofilm development. *P. aeruginosa* has two distinct QS systems, termed las and rhl [51,52]. The lack of las QS system allowed the formation of biofilms, however, does not allow them to achieve the mature stage. The *rhl* QS system has been reported as active in the early stages of biofilm development and its block may prevent biofilm formation [47,53]. Other regulatory systems can influence early stages of biofilm development, such as the global virulence regulator GacA [54], the catabolite repression control protein Crc [55], and the response regulator proteins AlgR [56]. The blockage by mutation of those factors has demonstrated a significant decreased of biofilm formation.

Gene expression may vary during biofilm development, which means that there is a stage-specific temporal and spatial gene expression patterns. This is particular relevant concerning the resistance of mature biofilms to antimicrobial treatment. The biofilm-specific phenotype can trigger mechanisms responsible for antimicrobial resistance and persistence and consequently enhanced pathogenicity. *P. aeruginosa* genome sequencing have revealed that a mature biofilm can express several cluster genes encoding efflux pump involved in resistance to some antibiotics [50].

The great variability or heterogeneity of phenotypes included and developed within biofilms is certainly one of the major contributors for sessile bacteria recalcitrance that it is not observed in planktonic state [57–59]. Within biofilms, various heterogeneous environments exist as a result of the distinct levels of nutrients and oxygen availability and accumulated metabolic wastes that bacteria have to face and adapt in a process similar to CF airway adaptation [60]. This range of microniches with specific biological activities may somewhat be translated by the several distinct colony morphologies that biofilm-growing bacteria adopt when grown in a solid media. Such trait diversification profits the whole population, with diverse abilities to face environmental challenges, as long as bacteria coordinate with each other. Bacterial cooperation and differentiation is facilitated through the production and perception of QS small signaling molecules called autoinducers. This interbacterial communication is mediated by two types of molecules, *N*-acylhomoserine lactones (AHL) and 4-quinolones, allowing bacteria to perceive their density and regulate their gene expressions properly. For instance, up-regulating genes encoding virulence factors such as those related to the production of enzymes or toxins, optimizes the metabolic and behavioral activities of bacteria within the community [61,62].

Biofilm heterogeneity is also reflected in distinct antibiotic susceptibility profiles. Due to the different biofilm-cell physiological states, biofilms have typically a top-to-bottom decreasing susceptibility profile. Antibiotics are effective against the cells located in the top of the biofilm, generally in active state, in contrast to the middle and bottom zones, in which cells have reduced or even an absence of metabolic activity. Even when antibiotics reach the middle and/or bottom biofilm zones, the majority of them have no activity against dormant cells and, thus, are unsuccessful in biofilm eradication [39,60,63].

Planktonic *P. aeruginosa* cells are also found in CF sputum [31]. Due to alterations in CF environment, such as pH and oxygen and nutrients availability, biofilm-cells dispersion may occur [64]. The dispersal of biofilm population provides to *P. aeruginosa* an opportunity to colonize new zones or niches and, thus, perpetuate infection. In fact, dispersal events can be responsible for the acute exacerbations observed in chronic infections [46,58,65].

The whole adaptation process to CF airways can be accelerated by the emergence of mutator phenotypes (or hypermutable phenotypes) which have high mutation rates up to 1000–fold than non-mutator phenotypes [66–68]. In extreme selective conditions, such as those occurring in CF airways, this sophisticated mechanism improves the microevolution of *P. aeruginosa* accelerating its intraclonal diversification. The emergence of phenotypic variants and mutators can be intrinsic, relying on mutations (or recombinations) caused by defects on one of the several DNA repair or error avoidance systems, combined, or not, with extrinsic or environmental factors, such as competition for different niches in a spatially heterogeneous environment as CF airways, and/or selection that favors any mutant as a better "fitter" to CF airways [67,69,70]. Mutators can also be stimulated by environmental factors, such as the presence of reactive oxygen species (ROS) generated from inflammatory responses [71]. ROS can trigger the generation of phenotypic variants damaging DNA and cause mutations in bacteria. Further, sub-inhibitory or sub-lethal concentrations of antibiotics can induce mutations and recombinations and, consequently, supporting the emergence of phenotypic variants and mutators [26,67,72]. The genes mainly affected are the antimutator genes *mutS*, *mutL*, and *uvrD* but it can be observed defects, as well in the genes *mutT*, *mutM*, and *mutY* [66,73,74].

The amount of mutators in biofilms is significantly higher than in planktonic state. This condition may explain why biofilm-associated bacteria exhibited enhanced antibiotic resistance, and frequently multidrug resistant, and high genetic diversity leading the emergence of diverse phenotypic variants [75,76].

The generation of various subclonal variants represents a huge biological advantage because it prepares the *P. aeruginosa* population for extreme and unpredictable stresses (insurance hypothesis) supporting the long-term survival of this pathogen [59,77]. Mutators achieve more quickly CF adaptation due to the expression of virulence traits, antibiotic resistance, metabolic functions, and increased ability to form biofilms, all these features representing a serious clinical problem [67,78,79]. In effect, mutators can increase the transcription of genes involved in the metabolism of fatty acids and amino acids crucial for obtaining energy in CF ecological niches where aerobic respiration is not possible [80]. On the other hand, mutators may have a reduced ability to survive in other distinct environments, indicating they can reach high levels of habitat- or niche-specialization spending their biological fitness [23,67]. During infection development non- and mutators coexist in CF airways, however, mutators prevail at chronic stage, which may be indicative that they have an adaptive advantage.

The combined action of all these sources of clonal diversification may achieve impressive levels of diversification, adaptation, and evolution, promoting the persistence of the bacterial populations in CF airways. Therefore, these sources should be intensively studied in order to understand the underlying mechanisms to further block them and combat the recalcitrant infections.

4. *P. aeruginosa* Evolution and Adaptation during Infection Development

The regular sampling of CF sputum has allowed performing a detailed characterization of *P. aeruginosa* over infection development through DNA sequencing and other approaches, such as transcriptomic, metabolomics and proteomic techniques. Therefore, it is now possible to start drawing an evolutionary trajectory of *P. aeruginosa* within CF airways.

During infection development genotypes and phenotypes differ markedly from those that initially colonized CF airways (Figure 2). Microbiological studies have reported changes in *P. aeruginosa* phenotypic and genetic traits, relevant in the context of bacterial pathogenesis, and different antibiotic resistance patterns along infection development, as well as after antibiotic treatments. Similar evolution and adaptation profiles were observed in distinct clonal linages of CF-adapted strains, suggesting that, in fact, there is a similar selective pressure in CF airways. This evolution and adaptation processes lead to the generation of several phenotypes varying in characteristics, such as colony morphology with distinct consistency, size, texture and color, the inactivation of QS, hypermutation, loss of the O-antigen components of the lipopolysaccharide (LPS), loss of motility, resistance to antibiotics, changes in nutritional requirements, and other virulence-associated traits [2,26,81,82]. In fact, some of those factors have been considered the hallmark of CF disease and can determine the infection stage, such as the conversion of *P. aeruginosa* to mucoid phenotype, loss of motility, and the emergence of SCV. However, many other characteristics have been described across all phenotypes isolated so far.

Figure 2. Representation of *P. aeruginosa* microevolution during infection in CF airways. At early stage of infection, *P. aeruginosa* is full equipped with cell-associated virulence factors, including flagella, pili, type 3 secretion systems (T3SS) and secreted virulence factors (e.g., proteases, pyoverdine, and rhamnolipid) and exhibit antibiotic sensitivity. At the chronic stage of infection, *P. aeruginosa* is fully adapted to CF environment and exhibits a variety of adaptations, including overproduction of alginate, loss of the implicated virulence factors for initial infection establishment, are resistant to antibiotics (expression of efflux pumps), and adapted metabolism. This microevolution occurs by the repeated interplay of mutation and selection.

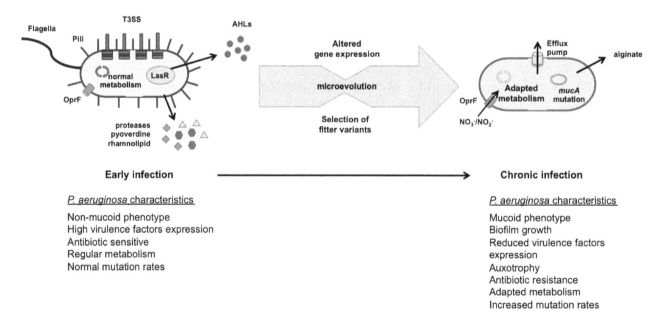

Antibiotics have provided significant control of bacterial infections in CF airways, however, the occurrence of antibiotic resistance and the lack of new drugs or therapeutic strategies make imperative the identification of alternative targets for treatment. For understanding the mechanisms underlying bacterial adaptation to CF environment and the resistance to antibiotic treatments, an overall picture of the actual knowledge about the *P. aeruginosa* populations, resident in CF lungs, is needed.

The compilation of the phenotypic traits exhibited by bacteria according the infection stage is a hard task due to the lack of agreement on the definitions of early, intermediate, and chronic colonization and infection stages. In this paper, the evolution, adaptation, and diversification profiles of *P. aeruginosa* were reviewed and compared agreed by the "European Consensus" that just considers two infection stages, early and chronic stages, according to the presence of *P. aeruginosa* being lower or higher than six months, respectively [83].

4.1. Early Infection

Most CF patients acquired pathogens mainly from environment, especially in clinical settings where CF patients remain for long periods of time. For this reason, respiratory infections associated to CF patients can be in somewhat considered nosocomial infections. As CF patients acquired environmental pathogens, early CF isolates exhibited identical microbial characteristics of their environmental or wild-phenotypes species (Figure 2) [21,84,85]. At the first colonization of CF airways, *P. aeruginosa* have to regulate properly its gene expression to quickly adapt to this new environment, including host immune defenses, antibiotics, and different substrate composition.

The bacterial characteristics among CF acute isolates significantly vary, however, there is a trend towards high virulence potential and cytotoxicity and lower frequency of mutators strains [86]. The expression of virulence factors, including cell-associated and secreted virulence factors, is considered to be fundamental at early stage for the success of infection establishment. For instance, (i) the increased production of pyoverdine, haemolysin, and phospholipase C; (ii) the augmented production of rhamnolipid, regulated by QS, helps biofilm formation that protects cells against oxidative stress, decreases liquid surface tension, due to its biosurfactant feature, and facilitates the access to nutrients within biofilms; (iii) the increased production of total protease that promotes mucoidy essential for long-term bacterial persistence; (iv) the swimming and twitching motilities; and (v) the expression of the type III secretion system that augments cell cytotoxicity potential and facilitates infection development [23,84,85,87,88].

Typically, *P. aeruginosa* exhibited a non-mucoid phenotype, sensibility to antibiotics and have low bacterial density in lungs in contrast to chronic infections [24,85]. Acute CF isolates produced AHL suggesting that QS circuit plays a role for *P. aeruginosa* pathogenesis at this stage of infection. Afterwards, QS seems be no longer needed and *lasR* mutants are frequently isolated. Mutator strains are not prevalent at this stage because they are not efficient to establish a primary infection [51,89].

At the early stage, eradication is still possible whether an antibiotic treatment was started as soon as possible. Otherwise, 20% of those first *P. aeruginosa* colonisations could become directly chronic infections and may persist up to the end of patient life [24,85]. Following *P. aeruginosa* eradication, it is common a new acquisition event with a different genotype or a re-colonization with the same genotype. Re-colonization with the same genotype may occur due to the persistence of the environmental source or due to the colonization of the upper airways, such as the paranasal sinuses [90,91]. Upper airways can function as reservoirs of pathogens, and interchange of *P. aeruginosa* can be possible. Colonization of the CF airways with mucoid strains is associated with an accelerated rate of decline in pulmonary function, however, there is some evidence that early acquisition of mucoid strains could be successfully achieved [24,92].

In summary, although the virulence potential of early CF isolates is higher than chronic isolates, they exhibited increased antibiotic sensitivity. Therefore, *P. aeruginosa* early detection and eradication are currently the main goal to avoid infection progression to chronic stage. Early infections are intensively treated with antimicrobial therapy resulting in *P. aeruginosa* eradication, at least temporal eradication in the majority of patients [24]. In cases of antimicrobial therapy failure, infection can shortly evolve to chronic infection. Identification of the CF patients who may evolve to chronic infections based on the acute bacterial characteristics is still not possible because of factors related to host-pathogen and pathogen-pathogen interactions may play a role and their impact is, thus far, unknown [86,93].

4.2. Chronic Infection

The continuous and selective pressure over the population leads to the emergence of diverse phenotypic and genetic variants specially adapted to CF airways. It has been observed, among chronic *P. aeruginosa* isolates, that there are alterations in colony morphology, namely the conversion to the mucoid morphotype, to SCV and non-pigmented variants, changes in surface antigens, lack of some virulence factors expression, increased antibiotic resistance, overproduction of exopolysaccharides, and modulation of microaerobic and anaerobic metabolic pathways (Figure 2). These alterations suggest a survival strategy to switch off or, at least, to reduce the expression of some traditional virulence factors. In fact, this *P. aeruginosa* strategy consists in saving or reducing energy costs with virulence factors expression in favor of alternative metabolic pathways crucial at this stage.

The repeated occurrence of these phenotypic features in chronic isolates of *P. aeruginosa* indicates that they may be a result of parallel evolution, which means that related microorganisms develop the same adaptive features in identical, but independent, environments [28]. Several transcriptomic studies have profiled isolates of *P. aeruginosa* in attempt to find the common route towards the chronic phenotype and the mechanisms underlying such a route. Longitudinal studies using transcriptomic approaches have provided relevant information regarding the genetic changes undergo by *P. aeruginosa* and allowed comparing the expression of specific set of genes among patients in different periods of time. Gene expression changes in multidrug efflux pumps and regulators of quorum sensing and alginate biosynthesis have been identified, being the two latter hotspots of mutations [21,28,94,95].

In the scope of genomic evolution in chronic CF lung infection, it should be highlighted that the notorious work performed by the Copenhagen and Hanover clinics, which had regularly collected *P. aeruginosa* from the CF lungs of all their patients in the 1970s and 1980s, and performed the genome sequencing of the isolates. They started their investigation with the most prevalent clones, the C and PA14, and observed that both clones convert their phenotype becoming deficient in the LPS O-antigen, with impaired motility and decreased siderophores secretion, as well as in other virulence factors expression and remaining non-mucoid [96]. Those isolates later collected just exhibited impaired competitive growth. These cases demonstrated that the evolutionary transition might be through the additive effects of various mutations. However, a single loss-of-function mutation can induce dramatic changes in *P. aeruginosa*, as those observed through the mucoid variant, due to the pleiotropic effects of *mucA* mutation [2,21].

Mucoid colony morphology results from alginate overproduction, absence of flagellin and pilin and expression of other virulence factors. Within the mucoid form, *P. aeruginosa* is more difficult to eradicate because it is highly resistance to antibiotics, as well as to the actions of host immune defenses, for instance, to phagocytosis, mediated by macrophages and neutrophils and to antibodies oponization [3,30,97]. Alginate overproduction is on the basis of such protection and resistance. Alginate promotes *P. aeruginosa* encapsulation and biofilm formation protecting sessile bacteria from the action of ROS, antibiotics and host immune defenses persisting in CF lungs [22,23]. Because mucoid *P. aeruginosa* raise a vigorous antibody response, its presence contributes to tissue damage, decreased lung function, and a decline in health [41,42]. The genetic mechanisms underlying *P. aeruginosa* transition to the mucoid form have been intensively studied and conversion is mainly caused by mutational inactivation of the *mucA* gene and rarely of *mucB* or *mucD* genes [98,99]. *mucA* gene encodes a cytoplasmatic membrane bound protein that acts as anti-σ-factor, σ^{22}, limiting the expression of the *algD* operon required for alginate synthesis. MucA binds to AlgT (also termed AlgU) that negatively controls the transcription of the *algD* gene. Inactivation of *mucA* results in upregulation of AlgT and production of alginate [2,100,101]. In fact, σ^{22} can also activate the transcription of several other genes related to virulence factor expression and to stress response, including heat shock, and osmotic and oxidative stress [21,102]. Additionally, it can repress the expression of type III secretion system (T3SS) genes through activation of AlgU that actives the regulatory genes *algP*, *algQ*, *algB*, and *algR*. AlgR, a global regulator, affects the expression of multiple genes including T3SS [103]. This suggests an impressive coordination of two high-cost energy systems in order to bacteria persist in CF airways.

Although mucoid phenotype is very successful at chronic infection stage, non- and mucoid phenotypes can coexist [31]. Non-mucoid isolates can occur from persistence of *P. aeruginosa* wild-type or re-conversion of mucoid phenotypes (revertants). Mucoid phenotypes can revert to non-mucoid form in the absence of *in vitro* selective pressure or through secondary mutations. Non-mucoid phenotypes can also carry *mucA* mutation, suggesting that mutation occurred when selective pressure occurs and when its vanished secondary mutation takes place [21,104]. This suggests that the production of alginate represents a high-energy cost and, thus, its unstable feature. At this stage, non-mucoid phenotypes have its alginate production at minimal levels [52].

The conversion to mucoid phenotype also promotes the biofilm mode of growth. The presence of biofilms is a key factor for the persistence of infection in CF airways. Biofilm-cell differentiation and dispersal events contribute to the generation of higher diversity that consequently increases the ability of *P. aeruginosa* to colonize new niches in CF airways, thus, perpetuating infection [46,58,59].

Another variant frequently isolated from chronic CF lung infections are the SCV. SCV designation comes from their small-colony size, typically 1–3 mm after 24–48 h of growth on agar media [105]. SCV are normally hyperpiliated, hyperadherent, excellent biofilm formers, and exhibit autoaggregative behavior and increased twitching motility [106–109]. In addition, SCV display augmented resistance to several classes of antibiotics, notably to aminoglycosides, contributing to their persistence in CF airways and poor lung function. SCV are generally selected after prolong antibiotic treatments [105,110]. In contrast with the mucoid phenotype, the mutations that arise in SCV appear to be very diverse and a challenge for the understanding of the underlying molecular mechanisms [111]. This phenotype may arise from the increased expression of the *pel* and *psl* polysaccharide gene loci and elevated intracellular c-di-GMP levels that enhance the ability to form biofilms, motility, and the expression of the type 3 secretion system, persisting, thus, more efficiently in the CF airways [109,111]. Until now,

SCV were mostly studied regarding *Staphylococcus aureus* but, currently, it has been equally assumed that *P. aeruginosa* SCV is, as well, a cause of infection persistence [35,112–114].

Other colony morphologies have been isolated from CF airways typically exhibiting rough texture due to alteration of the lipid A moiety of LPS. Those variants contain a few, short, or no O side chains and exhibited augmented proinflammatory activity [23].

In chronic infections, CF isolates typically exhibited impaired motility, namely swimming and twitching, due to the absence of flagella and pili, respectively. Lacking flagella (e.g., *fliC* mutant), *P. aeruginosa* isolates are hardly phagocytosed by alveolar macrophages and neutrophils helping to evade the host immune defenses, allowing its persistence in CF airways [23,52]. Moreover, *P. aeruginosa* lives in this chronic stage in biofilm-growth mode in which cells downregulate flagellum and type IV pili since they are no longer needed to move across sputum and along epithelial cell surfaces [115]. Nonpiliation may arise from mutations of *pilB*, encoding an ATPase needed for the extension and retraction of pili, or defects in *pilQ* gene, required to extrude the pilus through the bacterial outer membrane [116]. Nevertheless, the majority of CF isolates exhibited *rpoN* mutations that provoke the loss of both pili and flagella [117].

Chronic CF isolates show other attenuated virulence factors such as reduced production of AHL, proteases, phospholipase C, loss of pyoverdine, pyocyanin, and elastase and decreased cytotoxicity potential, due to the switching off of the T3SS. These alterations reduce the efficacy of the immune system to recognize *P. aeruginosa* helping, thus, its persistence in CF airways [23,52].

Chronic *P. aeruginosa* isolates are commonly *lasR* mutants. *lasR* gene encodes QS transcriptional regulator LasR and its downregulation may explain the reduced or absent production of AHL at this infection stage, the autolysis and the iridescent gloss of *P. aeruginosa* colonies, the growth advantage on amino acids and decreased virulence potential [94,118]. In addition, *lasR* mutants can use nitrate (NO_3^-) and nitrite (NO_2^-) as the terminal acceptor of electrons allowing *P. aeruginosa* growth in anaerobic niches. The loss of social and cooperative behavior may confer an adaptive advantage since the production of QS signal molecules, such as *N*-(3-oxo-dodecanoyl)-L-homoserine lactone (3-oxo-C12-HSL), *N*-butanoyl-L-homoserine lactone (C4-HSL), 2-heptyl-4(1H)-quinolone (C7-HHQ), and 2-heptyl-3-hydroxy-4(1H)-quinolone (PQS), are costly. Avoiding these costs, *P. aeruginosa* can ensure its persistence for the long-term [52,81]. QS seems just contribute to *P. aeruginosa* pathogenesis at colonization or acute stages [81,119].

To survive and adapt to CF airways, *P. aeruginosa* has, as well, to adapt its metabolic pathways. In fact, those alterations are also considered a marker of the chronic stage. The generation of energy is mainly based on oxidative substrate catabolism, however, *P. aeruginosa* is able to use alternative electron acceptors. The carbon metabolism of *P. aeruginosa* is mediated by catabolite repression control, which determines the catabolism of substrates in a preferred order. Short-chain fatty acids, amino acids, and polyamines are generally the preferred carbon sources and sugars the less favored [120].

CF sputum contains high amount of mucin, DNA, lipids, amino acids, and proteins that *P. aeruginosa* can uptake. Several studies have reported that peptides, amino acids, and fatty acids belonging to host defenses, such as prostaglandins and phosphatidylcholine, supports *P. aeruginosa* growth in CF airways [7,80]. The increased availability of those components is highlighted by the frequent isolation of auxotrophic variants for different amino acids, however the adaptive advantage of those variants in CF airways is unclear thus far [121]. Arginine and methionine are the most common auxotrophisms detected among CF isolates [122–124]. Auxotrophic variants may be more common than actually reported because those variants may be less cultivable *in vitro* and, consequently, under-estimated.

As mentioned earlier, the distinct oxygen availability in CF sputum represents a challenge for *P. aeruginosa*, which undergoes metabolic and physiologic changes with a high impact on antibiotic treatments. Along chronic infection progress, *P. aeruginosa* can face aerobic, microaerophilic, and anaerobic zones within the CF sputum and different enzymes, transporters, and regulators for different metabolic pathways are up-regulated to achieve this adaptation [86]. *P. aeruginosa* preferentially uses oxygen as terminal electron acceptor to obtain maximum energy. However, *P. aeruginosa* is able as well to survive and growth in hypoxic and anoxic CF niches adapting its metabolic pathways. Under anaerobic conditions, *P. aeruginosa* can obtain energy to grow from the denitrification or fermentation of arginine [30,80]. Denitrification or anaerobic respiration allows the detoxification of NO, generated during infection development. The outer membrane protein, OprF, represents a crucial factor in anaerobic metabolism since it allows the permeation of the ions NO_3^-/NO_2^- fundamental to perform denitrification [30,44,80]. In niches where oxygen and N-oxides are unavailable, but amino acids are in high amounts, *P. aeruginosa* can use fermentation of arginine, converting it into ornithine [80]. In cases of arginine limitation, *P. aeruginosa* can still convert pyruvate into acetate and, thus, obtain energy. In this way, anaerobic biofilms can be formed and support *P. aeruginosa* survival, growth, and persistence in CF airways. Anaerobic environments increase *P. aeruginosa* antibiotic tolerance and the robustness of biofilms through the increased production of alginate, typically via mutation in *algT/algU* [45,125–127]. Consequently, CF mucoid strains, that are alginate producers, are selected at this chronic stage. Despite all these findings about the metabolic pathways used by *P. aeruginosa* during chronic infections, information about the regulation and the mechanisms underlying each metabolic pathway and the specific effects on virulence, antibiotic resistance and persistence in CF lungs is still scarce. Certainly, the understanding of those mechanisms could help new therapeutic solutions to arise.

The presence of mutators within the populations are characteristic of chronic infections, considered a virulence determinant of *P. aeruginosa* and often associated with parallel occurrence of subpopulations with distinct phenotypic characteristics [66]. Mutators ensure *P. aeruginosa* survival against various CF stress conditions and other unpredictable stress factors, and being, moreover, a key factor in the development of multi-antimicrobial resistance [73]. At the chronic stage, hypermutability increases, also due to the presence of biofilms, in which the frequency of mutators is higher than the free-living mode of growth [75,128]. The transcriptome comparison of a non- and mutator revealed significantly transcriptional changes among them. In fact, it was observed that mutators exhibited increased levels of genes involved in amino acid and fatty acid metabolism [80].

Chronic infections are usually punctuated with acute exacerbations in which *P. aeruginosa* may regain the increased levels of acute virulence of early stages, suggesting that the expression of some virulence factors can be reversible [65].

Despite the intensive and long antibiotic treatment, chronic infections of *P. aeruginosa* are rarely eradicated due to the occurrence of antibiotic resistance. It is frequently observed β-lactam-resistant *P. aeruginosa* phenotypes, due to the derepression of chromosomal b-lactamase [129], as well as ciprofloxacin [130], colistin [131], and tobramycin-resistant phenotypes, and even multi-drug resistance [132]. The main reasons for such increased antibiotic resistance is the biofilm-growth style and the presence of mutators [73,133–136].

In summary, the exhibition of certain characteristics, including alginate overproduction (mucoid phenotype), slow growth, alternative metabolic pathways, antibiotic resistance, and loss of virulence factors expression, is currently considered a chronic phenotypic profile and the end-point result of *P. aeruginosa* evolution in CF airways. *P. aeruginosa* clearly adopts a strategy aiming to reduce its energy costs in favor of activation of other biological pathways that ensure its long-term persistence. The actual evolutionary "model" of *P. aeruginosa* within CF airways consists in an initial and rapid adaptation period dominated by positive selection and adaptive mutations, followed by a period with minor phenotypic changes dominated by negative selection and fewer adaptive mutations [2]. This evolutionary process ends with an advent of a lineage of highly adapted bacteria with impressive ability to persist in CF lungs for long-term. Despite the assumption of parallel evolution to CF-well adapted phenotypes and the limited number of adaptive features, it is important to highlight that the actual evolutionary route towards a common profile among different patients is still not well understood. In fact, genomic and transcriptomic studies have just begun tracking *P. aeruginosa* evolution.

5. Conclusions

The study of the adaptation process and dynamical evolution of *P. aeruginosa* within CF lungs, and its impact on bacterial pathogenicity and virulence, is currently a topic of most importance in disease management. In this paper, the most common evolutionary profile of *P. aeruginosa* reported by researchers and clinicians were reviewed, however, other evolutionary, phenotypic, and genotypic profiles can be found in different demographic locations, clinics, and patients.

Longitudinal studies of clonal variants of different CF patients have tried to identify a common "expression signature" of *P. aeruginosa* over time. Genome sequencing, transcriptomic, and proteomic analysis have advanced the understanding of *P. aeruginosa* evolution, epidemiology and response to CF stress conditions, however there is still limited information about such "expression signature". During adaptation, *P. aeruginosa* undergoes complex, structural and dynamic changes over the time. CF isolates from acute infections differs poorly from non-CF environment in contrast to the isolates from chronic infections that have been interpreted as the result of *P. aeruginosa* adaptation to CF airways. Depending on the early antibiotic treatment, infection, sooner or later, will evolve to chronic infection. The CF lung adaptation of *P. aeruginosa* is characterized by the transition from an acute environmental pathogen to a chronic CF-well-adapted pathogen, and the emergence of a phenotypically heterogeneous population. To establish chronic infections, *P. aeruginosa* loses some of its virulence potential (production of enzymes and toxins and lack of QS), slows down its growth rate, increases its antibiotic resistance (often multi-drug resistance), and/or reduces the stimulation of the immune system mainly due to a switch to the biofilm mode of growth, favored by overproduction of alginate. Typically, chronic *P. aeruginosa* isolates exhibited mucoid phenotype due to the overproduction of alginate and lack of flagella and pili. The presence of mutators in CF resident population is not strictly necessary to achieve adaptation, however, it represents a very large biological advantage in contrast with irreversible and accumulative mutations. Diversification of the metabolic pathways plays a fundamental role in the establishment of chronic infections in CF airways. In effect, *P. aeruginosa* can grow in microaerophilic and anaerobic zones by adjusting its metabolism. Denitrification, arginine fermentation and consumption of fatty acids are alternatives pathways to survive and growth in CF.

Future investigations should address the mechanisms underlying *P. aeruginosa* adaptation to CF airways to better understand them and to help design new therapeutic strategies. Studies about *P. aeruginosa* pathogenesis at early stages should be, especially, investigated more as the better way to avoid chronic infections is not allow their progression.

Acknowledgments

The authors thank the project FCT PTDC/SAUSAP/113196/2009/FCOMP-01-0124-FEDER-016012, the Strategic Project PEst-OE/EQB/LA0023/2013, the Project "BioHealth—Biotechnology and Bioengineering approaches to improve health quality", Ref. NORTE-07-0124-FEDER-000027, co-funded by the Programa Operacional Regional do Norte (ON.2—O Novo Norte), QREN, FEDER, the project "RECI/BBB-EBI/0179/2012—Consolidating Research Expertise and Resources on Cellular and Molecular Biotechnology at CEB/IBB", Ref. FCOMP-01-0124-FEDER-027462, FEDER. The authors also acknowledge PhD Grant of Ana Margarida Sousa SFRH/BD/72551/2010.

Author Contributions

Ana Margarida Sousa and Maria Olivia were all involved in the writing and editing of this manuscript.

References

1. Kreda, S.M.; Davis, C.W.; Rose, M.C. CFTR, mucins, and mucus obstruction in cystic fibrosis. *Cold Spring Harb. Perspect. Med.* **2012**, *2*, a009589.
2. Folkesson, A.; Jelsbak, L.; Yang, L.; Johansen, H.K.; Ciofu, O.; Hoiby, N.; Molin, S. Adaptation of *Pseudomonas aeruginosa* to the cystic fibrosis airway: An evolutionary perspective. *Nat. Rev. Microbiol.* **2012**, *10*, 841–851.
3. Ratjen, F.A. Cystic fibrosis: Pathogenesis and future treatment strategies. *Respir. Care* **2009**, *54*, 595–605.
4. Lubamba, B.; Dhooghe, B.; Noel, S.; Leal, T. Cystic fibrosis: Insight into CFTR pathophysiology and pharmacotherapy. *Clin. Biochem.* **2012**, *45*, 1132–1144.
5. Rubenstein, R.C. Targeted therapy for cystic fibrosis: Cystic fibrosis transmembrane conductance regulator mutation-specific pharmacologic strategies. *Mol. Diagn. Ther.* **2006**, *10*, 293–301.
6. Gomez, M.I.; Prince, A. Opportunistic infections in lung disease: *Pseudomonas* infections in cystic fibrosis. *Curr. Opin. Pharmacol.* **2007**, *7*, 244–251.
7. Palmer, K.L.; Mashburn, L.M.; Singh, P.K.; Whiteley, M. Cystic fibrosis sputum supports growth and cues key aspects of *Pseudomonas aeruginosa* physiology. *J. Bacteriol.* **2005**, *187*, 5267–5277.
8. Sriramulu, D.D.; Lunsdorf, H.; Lam, J.S.; Romling, U. Microcolony formation: A novel biofilm model of *Pseudomonas aeruginosa* for the cystic fibrosis lung. *J. Med. Microbiol.* **2005**, *54*, 667–676.

9. Schobert, M.; Jahn, D. Anaerobic physiology of *Pseudomonas aeruginosa* in the cystic fibrosis lung. *Int. J. Med. Microbiol. IJMM* **2010**, *300*, 549–556.

10. Bittar, F.; Richet, H.; Dubus, J.C.; Reynaud-Gaubert, M.; Stremler, N.; Sarles, J.; Raoult, D.; Rolain, J.M. Molecular detection of multiple emerging pathogens in sputa from cystic fibrosis patients. *PLoS One* **2008**, *3*, e2908.

11. Cystic Fibrosis Foundation. *Patient Registry 2011 Annual Report*; Cystic Fibrosis Foundation: Bethesda, MD, USA, 2011.

12. Narasimhan, M.; Cohen, R. New and investigational treatments in cystic fibrosis. *Ther. Adv. Respir. Dis.* **2011**, *5*, 275–282.

13. Jain, K.; Smyth, A.R. Current dilemmas in antimicrobial therapy in cystic fibrosis. *Exp. Rev. Respir. Med.* **2012**, *6*, 407–422.

14. Döring, G.; Flume, P.; Heijerman, H.; Elborn, J.S. Treatment of lung infection in patients with cystic fibrosis: Current and future strategies. *J. Cyst. Fibros.* **2012**, *11*, 461–479.

15. Ryan, G.; Singh, M.; Dwan, K. Inhaled antibiotics for long-term therapy in cystic fibrosis. *Cochrane Database Syst. Rev.* **2011**, *16*, CD001021.

16. Sawicki, G.S.; Signorovitch, J.E.; Zhang, J.; Latremouille-Viau, D.; von Wartburg, M.; Wu, E.Q.; Shi, L. Reduced mortality in cystic fibrosis patients treated with tobramycin inhalation solution. *Pediatr. Pulmonol.* **2012**, *47*, 44–52.

17. Ratjen, F.; Munck, A.; Kho, P.; Angyalosi, G. Treatment of early *Pseudomonas aeruginosa* infection in patients with cystic fibrosis: The ELITE trial. *Thorax* **2010**, *65*, 286–291.

18. Zobell, J.T.; Waters, C.D.; Young, D.C.; Stockmann, C.; Ampofo, K.; Sherwin, C.M.; Spigarelli, M.G. Optimization of anti-pseudomonal antibiotics for cystic fibrosis pulmonary exacerbations: II. cephalosporins and penicillins. *Pediatr. Pulmonol.* **2013**, *48*, 107–122.

19. Coutinho, H.D.; Falcao-Silva, V.S.; Goncalves, G.F. Pulmonary bacterial pathogens in cystic fibrosis patients and antibiotic therapy: A tool for the health workers. *Int. Arch. Med.* **2008**, *1*, 24.

20. Silby, M.W.; Winstanley, C.; Godfrey, S.A.; Levy, S.B.; Jackson, R.W. *Pseudomonas* genomes: Diverse and adaptable. *FEMS Microbiol. Rev.* **2011**, *35*, 652–680.

21. Rau, M.H.; Hansen, S.K.; Johansen, H.K.; Thomsen, L.E.; Workman, C.T.; Nielsen, K.F.; Jelsbak, L.; Hoiby, N.; Yang, L.; Molin, S. Early adaptive developments of *Pseudomonas aeruginosa* after the transition from life in the environment to persistent colonization in the airways of human cystic fibrosis hosts. *Environ. Microbiol.* **2010**, *12*, 1643–1658.

22. Hoiby, N.; Ciofu, O.; Bjarnsholt, T. *Pseudomonas aeruginosa* biofilms in cystic fibrosis. *Future Microbiol.* **2010**, *5*, 1663–1674.

23. Hogardt, M.; Heesemann, J. Adaptation of *Pseudomonas aeruginosa* during persistence in the cystic fibrosis lung. *Int. J. Med. Microbiol.* **2010**, *300*, 557–562.

24. Schelstraete, P.; Haerynck, F.; van Daele, S.; Deseyne, S.; de Baets, F. Eradication therapy for *Pseudomonas aeruginosa* colonization episodes in cystic fibrosis patients not chronically colonized by *P. aeruginosa*. *J. Cyst. Fibros.* **2013**, *12*, 1–8.

25. Bragonzi, A.; Paroni, M.; Nonis, A.; Cramer, N.; Montanari, S.; Rejman, J.; di Serio, C.; Doring, G.; Tummler, B. *Pseudomonas aeruginosa* microevolution during cystic fibrosis lung infection establishes clones with adapted virulence. *Am. J. Respir. Crit. Care Med.* **2009**, *180*, 138–145.

even continents. Numerous strategies have been used varying in route of antibiotic administration (systemic, oral, inhaled antibiotics, or routes combination), classes of antibiotics, and treatment duration. Inhaled antibiotics, mainly aminoglycosides, have high success rates in bacteria eradication, in particular against *Pseudomonas aeruginosa*, due to the direct delivery of high-dose of antibiotic to the bronchial lumen space with limited systemic toxicity. For instance, a tobramycin inhalation solution has been used to treat long-term and chronic bacterial infection with significant benefits for lung function delaying re-infection and reduce mortality [15–17]. Oral and intravenous antibiotics have also attracted interest and currently quinolones, in particular ciprofloxacin, are the most used. However, ciprofloxacin usage is somewhat limited due to the rapid emergence of resistance. As a solution, ciprofloxacin is frequently combined with other antibiotics through other routes of administration. Combination of inhaled colistin or inhaled tobramycin with oral ciprofloxacin has been used successfully [13]. Some authors had suggested the still used broad-spectrum penicillins and cephalosporins in efforts to improve outcomes for CF patients infected with *P. aeruginosa* [18].

Other antibiotics have been introduced and used as alternative agents, such as inhaled amikacin, aztreonam lysine, and the combination of fosfomycin and tobramycin [12–14]. However, it has assisted to the failure of these antibiotic courses, making urgent the comprehension of the mechanisms underlying antibiotic resistance to rapidly define effective strategies to eradicate those infections.

2. *Pseudomonas aeruginosa*

The microbial community resident in CF lungs is known to be complex and it has considerably changed, mainly due to alterations in antibiotic regimens. Nevertheless, *P. aeruginosa* is still the most common pathogen isolated from CF sputum, being more prevalent in adults [2,10,19].

P. aeruginosa is a versatile microorganism, ubiquitously distributed in different environments, including terrestrial, aquatic, animal, human, and plant. It is a Gram-negative opportunist pathogen in hospitalized or immune-compromised patients, causing infections, such as pneumonia, burn, wound, urinary tract and gastrointestinal infections, otitis media, and keratitis [19,20]. Its versatility arises from its large genome, with nearly 6000 genes that enclose, for instance, genes associated with diverse metabolic pathways, virulence factors, transport, efflux, and chemotaxis, conferring to *P. aeruginosa* great adaptive ability. Moreover, this bacterium is able to coordinate metabolic pathways, optimize nutritional and reproductive potential according to the surrounding conditions and resources and, thus, it can survive, grow and cause infection in different environments [20,21].

The presence of *P. aeruginosa* in CF airways is highly associated with poor lung function, morbidity and mortality of patients. Despite the inflammatory response and the long-term and intensive antibiotic treatments, infections caused by *P. aeruginosa* persist in CF lungs. Once entering in CF airways, *P. aeruginosa* is virtually impossible to eradicate due to its remarkable genome plasticity that allows it to rapidly adapt to the greatly stressful CF environment [2,22,23]. After *P. aeruginosa* colonization, patients may suffer of successive episodes of re-colonization until resulting in a chronic infection that can persist from years to decades, or even never eradicated [23,24]. Several factors can influence the infection course in CF airways and, unfortunately, there is limited knowledge about the characteristics of this microorganism that have impact on the severity of infection. Until now, it is just known that during CF infection development, *P. aeruginosa* switch from an acute environment

rgill, J.L.; Paterson, S.; Brockhurst, M.A.; Winstanley, C. Sub-inhibitory e antibiotics can drive diversification of *Pseudomonas aeruginosa* populations edium. *BMC Microbiol.* **2013**, *13*, 170.

rg, L.F.; Wang, H.; Hoiby, N. Phenotypes selected during chronic lung rosis patients: Implications for the treatment of *Pseudomonas aeruginosa* EMS Immunol. Med. Microbiol.* **2012**, *65*, 215–225.

T.; Zlosnik, J.E.; Speert, D.P.; Marcotte, E.M.; Whiteley, M. Parallel omonas aeruginosa* over 39,000 generations *in vivo. mBio* **2010**, 199-10.

ichel, J.B.; Aingaran, M.; Potter-Bynoe, G.; Roux, D.; Davis, M.R.J.; N.; LiPuma, J.J.; Goldberg, J.J.; *et.al*. Parallel bacterial evolution within tifies candidate pathogenicity genes. *Nat. Genet.* **2011**, *43*, 1275–1280.

M.D.; Schurr, M.J.; Herr, A.B.; Caldwell, C.C.; Matu, J.O. *Pseudomonas* anaerobic biofilm infections within cystic fibrosis airways. *Trends Microbiol.*

n, P.O.; Fiandaca, M.J.; Pedersen, J.; Hansen, C.R.; Andersen, C.B.; M.; Hoiby, N. *Pseudomonas aeruginosa* biofilms in the respiratory tract of . *Pediatr. Pulmonol.* **2009**, *44*, 547–558.

R.; Ulrich, M.; Schwab, U.; Cekici, A.; Meyer, K.C.; Birrer, P.; Bellon, G.; .; *et al*. Effects of reduced mucus oxygen concentration in airway ns of cystic fibrosis patients. *J. Clin. Investig.* **2002**, *109*, 317–325.

nan, V.; Palmer, J.N. Biofilms. *Otolaryngol. Clin. N. Am.* **2010**, *43*,

M.; Alhede, M.; Eickhardt-Sørensen, S.R.; Moser, C.; Kühl, M.; Jensen, vivo biofilm. *Trends Microbiol.* **2013**, *21*, 466–474.

lular signalling and growth of *Pseudomonas aeruginosa. Int. J. Med.* 544–548.

rangiskou, M.; Hultgren, S.J. Bacterial biofilms: Development, dispersal, ies in the dawn of the postantibiotic era. *Cold Spring Harb. Perspect. Med.*

ding biofilm resistance to antibacterial agents. *Nat. Rev. Drug Discov.*

T.; Givskov, M.; Molin, S.; Ciofu, O. Antibiotic resistance of bacterial crob. Agents* **2010**, *35*, 322–332.

ific antibiotic resistance. *Future Microbiol.* **2012**, *7*, 1061–1072.

nov, V.K. Biofilm—"City of microbes" or an analogue of multicellular gy* **2007**, *76*, 125–138.

ssen, T.B.; Jensen, P.O.; Stub, C.; Hentzer, M.; Molin, S.; Ciofu, O.; H.K.; Hoiby, N. Novel mouse model of chronic *Pseudomonas aeruginosa* g cystic fibrosis. *Infect. Immun.* **2005**, *73*, 2504–2514.

ffert, U.; Teran, L.M.; Schwichtenberg, L.; Bartels, J.; Maune, S.; *Pseudomonas aeruginosa*, TNF-alpha, and IL-1beta, but not IL-6, induce human beta-defensin-2 in respiratory epithelia. *Am. J. Respirat. Cell Mol. Biol.* **2000**, *22*, 714–721.

43. Goerke, C.; Wolz, C. Adaptation of *Staphylococcus aureus* to the cystic fibrosis lung. *Int. J. Med. Microbiol.* **2011**, *300*, 520–525.

44. Hassett, D.J.; Cuppoletti, J.; Trapnell, B.; Lymar, S.V.; Rowe, J.J.; Yoon, S.S.; Hilliard, G.M.; Parvatiyar, K.; Kamani, M.C.; Wozniak, D.J.; *et al.* Anaerobic metabolism and quorum sensing by *Pseudomonas aeruginosa* biofilms in chronically infected cystic fibrosis airways: Rethinking antibiotic treatment strategies and drug targets. *Adv. Drug Deliv. Rev.* **2002**, *54*, 1425–1443.

45. Yoon, S.S.; Hennigan, R.F.; Hilliard, G.M.; Ochsner, U.A.; Parvatiyar, K.; Kamani, M.C.; Allen, H.L.; DeKievit, T.R.; Gardner, P.R.; Schwab, U.; *et al. Pseudomonas aeruginosa* anaerobic respiration in biofilms: Relationships to cystic fibrosis pathogenesis. *Dev. Cell* **2002**, *3*, 593–603.

46. De la Fuente-Núñez, C.; Reffuveille, F.; Fernández, L.; Hancock, R.E.W. Bacterial biofilm development as a multicellular adaptation: Antibiotic resistance and new therapeutic strategies. *Curr. Opin. Microbiol.* **2013**, *16*, 580–589.

47. Sauer, K.; Camper, A.K.; Ehrlich, G.D.; Costerton, J.W.; Davies, D.G. *Pseudomonas aeruginosa* displays multiple phenotypes during development as a biofilm. *J. Bacteriol.* **2002**, *184*, 1140–1154.

48. Drenkard, E. Antimicrobial resistance of *Pseudomonas aeruginosa* biofilms. *Microbes. infect./Inst. Pasteur.* **2003**, *5*, 1213–1219.

49. Jouenne, T.; Vilain, S.; Cosette, P.; Junter, G.A. Proteomics of Biofilm Bacteria. *Curr. Proteomics* **2004**, *1*, 211–219.

50. Southey-Pillig, C.J.; Davies, D.G.; Sauer, K. Characterization of temporal protein production in *Pseudomonas aeruginosa* biofilms. *J. Bacteriol.* **2005**, *187*, 8114–8126.

51. Li, Y.H.; Tian, X. Quorum sensing and bacterial social interactions in biofilms. *Sensors* **2012**, *12*, 2519–2538.

52. Hassett, D.J.; Korfhagen, T.R.; Irvin, R.T.; Schurr, M.J.; Sauer, K.; Lau, G.W.; Sutton, M.D.; Yu, H.; Hoiby, N. *Pseudomonas aeruginosa* biofilm infections in cystic fibrosis: Insights into pathogenic processes and treatment strategies. *Exp. Opin. Ther. Targets* **2010**, *14*, 117–130.

53. Davies, D.G.; Parsek, M.R.; Pearson, J.P.; Iglewski, B.H.; Costerton, J.W.; Greenberg, E.P. The involvement of cell-to-cell signals in the development of a bacterial biofilm. *Science* **1998**, *280*, 295–298.

54. Parkins, M.D.; Ceri, H.; Storey, D.G. *Pseudomonas aeruginosa* GacA, a factor in multihost virulence, is also essential for biofilm formation. *Mol. Microbiol.* **2001**, *40*, 1215–1226.

55. O'Toole, G.A.; Gibbs, K.A.; Hager, P.W.; Phibbs, P.V.J.; Kolter, R. The global carbon metabolism regulator Crc is a component of a signal transduction pathway required for biofilm development by *Pseudomonas aeruginosa*. *J. Bacteriol.* **2000**, *182*, 425–431.

56. Whitchurch, C.B.; Erova, T.E.; Emery, J.A.; Sargent, J.L.; Harris, J.M.; Semmler, A.B.; Young, M.D.; Mattick, J.S.; Wozniak, D.J. Phosphorylation of the *Pseudomonas aeruginosa* response regulator AlgR is essential for type IV fimbria-mediated twitching motility. *J. Bacteriol.* **2002**, *184*, 4544–4554.

characteristic from early infection stages, to a CF-adapted pathogen, typical of
stages [6,21,25]. This review aimed to provide an overview of the successive
aeruginosa undergo, and to describe their impact on long-term persistence in the
cation of the genetic background, interactions, and strategies, used by *P. aeruginosa*
requisite to develop new approaches for effectively eradicate lung infections.

typic Diversification

persistence of *P. aeruginosa* infections in CF lung is associated with clonal
expansion, into specialized phenotypes (Figure 1). Driven by the challenging
imposed by the typical CF conditions, e.g., interspecies competition, deficient oxygen
growth, the immune system action, oxidative stress, and antibiotic treatment,
sively generates phenotypes specially adapted to CF airways conditions [2,9,26,27].
ces are evident when clinical isolates of *P. aeruginosa* are frequently mucoid and
tibiotics. Indeed, mucoid variants are rarely isolated from non-CF environments,
nce of specific CF selective pressure [2,23]. For this reason, *P. aeruginosa*
to mucoid form is considered the hallmark of CF airway.

course of *P. aeruginosa* infection development. (**a**) Sputum colonization
ginosa equipped with full virulence factors enter in CF sputum; (**b**) Early
—*P. aeruginosa*, which exhibit the environmental or wild-phenotypes
ristics, starts its adaptation to CF environmental conditions; (**c**) Chronic
—*P. aeruginosa* is full adapted to CF environment. At this stage, there is
and genotypic diversity and formation of biofilms.

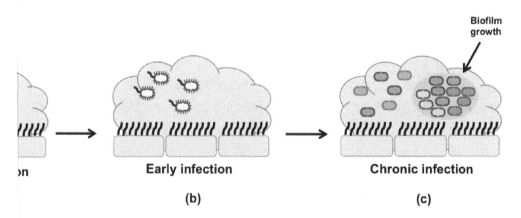

Early infection   **Chronic infection**

(**b**)   (**c**)

notypic features of clonal variants adapted to CF airways have been frequently
all colony variants (SCV), non-pigmented variants, increased antibiotic resistance,
ways, and attenuated virulence potential [3,22,27]. This phenotypic variation
the different niches in CF airways. The repeated occurrence of these particular
and/or gene expression in chronic isolates, sampled from different patients and
sts the existence of a parallel evolution of *P. aeruginosa* in CF airways [28,29].
in detail in Section 4.2.

57. Sousa, A.M.; Machado, I.; Nicolau, A.; Pereira, M.O. Improvements on colony morphology identification towards bacterial profiling. *J. Microbiol. Methods* **2013**, *95*, 327–335.

58. Kirov, S.M.; Webb, J.S.; O'May C, Y.; Reid, D.W.; Woo, J.K.; Rice, S.A.; Kjelleberg, S. Biofilm differentiation and dispersal in mucoid *Pseudomonas aeruginosa* isolates from patients with cystic fibrosis. *Microbiology* **2007**, *153*, 3264–3274.

59. Boles, B.R.; Thoendel, M.; Singh, P.K. Self-generated diversity produces "insurance effects" in biofilm communities. *Proc. Natl. Acad. Sci. USA* **2004**, *101*, 16630–16635.

60. Stewart, P.S.; Franklin, M.J. Physiological heterogeneity in biofilms. *Nat. Rev. Microbiol.* **2008**, *6*, 199–210.

61. Parsek, M.R.; Greenberg, E.P. Sociomicrobiology: The connections between quorum sensing and biofilms. *Trends Microbiol.* **2005**, *13*, 27–33.

62. Sharma, G.; Rao, S.; Bansal, A.; Dang, S.; Gupta, S.; Gabrani, R. *Pseudomonas aeruginosa* biofilm: Potential therapeutic targets. *Biologicals* **2014**, *42*, 1–7.

63. Fux, C.A.; Costerton, J.W.; Stewart, P.S.; Stoodley, P. Survival strategies of infectious biofilms. *Trends Microbiol.* **2005**, *13*, 34–40.

64. Sauer, K.; Cullen, M.C.; Rickard, A.H.; Zeef, L.A.; Davies, D.G.; Gilbert, P. Characterization of nutrient-induced dispersion in *Pseudomonas aeruginosa* PAO1 biofilm. *J. Bacteriol.* **2004**, *186*, 7312–7326.

65. Woo, J.K.K.; Webb, J.S.; Kirov, S.M.; Kjelleberg, S.; Rice, S.A. Biofilm dispersal cells of a cystic fibrosis *Pseudomonas aeruginosa* isolate exhibit variability in functional traits likely to contribute to persistent infection. *FEMS Immunol. Med. Microbiol.* **2012**, *66*, 251–264.

66. Oliver, A.; Canton, R.; Campo, P.; Baquero, F.; Blazquez, J. High frequency of hypermutable *Pseudomonas aeruginosa* in cystic fibrosis lung infection. *Science* **2000**, *288*, 1251–1253.

67. Rodriguez-Rojas, A.; Oliver, A.; Blazquez, J. Intrinsic and environmental mutagenesis drive diversification and persistence of *Pseudomonas aeruginosa* in chronic lung infections. *J. Infect. Dis.* **2012**, *205*, 121–127.

68. Mena, A.; Smith, E.E.; Burns, J.L.; Speert, D.P.; Moskowitz, S.M.; Perez, J.L.; Oliver, A. Genetic adaptation of *Pseudomonas aeruginosa* to the airways of cystic fibrosis patients is catalyzed by hypermutation. *J. Bacteriol.* **2008**, *190*, 7910–7917.

69. Spiers, A.J.; Buckling, A.; Rainey, P.B. The causes of *Pseudomonas* diversity. *Microbiology* **2000**, *146 Pt 10*, 2345–2350.

70. Jolivet-Gougeon, A.; Kovacs, B.; le Gall-David, S.; le Bars, H.; Bousarghin, L.; Bonnaure-Mallet, M.; Lobel, B.; Guille, F.; Soussy, C.J.; Tenke, P. Bacterial hypermutation: Clinical implications. *J. Med. Microbiol.* **2011**, *60*, 563–573.

71. Ciofu, O.; Riis, B.; Pressler, T.; Poulsen, H.E.; Hoiby, N. Occurrence of hypermutable *Pseudomonas aeruginosa* in cystic fibrosis patients is associated with the oxidative stress caused by chronic lung inflammation. *Antimicrob. Agents Chemother.* **2005**, *49*, 2276–2282.

72. Kohanski, M.A.; DePristo, M.A.; Collins, J.J. Sublethal antibiotic treatment leads to multidrug resistance via radical-induced mutagenesis. *Mol. Cell* **2010**, *37*, 311–320.

73. Macia, M.D.; Blanquer, D.; Togores, B.; Sauleda, J.; Perez, J.L.; Oliver, A. Hypermutation is a key factor in development of multiple-antimicrobial resistance in *Pseudomonas aeruginosa* strains causing chronic lung infections. *Antimicrob. Agents Chemother.* **2005**, *49*, 3382–3386.

74.   Ciofu, O.; Mandsberg, L.F.; Bjarnsholt, T.; Wassermann, T.; Hoiby, N. Genetic adaptation of *Pseudomonas aeruginosa* during chronic lung infection of patients with cystic fibrosis: Strong and weak mutators with heterogeneous genetic backgrounds emerge in mucA and/or lasR mutants. *Microbiology* **2010**, *156*, 1108–1119.

75.   Driffield, K.; Miller, K.; Bostock, J.M.; O'Neill, A.J.; Chopra, I. Increased mutability of *Pseudomonas aeruginosa* in biofilms. *J. Antimicrob. Chemother.* **2008**, *61*, 1053–1056.

76.   Lujan, A.M.; Macia, M.D.; Yang, L.; Molin, S.; Oliver, A.; Smania, A.M. Evolution and adaptation in *Pseudomonas aeruginosa* biofilms driven by mismatch repair system-deficient mutators. *PLoS One* **2011**, *6*, e27842.

77.   Yachi, S.; Loreau, M. Biodiversity and ecosystem productivity in a fluctuating environment: The insurance hypothesis. *Proc. Natl. Acad. Sci. USA* **1999**, *96*, 1463–1468.

78.   Hogardt, M.; Hoboth, C.; Schmoldt, S.; Henke, C.; Bader, L.; Heesemann, J. Stage-specific adaptation of hypermutable *Pseudomonas aeruginosa* isolates during chronic pulmonary infection in patients with cystic fibrosis. *J. Infect. Dis.* **2007**, *195*, 70–80.

79.   Oliver, A.; Mena, A. Bacterial hypermutation in cystic fibrosis, not only for antibiotic resistance. *Clin. Microbiol. Infect.* **2010**, *16*, 798–808.

80.   Hoboth, C.; Hoffmann, R.; Eichner, A.; Henke, C.; Schmoldt, S.; Imhof, A.; Heesemann, J.; Hogardt, M. Dynamics of adaptive microevolution of hypermutable *Pseudomonas aeruginosa* during chronic pulmonary infection in patients with cystic fibrosis. *J. Infect. Dis.* **2009**, *200*, 118–130.

81.   Jiricny, N.; Molin, S.; Foster, K.; Diggle, S.P.; Scanlan, P.D.; Ghoul, M.; Johansen, H.K.; Santorelli, L.A.; Popat, R.; West, S.A.; *et al.* Loss of social behaviours in populations of *Pseudomonas aeruginosa* infecting lungs of patients with cystic fibrosis. *PLoS One* **2014**, *9*, e83124.

82.   Workentine, M.L.; Sibley, C.D.; Glezerson, B.; Purighalla, S.; Norgaard-Gron, J.C.; Parkins, M.D.; Rabin, H.R.; Surette, M.G. Phenotypic heterogeneity of *Pseudomonas aeruginosa* populations in a cystic fibrosis patient. *PLoS One* **2013**, *8*, e60225.

83.   Doring, G.; Conway, S.P.; Heijerman, H.G.; Hodson, M.E.; Hoiby, N.; Smyth, A.; Touw, D.J. Antibiotic therapy against *Pseudomonas aeruginosa* in cystic fibrosis: A European consensus. *Eur. Respirat. J.* **2000**, *16*, 749–767.

84.   Manos, J.; Hu, H.; Rose, B.R.; Wainwright, C.E.; Zablotska, I.B.; Cheney, J.; Turnbull, L.; Whitchurch, C.B.; Grimwood, K.; *et al.* Virulence factor expression patterns in *Pseudomonas aeruginosa* strains from infants with cystic fibrosis. *Eur. J. Clin. Microbiol. Infect. Dis.* **2013**, *32*, 1583–1592.

85.   Burns, J.L.; Gibson, R.L.; McNamara, S.; Yim, D.; Emerson, J.; Rosenfeld, M.; Hiatt, P.; McCoy, K.; Castile, R.; Smith, A.L.; *et al.* Longitudinal assessment of *Pseudomonas aeruginosa* in young children with cystic fibrosis. *J. Infect. Dis.* **2001**, *183*, 444–452.

86.   Tramper-Stranders, G.A.; van der Ent, C.K.; Molin, S.; Yang, L.; Hansen, S.K.; Rau, M.H.; Ciofu, O.; Johansen, H.K.; Wolfs, T.F. Initial *Pseudomonas aeruginosa* infection in patients with cystic fibrosis: Characteristics of eradicated and persistent isolates. *Clin. Microbiol. Infect.* **2012**, *18*, 567–574.

87. Pacheco, G.J.; Reis, R.S.; Fernandes, A.C.; da Rocha, S.L.; Pereira, M.D.; Perales, J.; Freire, D.M. Rhamnolipid production: Effect of oxidative stress on virulence factors and proteome of *Pseudomonas aeruginosa* PA1. *Appl. Microbiol. Biotechnol.* **2012**, *95*, 1519–1529.

88. Abdel-Mawgoud, A.M.; Lepine, F.; Deziel, E. Rhamnolipids: Diversity of structures, microbial origins and roles. *Appl. Microbiol. Biotechnol.* **2010**, *86*, 1323–1336.

89. Montanari, S.; Oliver, A.; Salerno, P.; Mena, A.; Bertoni, G.; Tummler, B.; Cariani, L.; Conese, M.; Doring, G.; Bragonzi, A. Biological cost of hypermutation in *Pseudomonas aeruginosa* strains from patients with cystic fibrosis. *Microbiol. Sgm* **2007**, *153*, 1445–1454.

90. Hansen, S.K.; Rau, M.H.; Johansen, H.K.; Ciofu, O.; Jelsbak, L.; Yang, L.; Folkesson, A.; Jarmer, H.O.; Aanaes, K.; von Buchwald, C.; *et al.* Evolution and diversification of *Pseudomonas aeruginosa* in the paranasal sinuses of cystic fibrosis children have implications for chronic lung infection. *ISME J.* **2012**, *6*, 31–45.

91. Berkhout, M.C.; Rijntjes, E.; el Bouazzaoui, L.H.; Fokkens, W.J.; Brimicombe, R.W.; Heijerman, H.G.M. Importance of bacteriology in upper airways of patients with Cystic Fibrosis. *J. Cyst. Fibros.* **2013**, *12*, 525–529.

92. Troxler, R.B.; Hoover, W.C.; Britton, L.J.; Gerwin, A.M.; Rowe, S.M. Clearance of initial mucoid *Pseudomonas aeruginosa* in patients with cystic fibrosis. *Pediatr. Pulmonol.* **2012**, *47*, 1113–1122.

93. Williams, B.J.; Dehnbostel, J.; Blackwell, T.S. *Pseudomonas aeruginosa*: Host defence in lung diseases. *Respirology* **2010**, *15*, 1037–1056.

94. Smith, E.E.; Buckley, D.G.; Wu, Z.; Saenphimmachak, C.; Hoffman, L.R.; D'Argenio, D.A.; Miller, S.I.; Ramsey, B.W.; Speert, D.P.; Moskowitz, S.M.; *et al.* Genetic adaptation by *Pseudomonas aeruginosa* to the airways of cystic fibrosis patients. *Proc. Natl. Acad. Sci. USA* **2006**, *103*, 8487–8492.

95. Döring, G.; Parameswaran, I.G.; Murphy, T.F. Differential adaptation of microbial pathogens to airways of patients with cystic fibrosis and chronic obstructive pulmonary disease. *FEMS Microbiol. Rev.* **2011**, *35*, 124–146.

96. Cramer, N.; Klockgether, J.; Wrasman, K.; Schmidt, M.; Davenport, C.F.; Tummler, B. Microevolution of the major common *Pseudomonas aeruginosa* clones C and PA14 in cystic fibrosis lungs. *Environ. Microbiol.* **2011**, *13*, 1690–1704.

97. Qiu, D.; Eisinger, V.M.; Rowen, D.W.; Yu, H.D. Regulated proteolysis controls mucoid conversion in *Pseudomonas aeruginosa*. *Proc. Natl. Acad. Sci. USA* **2007**, *104*, 8107–8112.

98. Govan, J.R.; Deretic, V. Microbial pathogenesis in cystic fibrosis: Mucoid *Pseudomonas aeruginosa* and *Burkholderia cepacia*. *Microbiol. Rev.* **1996**, *60*, 539–574.

99. Deretic, V.; Schurr, M.J.; Yu, H. *Pseudomonas aeruginosa*, mucoidy and the chronic infection phenotype in cystic fibrosis. *Trends Microbiol.* **1995**, *3*, 351–356.

100. Ramsey, D.M.; Wozniak, D.J. Understanding the control of *Pseudomonas aeruginosa* alginate synthesis and the prospects for management of chronic infections in cystic fibrosis. *Mol. Microbiol.* **2005**, *56*, 309–322.

101. Martin, D.W.; Schurr, M.J.; Mudd, M.H.; Govan, J.R.; Holloway, B.W.; Deretic, V. Mechanism of conversion to mucoidy in *Pseudomonas aeruginosa* infecting cystic fibrosis patients. *Proc. Natl. Acad. Sci. USA* **1993**, *90*, 8377–8381.

102. Wood, L.F.; Ohman, D.E. Identification of genes in the σ^{22} regulon of *Pseudomonas aeruginosa* required for cell envelope homeostasis in either the planktonic or the sessile mode of growth. *mBio* **2012**, *3*, e00094-12.

103. Wu, W.; Badrane, H.; Arora, S.; Baker, H.V.; Jin, S. MucA-mediated coordination of type III secretion and alginate synthesis *in Pseudomonas aeruginosa*. *J. Bacteriol.* **2004**, *186*, 7575–7585.

104. Bragonzi, A.; Wiehlmann, L.; Klockgether, J.; Cramer, N.; Worlitzsch, D.; Doring, G.; Tummler, B. Sequence diversity of the mucABD locus in *Pseudomonas aeruginosa* isolates from patients with cystic fibrosis. *Microbiology* **2006**, *152*, 3261–3269.

105. Haussler, S.; Tummler, B.; Weissbrodt, H.; Rohde, M.; Steinmetz, I. Small-colony variants of *Pseudomonas aeruginosa* in cystic fibrosis. *Clin. Infect. Dis.* **1999**, *29*, 621–625.

106. Haussler, S.; Ziegler, I.; Lottel, A.; von Gotz, F.; Rohde, M.; Wehmhohner, D.; Saravanamuthu, S.; Tummler, B.; Steinmetz, I. Highly adherent small-colony variants of *Pseudomonas aeruginosa* in cystic fibrosis lung infection. *J. Med. Microbiol.* **2003**, *52*, 295–301.

107. Haussler, S. Biofilm formation by the small colony variant phenotype of *Pseudomonas aeruginosa*. *Environ. Microbiol.* **2004**, *6*, 546–551.

108. Deziel, E.; Comeau, Y.; Villemur, R. Initiation of biofilm formation by *Pseudomonas aeruginosa* 57RP correlates with emergence of hyperpiliated and highly adherent phenotypic variants deficient in swimming, swarming, and twitching motilities 1. *J. Bacteriol.* **2001**, *183*, 1195–1204.

109. Kirisits, M.J.; Prost, L.; Starkey, M.; Parsek, M.R. Characterization of colony morphology variants isolated from *Pseudomonas aeruginosa* biofilms. *Appl. Environ. Microbiol.* **2005**, *71*, 4809–4821.

110. Kahl, B.C. Small colony variants (SCVs) of *Staphylococcus aureus*—A bacterial survival strategy. *Infect. Genet. Evol.* **2014**, *21*, 515–522.

111. Starkey, M.; Hickman, J.H.; Ma, L.; Zhang, N.; de Long, S.; Hinz, A.; Palacios, S.; Manoil, C.; Kirisits, M.J.; Starner, T.D.; *et al. Pseudomonas aeruginosa* rugose small-colony variants have adaptations that likely promote persistence in the cystic fibrosis lung. *J. Bacteriol.* **2009**, *191*, 3492–3503.

112. Tuchscherr, L.; Medina, E.; Hussain, M.; Volker, W.; Heitmann, V.; Niemann, S.; Holzinger, D.; Roth, J.; Proctor, R.A.; Becker, K.; *et al. Staphylococcus aureus* phenotype switching: An effective bacterial strategy to escape host immune response and establish a chronic infection. *EMBO Mol. Med.* **2011**, *3*, 129–141.

113. Sendi, P.; Proctor, R.A. *Staphylococcus aureus* as an intracellular pathogen: The role of small colony variants. *Trends Microbiol.* **2009**, *17*, 54–58.

114. Proctor, R.A.; von Eiff, C.; Kahl, B.C.; Becker, K.; McNamara, P.; Herrmann, M.; Peters, G. Small colony variants: A pathogenic form of bacteria that facilitates persistent and recurrent infections. *Nat. Rev. Microbiol.* **2006**, *4*, 295–305.

115. Willcox, M.D.; Zhu, H.; Conibear, T.C.; Hume, E.B.; Givskov, M.; Kjelleberg, S.; Rice, S.A. Role of quorum sensing by *Pseudomonas aeruginosa* in microbial keratitis and cystic fibrosis. *Microbiology* **2008**, *154*, 2184–2194.

116. Chang, Y.S.; Klockgether, J.; Tummler, B. An intragenic deletion in pilQ leads to nonpiliation of a *Pseudomonas aeruginosa* strain isolated from cystic fibrosis lung. *FEMS Microbiol. Lett.* **2007**, *270*, 201–206.

117. Kresse, A.U.; Dinesh, S.D.; Larbig, K.; Romling, U. Impact of large chromosomal inversions on the adaptation and evolution of *Pseudomonas aeruginosa* chronically colonizing cystic fibrosis lungs. *Mol. Microbiol.* **2003**, *47*, 145–158.

118. D'Argenio, D.A.; Wu, M.; Hoffman, L.R.; Kulasekara, H.D.; Deziel, E.; Smith, E.E.; Nguyen, H.; Ernst, R.K.; Larson Freeman, T.J.; Spencer, D.H.; *et al.* Growth phenotypes of *Pseudomonas aeruginosa* lasR mutants adapted to the airways of cystic fibrosis patients. *Mol. Microbiol.* **2007**, *64*, 512–533.

119. Schaber, J.A.; Carty, N.L.; McDonald, N.A.; Graham, E.D.; Cheluvappa, R.; Griswold, J.A.; Hamood, A.N. Analysis of quorum sensing-deficient clinical isolates of *Pseudomonas aeruginosa*. *J. Med. Microbiol.* **2004**, *53*, 841–853.

120. Frimmersdorf, E.; Horatzek, S.; Pelnikevich, A.; Wiehlmann, L.; Schomburg, D. How *Pseudomonas aeruginosa* adapts to various environments: A metabolomic approach. *Environ. Microbiol.* **2010**, *12*, 1734–1747.

121. Thomas, S.R.; Ray, A.; Hodson, M.E.; Pitt, T.L. Increased sputum amino acid concentrations and auxotrophy of *Pseudomonas aeruginosa* in severe cystic fibrosis lung disease. *Thorax* **2000**, *55*, 795–797.

122. Barth, A.L.; Pitt, T.L. Auxotrophic variants of *Pseudomonas aeruginosa* are selected from prototrophic wild-type strains in respiratory infections in patients with cystic fibrosis. *J. Clin. Microbiol.* **1995**, *33*, 37–40.

123. Mowat, E.; Paterson, S.; Fothergill, J.L.; Wright, E.A.; Ledson, M.J.; Walshaw, M.J.; Brockhurst, M.A.; Winstanley, C. *Pseudomonas aeruginosa* population diversity and turnover in cystic fibrosis chronic infections. *Am. J. Respir. Crit. Care Med.* **2011**, *183*, 1674–1679.

124. Agarwal, G.; Kapil, A.; Kabra, S.K.; Das, B.K.; Dwivedi, S.N. Characterization of *Pseudomonas aeruginosa* isolated from chronically infected children with cystic fibrosis in India. *BMC Microbiol.* **2005**, *5*, 43.

125. Borriello, G.; Werner, E.; Roe, F.; Kim, A.M.; Ehrlich, G.D.; Stewart, P.S. Oxygen limitation contributes to antibiotic tolerance of *Pseudomonas aeruginosa* in biofilms. *Antimicrob. Agents Chemother.* **2004**, *48*, 2659–2664.

126. Field, T.R.; White, A.; Elborn, J.S.; Tunney, M.M. Effect of oxygen limitation on the *in vitro* antimicrobial susceptibility of clinical isolates of *Pseudomonas aeruginosa* grown planktonically and as biofilms. *Eur.J. Clin. Microbiol. Infect. Dis.* **2005**, *24*, 677–687.

127. Bragonzi, A.; Worlitzsch, D.; Pier, G.B.; Timpert, P.; Ulrich, M.; Hentzer, M.; Andersen, J.B.; Givskov, M.; Conese, M.; Doring, G. Nonmucoid *Pseudomonas aeruginosa* expresses alginate in the lungs of patients with cystic fibrosis and in a mouse model. *J. Infect. Dis.* **2005**, *192*, 410–419.

128. Boles, B.R.; Singh, P.K. Endogenous oxidative stress produces diversity and adaptability in biofilm communities. *Proc. Natl. Acad. Sci. USA* **2008**, *105*, 12503–12508.

129. Giwercman, B.; Meyer, C.; Lambert, P.A.; Reinert, C.; Hoiby, N. High-level beta-lactamase activity in sputum samples from cystic-fibrosis patients during antipseudomonal treatment. *Antimicrob. Agents Chemother.* **1992**, *36*, 71–76.

130. Jalal, S.; Ciofu, O.; Hoiby, N.; Gotoh, N.; Wretlind, B. Molecular mechanisms of fluoroquinolone resistance in *Pseudomonas aeruginosa* isolates from cystic fibrosis patients. *Antimicrob. Agents Chemother.* **2000**, *44*, 710–712.

131. Johansen, H.K.; Moskowitz, S.M.; Ciofu, O.; Pressler, T.; Høiby, N. Spread of colistin resistant non-mucoid *Pseudomonas aeruginosa* among chronically infected Danish cystic fibrosis patients. *J. Cyst. Fibros.* **2008**, *7*, 391–397.

132. Islam, S.; Oh, H.; Jalal, S.; Karpati, F.; Ciofu, O.; Hoiby, N.; Wretlind, B. Chromosomal mechanisms of aminoglycoside resistance in *Pseudomonas aeruginosa* isolates from cystic fibrosis patients. *Clin. Microbiol. Infect.* **2009**, *15*, 60–66.

133. Giwercman, B.; Jensen, E.T.; Hoiby, N.; Kharazmi, A.; Costerton, J.W. Induction of beta-lactamase production in *Pseudomonas aeruginosa* biofilm. *Antimicrob. Agents Chemother.* **1991**, *35*, 1008–1010.

134. Bagge, N.; Hentzer, M.; Andersen, J.B.; Ciofu, O.; Givskov, M.; Hoiby, N. Dynamics and spatial distribution of beta-lactamase expression in *Pseudomonas aeruginosa* biofilms. *Antimicrob. Agents Chemother.* **2004**, *48*, 1168–1174.

135. Hengzhuang, W.; Ciofu, O.; Yang, L.; Wu, H.; Song, Z.; Oliver, A.; Hoiby, N. High beta-lactamase levels change the pharmacodynamics of beta-lactam antibiotics in *Pseudomonas aeruginosa* biofilms. *Antimicrob. Agents Chemother.* **2013**, *57*, 196–204.

136. Plasencia, V.; Borrell, N.; Macia, M.D.; Moya, B.; Perez, J.L.; Oliver, A. Influence of high mutation rates on the mechanisms and dynamics of *in vitro* and *in vivo* resistance development to single or combined antipseudomonal agents. *Antimicrob. Agents Chemother.* **2007**, *51*, 2574–2581.

11

Role of Daptomycin in the Induction and Persistence for Biomaterial Applications of the Viable but Non-Culturable State of Staphylococcus Aureus Biofilms

Sonia Pasquaroli [1], Barbara Citterio [2], Andrea Di Cesare [1], Mehdi Amiri [1], Anita Manti [3], Claudia Vuotto [4] and Francesca Biavasco [1,*]

[1] Department of Life and Environmental Sciences, Polytechnic University of Marche, Ancona 60131, Italy; E-Mails: s.pasquaroli@univpm.it (S.P.); andrix.di.cesare@alice.it (A.D.C.); amiri.m1983@gmail.com (M.A.)

[2] Department of Biomolecular Sciences, Sect. Toxicological, Hygiene, and Environmental Sciences, University of Urbino Carlo Bo, Urbino 61029, Italy; E-Mail: barbara.citterio@uniurb.it

[3] Department of Earth, Life and Environmental Sciences, University of Urbino Carlo Bo, Urbino 61029, Italy; E-Mail: anita.manti@uniurb.it

[4] Microbial Biofilm Laboratory, IRCCS Fondazione Santa Lucia, Rome 00179, Italy; E-Mail: c.vuotto@hsantalucia.it

* Author to whom correspondence should be addressed; E-Mail: f.biavasco@univpm.it;

Abstract: We have recently demonstrated that antibiotic pressure can induce the viable but non-culturable (VBNC) state in *Staphylococcus aureus* biofilms. Since dormant bacterial cells can undermine anti-infective therapy, a greater understanding of the role of antibiotics of last resort, including daptomycin, is crucial. Methicillin-resistant *S. aureus* 10850 biofilms were maintained on non-nutrient (NN) agar in the presence or absence of the MIC of daptomycin until loss of culturability. Viable cells were monitored by epifluorescence microscopy and flow cytometry for 150 days. All biofilms reached non-culturability at 40 days and showed a similar amount of viable cells; however, in biofilms exposed to daptomycin, their number remained unchanged throughout the experiment, whereas in those maintained on NN agar alone, no viable cells were detected after 150 days. Gene expression assays showed that after achievement of non-culturability, 16S rDNA and *mecA* were expressed by all biofilms, whereas *glt* expression was found only in daptomycin-exposed biofilms. Our findings suggest that low daptomycin concentrations, such as those that are likely to obtain within biofilms, can influence the viability and gene expression of non-culturable *S. aureus* cells. Resuscitation experiments are needed to establish the VBNC state of daptomycin-exposed biofilms.

Keywords: *Staphylococcus aureus* biofilm; VBNC; daptomycin

1. Introduction

Biofilm production protects bacteria from a number of stress conditions [1,2], it promotes antibiotic resistance [2,3] and is often related to the onset of persistent infections [1,2], especially those associated with indwelling medical devices [3,4].

The continuous increase in antimicrobial resistance hampers the treatment of infections. The success of multidrug-resistant Gram-positive pathogens, such as methicillin-resistant *Staphylococcus aureus* (MRSA) [5–7], vancomycin-resistant enterococci (VRE) [8] and coagulase-negative staphylococci [9], emphasizes the need for new antimicrobials with alternative mechanisms of action. Daptomycin is a cyclic anionic lipopeptide antibiotic produced by *Streptomyces roseosporus* that, in the EU, has been approved to treat skin and soft-tissue infections since 2006 [10]. Daptomycin has bactericidal activity against Gram-positive bacteria, including MRSA [11,12] and VRE [13], and is currently the last line of defense against severe Gram-positive infections. It has a unique, but not completely elucidated, mechanism of action, where a calcium-dependent dissipation of membrane potential leads to the release of intracellular ions from the cell and, ultimately, to death [14]. Daptomycin is effective in treating skin infections, endocarditis and bacteremia [15] and in counteracting biofilm-based infections associated with medical devices [16,17], which frequently require combination therapy [18]. The combination with rifampicin or beta-lactams has been reported to be effective in treating biofilm-related enterococcal [18] and staphylococcal [12] infections.

The viable but non-culturable (VBNC) state is a survival strategy characterized by low-level metabolic activity and bacterial growth failure on standard media [19]. It protects bacterial cells from environmental stress, such as nutrient depletion, changes in temperature, pH or salinity [20], and presence of antibiotics [21]. The VBNC state has been reported for several human pathogens [19], including biofilm-producing staphylococci [21]. The critical feature of cells in the VBNC state is their ability to regain culturability in the presence of resuscitation-promoting factors [22]. In a recent *in vitro* study by our group, vancomycin and quinupristin-dalfopristin, which are often used to treat biofilm-associated chronic infections [23], have been demonstrated to promote the emergence of persistent VBNC forms in *S. aureus* biofilms [22]. These findings prompted us to establish whether daptomycin, which is considered as a last line of defense antibiotic, also induces the VBNC state.

2. Results and Discussion

2.1. Biofilm Production, Stress Exposure and Non-Culturability

The strong biofilm producer, *S. aureus* 10850 [21,24], was analyzed for susceptibility to daptomycin by MIC determination and showed low-level resistance with a MIC value of 2 µg/mL (European Committee on Antimicrobial Susceptibility Testing (EUCAST) susceptibility breakpoint ≤1 µg/mL).

To induce the VBNC state, *S. aureus* 10850 biofilms developed on membrane filters were placed on non-nutrient (NN) agar plates without or with daptomycin (at a concentration equal to the MIC) to induce the largest possible amount of VBNC cells [21] and incubated at 37 °C. Culturability was tested every two days.

All biofilms reached non culturability in 40 days. They were then detached from the filters, stained by the live/dead method, and examined for viable cells by epifluorescence microscopy. All filters were culture-negative and contained green coccoid cells whose average counts were 3.8×10^4/mL (starved biofilms) and 2.7×10^4/mL (starved + daptomycin-exposed biofilms).

2.2. Persistence of the VBNC State

After achievement of non-culturability on the 40th day, the persistence of the VBNC state was monitored by epifluorescence microscopy for 150 days in biofilms maintained on NN agar plates without or with daptomycin (Figure 1). Live/dead staining of a non-culturable daptomycin-exposed biofilm on the 15th day followed by flow cytometry demonstrated a viable subpopulation (Table 1), whose abundance was comparable to that documented by epifluorescence counts (differences ≤0.5 log).

The number of viable cells remained substantially unchanged throughout the experiment in starved and daptomycin-exposed biofilms; in those maintained on NN agar alone, it did not change significantly over the first 90 days, but no viable cells were left on the 150th day (Figure 1, Table 1).

These findings indicate that daptomycin exposure extended the viability of non-culturable cells compared with starvation alone, whereas nutrient depletion rather seemed to give rise to premortem VBNC forms, supporting previous data by our group [21].

Figure 1. Epifluorescence counts after live-dead staining of viable and total cells in detached non-culturable *S. aureus* 10850 biofilms exposed to nutrient depletion with (D) or without (NN) daptomycin. Counts were performed at various intervals (0–150 days) from the loss of culturability. The results are the means of two counts. VBNC, viable but non-culturable.

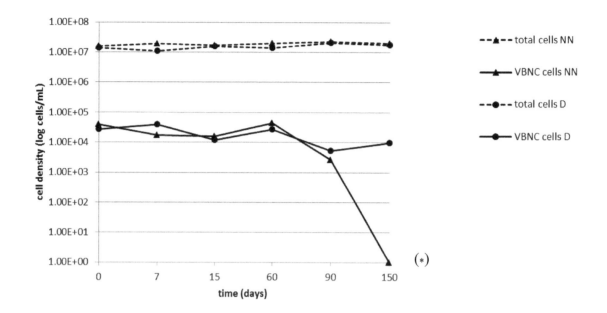

* No viable cells detected by epifluorescence microscopy (< 60 cells/mL).

Table 1. Total and viable cells counts in biofilms exposed to nutrient depletion or nutrient depletion with daptomycin.

Stress Condition	Days Since Achievement of Non-Culturability	Cells/mL	
		Total	**Viable**
Nutrient depletion	0	1.6×10^7	3.8×10^4
	7	1.9×10^7	1.7×10^4
	15	$1.7 \times 10^7/1.5 \times 10^8$ *	$1.6 \times 10^4/8.2 \times 10^4$ *
	60	2.0×10^7	4.4×10^4
	90	2.3×10^7	2.6×10^3
	150	2.0×10^7	<60
Nutrient depletion + daptomycin	0	1.4×10^7	2.7×10^4
	7	1.1×10^7	3.9×10^4
	15	$1.6 \times 10^7/1.4 \times 10^8$ *	$1.2 \times 10^4/7.6 \times 10^4$ *
	60	1.4×10^7	2.7×10^4
	90	2.1×10^7	5.3×10^3
	150	1.8×10^7	9.8×10^3

* Flow cytometric analysis.

2.3. Gene Expression of VBNC Cells

The presence of viable subpopulations after loss of culturability was tested by gene expression experiments. Non-culturable biofilms, either starved and starved and daptomycin-exposed, were tested for the expression of two *S. aureus* housekeeping genes, 16S rDNA and *glt* (coding for glutamate synthase). Aliquots of non-culturable biofilms detached 0, 7, 15 and 60 days from the loss of culturability were analyzed by real-time RT–PCR. The expression of 16S rRNA was detected in all biofilms tested, whereas *glt* was expressed exclusively in daptomycin-exposed biofilms at 0, 7 and 15 days (Table 2). Since 16S rRNA quantification is considered a reliable assay of viability [25], these findings support the epifluorescence and cytofluorimetric evidence of the presence of VBNC cells, in line with data from an earlier study by our group [21]. Given that glutamate synthase is involved in the incorporation of ammonium ions into organic compounds, which is a key step in amino acid production [26], it could have a role in the persistence of a true viable state in non-culturable biofilms via continued amino acid uptake and incorporation [27].

The ability of non-culturable biofilms to express virulence and antibiotic resistance genes was explored by further real-time RT-PCR assays targeting the thermonuclease (*nuc*) and the methicillin resistance penicillin binding protein 2a (PBP2a) (*mecA*) genes. *nuc* expression was detected in none of the biofilms analyzed and *mecA* expression in all of them (Table 2). These findings suggest that thermonuclease may not be essential for biofilm survival *in vitro*. Moreover, the paucity of metabolically active cells suggests that its expression could be inhibited by quorum sensing [28]. Conversely, the *mecA* gene encodes a PBP involved in cell wall formation [5] that could play an important role in maintaining the wall of VBNC cells intact and functional.

Table 2. Expression of key genes in non-culturable *S. aureus* 10850 biofilms exposed to nutrient depletion with or without daptomycin.

Stress Condition	Time from non Culturability	Gene Analysis			
		16SrDNA	*glt*	*nuc*	*mecA*
Nutrient depletion	T0	+	ND	ND	ND
	T7	+	-	-	+
	T15	+	-	-	+
	T60	+	-	-	+
Nutrient depletion + daptomycin	T0	+	ND	ND	ND
	T7	+	+	-	+
	T15	+	+	-	+
	T60	+	-	-	+

ND: not determined.

Taken together, the findings of our experiments seem to indicate that daptomycin acts as an inducer of the VBNC state of *S. aureus* by modulating gene expression, activating or repressing the transcription of specific genes. This effect may be explained by a poor penetration of daptomycin and the achievement of subinhibitory concentrations in the deep layers of the *S. aureus* biofilm matrix.

Indeed, low concentrations of a number of antibiotics exert biological activities other than inhibition, with major effects on transcription patterns [29]. The phenomenon, known as hormesis, involves biological responses to environmental signals or stress conditions that are characterized by biphasic dose-response relationships exhibiting low-dose stimulation and high-dose inhibition [30]. Subinhibitory concentrations of antimicrobial peptides, such as the cyclic lipopeptide daptomycin, which causes rapid membrane depolarization and potassium ion efflux, can thus increase the transcription levels of osmoprotectants, countering the osmotic stress, and downregulate the ribose transport system [30]. Given that ribose is a key element for ATP and RNA synthesis, this condition could be a stress factor for bacterial cells, contributing to VBNC state induction and persistence.

Since increased cell wall thickness is typical of the VBNC state [19], it may be hypothesized that low daptomycin concentrations stimulate the synthesis of peptidoglycan genes, as reported for imipenem in studies of the *Pseudomonas aeruginosa* transcriptome [30]. On the other hand, an involvement of daptomycin in the regulation of cell wall synthesis is quite likely, given that PBPs are membrane proteins. A role for daptomycin may also be inferred based on its reported synergism with beta-lactams against staphylococcal biofilms [12].

3. Experimental Section

3.1. Bacterial Strains, Media, Antibiotics and Enzymes

The strong biofilm producer, *S. aureus* 10850 [24], was routinely grown in tryptic soy broth (TSB) or agar (TSA) (Oxoid, Basingstoke, U.K.), supplemented with 1% (v/v) glucose (TSBG or TSAG) to promote biofilm production. M9 minimal medium without glucose was used as NN agar in VBNC induction assays, as described by Pasquaroli *et al.* [21]. The following antibiotics and enzymes were used: daptomycin (Cubicin, Novartis Pharma SpA, Italy) and lysozyme and lysostaphin (Sigma-Aldrich St Louis, MO, USA).

3.2. MIC Determination

The MIC of daptomycin was determined by a broth microdilution method, and *S. aureus* susceptibility was defined according to the European Committee on Antimicrobial Susceptibility Testing (EUCAST) breakpoints [31]. The test medium was MHII broth (Becton-Dickinson, Milan, Italy) supplemented with $CaCl_2$ (calcium chloride; Merck KGaA, Darmstadt, Germany) to a final Ca^{2+} concentration of 50 µg/mL. *S. aureus* ATCC 29213 was used as the control strain.

3.3. Biofilm Production, Stress Exposure and Culturability Assays

In vitro biofilm production, stress exposure and culturability assays were performed as described by Pasquaroli *et al.* [21]. Briefly, 100 µL of a late-log culture of *S. aureus* 10850 grown in TSBG was spotted on 0.22-µm sterile nitrocellulose filters (Millipore Corporation, Billerica, MA, USA); the filters were placed onto TSAG plates for 48 h at 37 °C to allow biofilm development at the filter-air interface. They were then moved to NN agar plates, unsupplemented or supplemented with daptomycin (2 µg/mL), and incubated at 37 °C until loss of culturability. Filter cultures were transferred weekly to fresh agar plates without washing. Culturability was assessed every 2 days by placing a loop of filter cultures in TSB and onto TSA, followed by incubation for 48 h at 37 °C. Filter cultures testing negative on culturability assays were placed in 5 mL saline, detached by 3 cycles of sonication and vortexing, washed and resuspended in the same volume of saline.

3.4. Epifluorescence Microscopy and Flow Cytometry

Epifluorescence microscopy and flow cytometry counts were performed as described previously [21]; each count was carried out in duplicate. The limit of detection of epifluorescence counts was 60 cells/mL of detached biofilm.

3.5. Real-Time RT–PCR Assays

Total RNA was extracted from 5 mL of detached biofilm using the RNeasy Mini Kit (Qiagen, Hilden, Germany), as described previously [21]. Total RNA was retro-transcribed using Qiagen's QuantiTect Reserve Transcription kit.

Real-time PCRs were carried out in a total volume of 20 µL containing 0.25 µM of each primer (Table 3), 10 µL of 2× Supermix (Qiagen) and 2 µL of reverse transcription mixture. Cycling conditions were 95 °C for 3 min, followed by 40 cycles of 95 °C for 10 s, different annealing temperatures (Table 3) for 20 s and 72 °C for 20 s. Amplification reactions and melt-curve analysis were performed using the Rotor-Gene Q MDx (Qiagen). cDNA obtained starting from a broth culture of *S. aureus* 10850 was used as a positive control.

Table 3. Target genes and primer pairs used in gene expression assays.

Target Gene	Gene Function	Primer Pair (5′-3′)	Annealing Temperature (°C)	Product Size (bp)	Reference
16S rDNA	Housekeeping	F-TGGAGCATGTGGTTTAATTCGA R-TGCGGGACTTAACCCAACA	60	159	[32]
glt	Species specific, coding for glutamate synthase	F-AATCTTTGTCGGTACA CGATATTCTTCACG R-CGTAATGAGATTTCA GTAGATAATACAACA	58	108	[33]
nuc	Virulence factor, coding for thermonuclease	F-GACTATTATTGGTTGATCCACCTG R- GCCTTGACGAACTAAAGCTTCG	60	218	[34]
mecA	Methicillin resistance	F-TCCAGATTACAACTTCACCAGG R-CCACTTCATATCTTGTAACG	57	162	[35]

4. Conclusions

The present findings provide evidence that daptomycin may play a role in the induction and persistence of VBNC *S. aureus* biofilms by showing cell viability and gene expression for months after achievement of non-culturability. Infections caused by staphylococcal biofilms should be treated by carefully selected and dosed antibiotics, to maintain drug concentrations capable of exerting full inhibitory activity. The ability of non-culturable daptomycin-exposed staphylococcal biofilms to resuscitate requires additional testing. Further experiments are under way in our laboratory.

Acknowledgments

The authors are grateful to Sofia Giaconi for biofilm preparation and technical assistance.

Author Contributions

Sonia Pasquaroli designed the experiments, cultured the biofilms, performed RNA extractions, epifluorescence and cytofluorimetric counts and wrote the paper draft. Barbara Citterio contributed to monitoring non-culturability, to extracting RNA from non-culturable biofilms and to performing retro-transcription assays. Andrea Di Cesare and Mehdi Amiri performed the RT-PCR assays and analyzed the data. Anita Manti performed the cytofluorimetric analyses. Claudia Vuotto analyzed the biofilm production by SEM. Francesca Biavasco conceived of the experiments, analyzed the data and wrote the paper.

References

1. Donlan, R.; Costerton, J. Biofilms: survival mechanisms of clinically relevant microorganisms. *Clin. Microbiol. Rev.* **2002**, *15*, 167–193.
2. Hall-Stoodley, L.; Stoodley, P. Evolving concepts in biofilm infections. *Cell. Microbiol.* **2009**, *11*, 1034–1043.
3. Francolini, I.; Donelli, G. Prevention and control of biofilm-based medical- device-related infections. *FEMS Immunol. Med. Microbiol.* **2010**, *59*, 227–238.
4. Zandri, G.; Pasquaroli, S.; Vignaroli, C.; Talevi, S.; Manso, E.; Donelli, G.; Biavasco, F. Detection of viable but non-culturable staphylococci in biofilms from central venous catheters negative on standard microbiological assays. *Clin. Microbiol. Infect.* **2012**, *18*, 259–261.
5. Chambers, H.F. Methicillin resistance in staphylococci: Molecular and biochemical basis and clinical implications. *Clin. Microbiol. Rev.* **1997**, *10*, 781–791.
6. Enoch, D.A.; Bygott, J.M.; Daly, M.L.; Karas, J.A. Daptomycin. *J. Infect.* **2007**, *55*, 205–213.
7. Tarai, B.; Das, P.; Kumar, D. Recurrent challenges for clinicians: Emergence of methicillin-resistant Staphylococcus aureus, vancomycin resistance, and current treatment options. *J. Lab. Phys.* **2013**, *5*, 71–78.
8. Popiel, K.Y.; Miller, M.A. Evaluation of Vancomycin-Resistant Enterococci (VRE)-associated morbidity following relaxation of VRE screening and isolation precautions in a tertiary care hospital. *Infect. Control Hosp. Epidemiol.* **2014**, *35*, 818–825.
9. Carugati, M.; Bayer, A.S.; Miró, J.M.; Park, L.P.; Guimarães, A.C.; Skoutelis, A.; Fortes, C.Q.; Durante-Mangoni, E.; Hannan, M.M.; Nacinovich, F.; *et al.* High-Dose daptomycin therapy for left-sided infective endocarditis: A prospective study from the international collaboration on endocarditis. *Antimicrob. Agents Chemother.* **2013**, *57*, 6213–6222.
10. Robbel, L.; Marahiel, M.A. Daptomycin, a bacterial lipopeptide synthesized by a nonribosomal machinery. *J. Biol. Chem.* **2010**, *285*, 27501–27508.

11. Raad, I.; Hanna, H.; Jiang, Y.; Dvorak, T.; Reitzel, R.; Chaiban, G.; Sherertz, R.; Hachem, R. Comparative activities of daptomycin, linezolid, and tigecycline against catheter-related methicillin-resistant *Staphylococcus* bacteremic isolates embedded in biofilm. *Antimicrob. Agents Chemother.* **2007**, *51*, 1656–1660.

12. Barber, K.E.; Werth, B.J.; McRoberts, J.P.; Rybak, M.J. A novel approach utilizing biofilm time-kill curves to assess the bactericidal activity of ceftaroline combinations against biofilm-producing methicillin-resistant *Staphylococcus aureus*. *Antimicrob. Agents Chemother.* **2014**, *58*, 2989–2992.

13. Len, O.; Montejo, M.; Cervera, C.; Fariñas, M.C.; Sabé, N.; Ramos, A.; Cordero, E.; Torre-Cisneros, J.; Martín-Dávila, P.; Azanza, J.R.; *et al.* Daptomycin is safe and effective for the treatment of gram-positive cocci infections in solid organ transplantation. *Transpl. Infect. Dis.* **2014**, doi:10.1111/tid.12232.

14. Vilhena, C.; Bettencourt, A. Daptomycin: A review of properties, clinical use, drug delivery and resistance. *Mini Rev. Med. Chem.* **2012**, *12*, 202–209.

15. Kelesidis, T. The interplay between daptomycin and the immune system. *Front. Immunol.* **2014**, *5*, 52.

16. Agarwal, A.; Singh, K.P.; Jain, A. Medical significance and management of staphylococcal biofilm. *FEMS Immunol. Med. Microbiol.* **2010**, *58*, 147–160.

17. Meije, Y.; Almirante, B.; del Pozo, J.L.; Martín, M.T.; Fernández-Hidalgo, N.; Shan, A.; Basas, J.; Pahissa, A.; Gavaldà, J. Daptomycin is effective as antibiotic-lock therapy in a model of *Staphylococcus aureus* catheter-related infection. *J. Infect.* **2014**, *68*, 548–552.

18. Holmberg, A.; Rasmussen, M. Antibiotic regimens with rifampicin for treatment of Enterococcus faecium in biofilms. *Int. J. Antimicrob. Agents* **2014**, *44*, 78–80.

19. Oliver, J.D. Recent findings on the viable but non-culturable state in pathogenic bacteria. *FEMS Microbiol. Rev.* **2009**, *34*, 415–425.

20. Nowakowska, J.; Oliver, J.D. Resistance to environmental stresses by *Vibrio vulnificus* in the viable but non-culturable state. *FEMS Microbiol. Ecol.* **2013**, *84*, 213–222.

21. Pasquaroli, S.; Zandri, G.; Vignaroli, C.; Vuotto, C.; Donelli, G.; Biavasco, F. Antibiotic pressure can induce the viable but non-culturable state in *Staphylococcus aureus* growing in biofilms. *J. Antimicrob. Chemother.* **2013**, *68*, 1812–1817.

22. Pascoe, B.; Dams, L.; Wilkinson, T.S.; Harris, L.G.; Bodger, O.; Mack, D.; Davies, A.P. Dormant cells of *Staphylococcus aureus* are resuscitated by spent culture supernatant. *PLoS One* **2014**, *9*, e85998.

23. El-Azizi, M.; Rao, S.; Kanchanapoom, T.; Khardori, N. *In vitro* activity of vancomycin, quinupristin/dalfopristin, and linezolid against intact and disrupted biofilms of staphylococci. *Ann. Clin. Microbiol. Antimicrob.* **2005**, *4*, 2.

24. Donelli, G.; Francolini, I.; Romoli, D.; Guaglianone, E.; Piozzi, A.; Ragunath, C.; Kaplan, J.B. Synergistic activity of dispersin B and cefamandole nafate in inhibition of staphylococcal biofilm growth on polyurethanes. *Antimicrob. Agents Chemother.* **2007**, *51*, 2733–2740.

25. Lahtinen, S.J.; Ahokoski, H.; Reinikainen, J.P.; Gueimonde, M.; Nurmi, J.; Ouwehand, A.C.; Salminen, S.J. Degradation of 16S rRNA and attributes of viability of viable but non-culturable probiotic bacteria. *Lett. Appl. Microbiol.* **2008**, *46*, 693–698.

26. Wiltshire, M.D.; Foster, S.J. Identification and analysis of *Staphylococcus aureus* components expressed by a model system of growth in serum. *Infect. Immun.* **2001**, *69*, 5198–5202.

27. Rahman, I.; Shahamat, M.; Kirchman, P.A.; Russek-Cohen, E.; Colwell, R.R. Methionine uptake and cytopathogenicity of viable but non-culturable *Shigella dysenteriae* type 1. *Appl. Environ. Microb.* **1994**, *60*, 3573–3578.

28. Kiedrowski, M.R.; Kavanaugh, J.S.; Malone, C.L.; Mootz, J.M.; Voyich, J.M.; Smeltzer, M.S.; Bayles, K.W.; Horswill, A.R. Nuclease modulates biofilm formation in community-associated methicillin-resistant *Staphylococcus aureus*. *PLoS One* **2011**, *6*, e26714.

29. Sengupta, S.; Chattopadhyay, M.K.; Grossart, H.P. The multifaceted roles of antibiotics and antibiotic resistance in nature. *Front. Microbiol.* **2013**, *4*, 47.

30. Davies, J.; Spiegelman, G.B.; Yim, G. The world of subinhibitory antibiotic concentrations. *Curr. Opin. Microbiol.* **2006**, *9*, 445–453.

31. The European Committee on Antimicrobial Susceptibility Testing. Breakpoint tables for interpretation of MICs and zone diameters.Version 4.0, 2014. Available online: http://www.eucast.org (accessed on 17 September 2014).

32. Warwick, S.; Wilks, M.; Hennessy, E.; Powell-Tuck, J.; Small, M.; Sharp, J.; Millar, M.R. Use of quantitative 16S ribosomal DNA detection for diagnosis of central vascular catheter-associated bacterial infection. *J. Clin. Microbiol.* **2004**, *42*, 1402–1408.

33. Martineau, F.; Picard, F.J.; Roy, P.H.; Ouellette, M.; Bergeron, M.G. Species-Specific and ubiquitous-DNA-based assays for rapid identification of *Staphylococcus aureus*. *J. Clin. Microbiol.* **1998**, *36*, 618–623.

34. Depardieu, F.; Perichon, B.; Courvalin, P. Detection of the van alphabet and identification of enterococci and staphylococci at the species level by multiplex PCR. *J. Clin. Microbiol.* **2004**, *42*, 5857–5860.

35. Oliveira, D.C.; Milheiric, C.; de Lencastre, H. Update to the multiplex PCR strategy for assignment of *mec* element types in *Staphylococcus aureus*. *Antimicrob. Agents Chemother.* **2007**, *51*, 3374–3377.

Permissions

List of Contributors

Robert D. Wojtyczka, Kamila Orlewska, Małgorzata Kępa, Danuta Idzik, Tomasz Mularz, Michał Krawczyk, Maria Miklasińska and Tomasz J. Wąsik
Department and Institute of Microbiology and Virology, School of Pharmacy with the Division of Laboratory Medicine, Medical University of Silesia, ul. Jagiellońska 4, 41-200 Sosnowiec, Poland

Arkadiusz Dziedzic
Department of Conservative Dentistry with Endodontics, School of Medicine with the Division of Dentistry, Medical University of Silesia, Pl. Akademicki 17, 41-902 Bytom, Poland

Céline Lucchetti-Miganeh and François Rechenmann
Genostar, 60 rue Lavoisier, Montbonnot 38330, France

David Redelberger, Gaël Chambonnier, Christophe Bordi and Sophie de Bentzmann
UMR7255-Laboratoire d'Ingénierie des Systèmes Macromoléculaires, CNRS—Aix Marseille University, Marseille 13402, France

Sylvie Elsen and Ina Attrée
INSERM, UMR-S 1036, Biology of Cancer and Infection, Grenoble 38054, France

Katy Jeannot and Patrick Plésiat
Laboratoire de Bactériologie, Faculté de Médecine-Pharmacie, Université de Franche-Comté, Besançon 25030, France

Eduardo Costa, Sara Silva, Freni Tavaria and Manuela Pintado
Universidade Católica Portuguesa/Porto, Rua Arquiteto Lobão Vital, Apartado 2511, 4202-401 Porto, Portugal

Valentina Gentile, Emanuela Frangipani, Carlo Bonchi, Fabrizia Minandri, Federica Runci and Paolo Visca
Department of Sciences, Roma Tre University, Viale Marconi 446, 00146 Rome, Italy

Alice P. McCloskey
Biomaterials, Biofilm and Infection Control Research Group, School of Pharmacy, Queen's University Belfast, Medical Biology Centre, 97 Lisburn Road, Belfast BT9 7BL, N. Ireland

Garry Laverty, Sean P. Gorman and Brendan F. Gilmore
Biomaterials, Biofilm and Infection Control Research Group, School of Pharmacy, Queen's University Belfast, Medical Biology Centre, 97 Lisburn Road, Belfast BT9 7BL, UK

Claudia Vuotto
Microbial Biofilm Laboratory, IRCCS Fondazione Santa Lucia, Rome 00179, Italy
Department of Biomedical Sciences and Public Health, Section of Microbiology, Polytechnic University of Marche, Ancona 60126, Italy

Francesca Longo and Gianfranco Donelli
Microbial Biofilm Laboratory, IRCCS Fondazione Santa Lucia, Rome 00179, Italy

Maria Pia Balice
Clinical Microbiology Laboratory, IRCCS Fondazione Santa Lucia, Rome 00179, Italy

Pietro E. Varaldo
Department of Biomedical Sciences and Public Health, Section of Microbiology, Polytechnic University of Marche, Ancona 60126, Italy

Paulo J. M. Bispo, Wolfgang Haas and Michael S. Gilmore
Departments of Ophthalmology, Microbiology and Immunology, Massachusetts Eye and Ear Infirmary, Harvard Medical School, Boston, MA, 02114 USA

Mary Anne Roshni Amalaradjou and Kumar Venkitanarayanan
Department of Animal Science, University of Connecticut, 3636 Horse Barn Hill Road Ext., Unit 4040, Storrs, CT 06269, USA

Ana Margarida Sousa and Maria Olívia Pereira
CEB—Centre of Biological Engineering, LIBRO—Laboratório de Investigação em Biofilmes Rosário Oliveira, University of Minho, Campus de Gualtar, 4710-057 Braga, Portugal

Sonia Pasquaroli, Andrea Di Cesare, Mehdi Amiri and Francesca Biavasco
Department of Life and Environmental Sciences, Polytechnic University of Marche, Ancona 60131, Italy

Barbara Citterio
Department of Biomolecular Sciences, Sect. Toxicological, Hygiene, and Environmental Sciences, University of Urbino Carlo Bo, Urbino 61029, Italy

Anita Manti
Department of Earth, Life and Environmental Sciences, University of Urbino Carlo Bo, Urbino 61029, Italy

Index

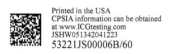
Printed in the USA
CPSIA information can be obtained
at www.ICGtesting.com
JSHW051342041223
53221JS00006B/60

9 781639 276929